KU-659-523

Guyton & Hall

Physiology

Review

Guyton &
Hall
Physiology
Review

Edited by
John E. Hall, PhD

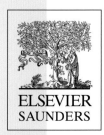

ELSEVIER
SAUNDERS

ELSEVIER
SAUNDERS

1600 John F. Kennedy Blvd.
Suite 1800
Philadelphia, PA 19103-2899

GUYTON & HALL PHYSIOLOGY REVIEW   ISBN 0-7216-8307-x
Copyright © 2006, Elsevier Inc.

All rights reserved. No part of this publication may be reproduced or transmitted in any form or by
any means, electronic or mechanical, including photocopying, recording, or any information storage and
retrieval system, without permission in writing from the publisher. Permissions may be sought directly from
Elsevier's Health Sciences Rights Department in Philadelphia, PA, USA: phone: (+1) 215 239 3804, fax:
(+1) 215 239 3805, e-mail: healthpermissions@elsevier.com. You may also complete your request on-line via
the Elsevier homepage (http://www.elsevier.com), by selecting 'Customer Support' and then 'Obtaining
Permissions'.

Notice

Knowledge and best practice in this field are constantly changing. As new research and experience
broaden our knowledge, changes in practice, treatment and drug therapy may become necessary or
appropriate. Readers are advised to check the most current information provided (i) on procedures featured
or (ii) by the manufacturer of each product to be administered, to verify the recommended dose or
formula, the method and duration of administration, and the contraindications. It is the responsibility of
the practitioner, relying on their own experience and knowledge of the patient, to take diagnoses, to
determine dosages and the best treatment for each individual patient, and to take all appropriate safety
precautions. To the fullest extent of the law, neither the Publisher nor the Authors assume any liability for
any injury and/or damage to persons or property arising out or related to any use of the material contained
in this book.

The Publisher

Library of Congress Cataloging-in-Publication Data
Hall, John E. (John Edward)
  Guyton & Hall physiology review / John E. Hall.
    p. ; cm.
  ISBN 0-7216-8307-X
  1. Human physiology–Examinations, questions, etc.   I. Title: Physiology review.   II. Guyton, Arthur C.
Textbook of medical physiology.   III. Title.
  [DNLM: 1. Physiology–Examination Questions. QT 18.2 H177g 2006]
  QP40.H268 2006
  612′.0076–dc22

                                                                            2005042826

Acquisitions Editor: William R. Schmitt
Developmental Editor: Katie Miller
Publishing Services Manager: Tina Rebane
Project Manager: Mary Anne Folcher
Design Direction: Steven Stave

Printed in China

Last digit is the print number: 9   8   7   6   5   4   3   2   1

Working together to grow
libraries in developing countries

www.elsevier.com | www.bookaid.org | www.sabre.org

ELSEVIER   **BOOK AID** International   Sabre Foundation

CONTRIBUTORS

Thomas H. Adair, PhD
Professor of Physiology and Biophysics
  Department of Physiology and Biophysics
  University of Mississippi School of Medicine
  University of Mississippi Medical Center
  Jackson, Mississippi
  Unit VII, Unit VIII and Unit XIII

David J. Dzielak, PhD
Associate Professor of Physiology and Biophysics
  Department of Physiology and Biophysics
  University of Mississippi School of Medicine
Professor of Surgery
  University of Mississippi Medical Center
  Jackson, Mississippi
  Unit XII

Joey P. Granger, PhD
Professor of Physiology and Biophysics
  Department of Physiology and Biophysics
  University of Mississippi School of Medicine
  University of Mississippi Medical Center
  Jackson, Mississippi
  Unit IV

John E. Hall, PhD
Guyton Professor and Chair of Physiology and
Biophysics
  Department of Physiology and Biophysics
  University of Mississippi School of Medicine
  University of Mississippi Medical Center
  Jackson, Mississippi
  Unit V and Unit XIII

Robert L. Hester, PhD
Professor of Physiology and Biophysics
  Department of Physiology and Biophysics
  University of Mississippi School of Medicine
  University of Mississippi Medical Center
  Jackson, Mississippi
  Unit VI

Thomas E. Lohmeier, PhD
Professor of Physiology and Biophysics
  Department of Physiology and Biophysics
  University of Mississippi School of Medicine
  University of Mississippi Medical Center
  Jackson, Mississippi
  Unit XIV

R. Davis Manning, PhD
Professor of Physiology and Biophysics
  Department of Physiology and Biophysics
  University of Mississippi School of Medicine
  University of Mississippi Medical Center
  Jackson, Mississippi
  Unit III, Unit IV and Unit XV

Gregory Mihailoff, PhD
Professor of Neuroscience and Anatomy
Director of Research Affairs
  Arizona College of Osteopathic Medicine
  Glendale, Arizona
  Unit IX, Unit X and Unit XI

Louise C. Nuttle, PhD
Assistant Professor of Physiology and Biophysics
  Department of Physiology and Biophysics
  University of Mississippi School of Medicine
  University of Mississippi Medical Center
  Jackson, Mississippi
  Unit I and Unit II

David B. Young, PhD
Professor of Physiology and Biophysics
  Department of Physiology and Biophysics
  University of Mississippi School of Medicine
  University of Mississippi Medical Center
  Jackson, Mississippi
  Unit XIV

TABLE OF CONTENTS

PREFACE

Self-assessment is an important component of effective learning, especially when studying a subject as complex as medical physiology. *Guyton & Hall Physiology Review* is designed to assist students in learning medical physiology by providing a comprehensive review of the subject through multiple-choice questions and explanations of the answers. Medical students preparing for the United States Medical Licensure Examinations (USMLE) will find this book useful since test questions have been constructed according to the USMLE format.

The questions and answers in this review are based on *Guyton and Hall's Textbook of Medical Physiology*, 11th edition (**TMP 11**). More than 1000 questions and answers are provided, and each answer is referenced to the *Textbook of Medical Physiology* to facilitate a more complete understanding of the topic. Illustrations are used to reinforce basic concepts. Some of the questions incorporate information from multiple chapters in the *Textbook of Medical Physiology* to permit assessment of your ability to apply and integrate the principles necessary for the mastery of medical physiology.

An effective way to use the review is to allow about one minute for each question in a given unit, approximating the time limit for a question in the USMLE examination. As you proceed, indicate your answer next to each question. After finishing the questions and answers, spend as much time as necessary to verify your answers and to carefully read the explanations provided. Read the additional material referred to in the *Textbook of Medical Physiology*, especially for questions where incorrect answers were chosen.

Guyton & Hall Physiology Review cannot serve as a substitute for the *Textbook of Medical Physiology*, however. It is intended mainly as a means of assessing your knowledge of physiology and of strengthening your ability to apply and integrate this knowledge.

We have attempted to make this review as accurate as possible, and we hope that it will be a valuable tool for your study of physiology. Your critiques and suggestions for improvement of the textbook will be greatly appreciated.

I am grateful to each of the contributors for their careful work on this book. I also wish to express my thanks to William Schmitt, Katie Miller, Mary Anne Folcher, Susan Kelly, and the rest of the Elsevier staff for their editorial and production excellence. I am especially indebted to the late Dr. Arthur C. Guyton who wrote the first eight editions of the *Textbook of Medical Physiology*, beginning nearly 50 years ago, and gave me the privilege of contributing to the last three editions.

John E. Hall, PhD
Jackson, Mississippi

The Cell and General Physiology

Questions 1-3

    (A) Nucleolus
    (B) Nucleus
    (C) Agranular endoplasmic reticulum
    (D) Granular endoplasmic reticulum
    (E) Golgi apparatus
    (F) Endosomes
    (G) Peroxisomes
    (H) Lysosomes
    (I) Cytosol
    (J) Cytoskeleton
    (K) Glycocalyx
    (L) Microtubules

For each of the scenarios described below, identify the most likely subcellular site listed above for the deficient or mutant protein.

1. Studies completed on a 5-year-old boy show an accumulation of cholesteryl esters and triglycerides in his liver, spleen, and intestines and calcification of both adrenal glands. Additional studies indicate the cause to be a deficiency in acid lipase A activity. ( )

2. The abnormal cleavage of mannose residues during the post-translational processing of glycoproteins results in the development of a lupus-like autoimmune disease in mice. The abnormal cleavage is due to a mutation of the enzyme α-mannosidase II. ( )

3. The observation that abnormal cleavage of mannose residues from glycoproteins causes an autoimmune disease in mice supports the role of this structure in the normal immune response. ( )

Questions 4 and 5

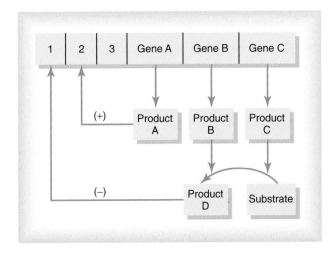

The diagram above is of a hypothetical operon containing three structural genes (A, B, and C) and three upstream sequences (1, 2, and 3).

4. The protein product of gene A binds to sequence 2 and enhances further transcription of the operon. What is this mode of regulation called?
    (A) Feed-forward
    (B) Positive feedback
    (C) Negative feedback
    (D) Promoter activation
    (E) Repression

5. The protein products of genes B and C participate in the enzymatic conversion of substrate into product D. Product D binds to sequence 1 and inhibits transcription of the operon. In this example, what does product D function as?
    (A) Repressor operator
    (B) Repressor protein
    (C) Activator operator
    (D) Activator protein
    (E) Promoter

6. Facioscapulohumeral muscular dystrophy (FSHD) is characterized by a deletion of tandem 3.3-kilobase repeats on chromosome 4q35. This deletion results in the inability of a protein complex to bind to DNA and an overexpression of genes upstream of the deletion. Normally, what does the sequence deleted in FSHD most likely function as?
    (A) Activator protein
    (B) Repressor protein
    (C) Activator element
    (D) Repressor element
    (E) Promoter sequence

Questions 7-9

    (A) Nucleolus
    (B) Nucleus
    (C) Agranular endoplasmic reticulum
    (D) Granular endoplasmic reticulum
    (E) Golgi apparatus
    (F) Endosomes
    (G) Peroxisomes
    (H) Lysosomes
    (I) Cytosol
    (J) Cytoskeleton
    (K) Glycocalyx
    (L) Microtubules

Match the cellular location for each of the steps involved in the synthesis and packaging of a secreted protein listed below with a term listed above.

7. Initiation of translation ( )

8. Protein condensation and packaging ( )

9. Gene transcription ( )

10. "Redundancy" or "degeneration" of the genetic code occurs during which of the following steps of protein synthesis?
    (A) DNA replication
    (B) Transcription
    (C) Post-transcriptional modification
    (D) Translation
    (E) Protein glycosylation

11. Which of the following characteristics is shared by the events of pinocytosis and phagocytosis?
    (A) Involve the recruitment of actin filaments
    (B) Occur spontaneously and nonselectively
    (C) Permit the uptake of bacterium into the cytosol
    (D) Are observed only in macrophages and neutrophils
    (E) Do not require adenosine triphosphate (ATP)

12. Which of the following does not play a direct role in the process of transcription?
    (A) Helicase
    (B) RNA polymerase
    (C) Chain terminating sequence
    (D) "Activated" RNA molecules
    (E) Promoter sequence

13. Which of the following proteins is most likely to be the product of a proto-oncogene?
    (A) Growth factor receptor
    (B) Cytoskeletal protein
    (C) Na^+ channel
    (D) Ca^{++}-ATPase
    (E) Myosin light chain

14. A pure phospholipid bilayer is most permeable to which of the following?
    (A) Sodium
    (B) Calcium
    (C) Chloride
    (D) Water
    (E) Oxygen

15. Which of the following events does not occur during the process of mitosis?
    (A) Condensation of the chromosomes
    (B) Replication of the genome
    (C) Fragmentation of the nuclear envelope
    (D) Alignment of the chromatids along the equatorial plate
    (E) Separation of the chromatids into two sets of 46 "daughter" chromosomes

16. When comparing two types of cells from the same person, what does the variation in the proteins expressed by each cell type reflect?
    (A) Differences in the DNA contained in the nucleus of each cell
    (B) Differences in the number of specific genes in their genomes
    (C) Cell-specific expression and repression of specific genes
    (D) Differences in the number of chromosomes in each cell
    (E) Age of the cells

17. Which of the following characteristics of a biological membrane is most influenced by its cholesterol content?
    (A) Thickness
    (B) Ion permeability
    (C) Fluidity
    (D) Glycosylation
    (E) Hydrophobicity

18. The appearance of which of the following distinguishes eukaryotic cells from lower units of life?
    (A) DNA
    (B) RNA
    (C) Membranes
    (D) Protein
    (E) Nucleus

Answers

1. (H) Acid lipases, along with other acid hydrolases, are localized to lysosomes. Fusion of endocytotic and autolytic vesicles with lysosomes initiates the intracellular process that allows cells to digest cellular debris and particles ingested from the extracellular milieu, including bacteria. In the normal acidic environment of the lysosome, acid lipases use hydrogen to convert lipids into fatty acids and glycerol. Other acid lipases include a variety of nucleases, proteases, and polysaccharide-hydrolyzing enzymes.
   TMP11 16

2. (E) Membrane proteins are glycosylated during their synthesis in the lumen of the rough endoplasmic reticulum. Most post-translational modification of the oligosaccharide chains, however, occurs during the transport of the protein through the layers of the Golgi apparatus matrix, where enzymes such as α-mannosidase II are localized.
   TMP11 15

3. (K) The oligosaccharide chains that are added to glycoproteins on the luminal side of the rough endoplasmic reticulum, and subsequently modified during their transport through the Golgi apparatus, are attached to the extracellular surface of the cell. This negatively charged layer of carbohydrate moieties is collectively called the glycocalyx. It participates in cell-cell interactions, cell-ligand interactions, and the immune response.
   TMP11 14; SEE ALSO CHAPTER 34

4. (B) Positive feedback refers to a situation in which the product of an action, in this case product A, acts on the system to perpetuate that action. In many cases, such an effect creates a "vicious circle." However, in some cases, the perpetuation is temporary and is ultimately controlled by an overriding negative feedback mechanism. Unlike feed-forward regulation, the substance regulating the action is a product of the same action.
   TMP11 8

5. (B) One of the simplest mechanisms of transcriptional regulation involves the specific binding of a protein to a DNA sequence adjacent to the promoter, either facilitating or prohibiting the binding of RNA polymerase to the promoter sequence. Such binding is said to "activate" or "repress" transcription, respectively. In this case, the binding of product D inhibits or represses transcription. Product D is therefore considered to be a repressor protein, and the DNA sequence to which it binds would be a repressor operator or repressor element.
   TMP11 35

6. (D) The deletion that is characteristic of facioscapulohumeral muscular dystrophy both prevents protein-DNA binding and results in the overexpression of genes downstream of the deleted sequences. It is reasonable to assume that protein binding to this deleted region, under normal conditions, represses the transcription of these genes. The deleted sequence would therefore include a repressor element. The DNA-binding protein that binds to this region would be a repressor protein.
   TMP11 35

7. (I) Initiation of translation, whether of a cytosolic protein, a membrane-bound protein, or a secreted protein, occurs in the cytosol and involves a common pool of ribosomes. Only after the appearance of the N-terminus of the polypeptide is it identified as a protein destined for secretion. At this point, the ribosome attaches to the cytosolic surface of the rough endoplasmic reticulum. Translation continues, and the new polypeptide is extruded into the matrix of the endoplasmic reticulum.
   TMP11 33

8. (E) Secreted proteins are condensed, sorted, and packaged into secretory vesicles in the terminal portions of the Golgi apparatus, also known as the trans-Golgi network. It is here that proteins destined for secretion are separated from those destined for intracellular compartments or cellular membranes.
   TMP11 15

9. (B) All transcription events occur in the nucleus, regardless of the final destination of the protein product. The resulting messenger RNA molecule is transported through the nuclear pores in the nuclear membrane and translated into either the cytosol or the lumen of the rough endoplasmic reticulum.
   TMP11 31

10. (D) During both replication and transcription, the new nucleic acid molecule is an exact complement of the parent DNA molecule. This is a result of predictable, specific, one-to-one base pairing. During the process of translation, however, each amino acid in the new polypeptide is encoded by a codon, a series of three consecutive nucleotides. Whereas each codon encodes a specific amino acid, most amino acids can be encoded for by multiple codons. Redundancy results because 60 codons encode a mere 20 amino acids.
    TMP11 31

11. (A) The events of pinocytosis and phagocytosis involve a movement of the plasma membrane—in one case an invagination, in the other an evagination. Generally, such events involve the recruitment of actin and other cytoskeletal elements. Pinocytosis occurs in all cells to some extent, but it cannot accommodate large particles such as bacteria. Phagocytosis is neither spontaneous nor nonselective and is triggered by specific receptor-ligand interactions. Neither is ATP-independent.
    TMP11 19

12. (A) Helicase is one of the many proteins involved in the process of DNA replication. It does not play a role in transcription. RNA polymerase binds to the promoter sequence and facilitates the addition of "activated" RNA molecules to the growing RNA molecule until the polymerase reaches the chain terminating sequence on the template DNA molecule.
    TMP11 30-31

13. (A) An oncogene is a gene that is either abnormally activated or mutated in such a way that its product causes uncontrolled cell growth. A proto-oncogene is simply the "normal" version of an oncogene. By definition, proto-oncogenes are divided into several families of proteins, all of which participate in the control of cell growth. These families include, but are not limited to, growth factors and their receptors, protein kinases, transcription factors, and proteins that regulate cell proliferation.
    TMP11 40-41

14. (E) A "naked" phospholipid bilayer, devoid of protein, is virtually impermeable to charged, water-soluble molecules such as ions; slightly more permeable to large polar molecules such as water; and very permeable to lipophilic or fat-soluble molecules such as gases and alcohol.
    TMP11 47

15. (B) DNA replication occurs during the S phase of the cell cycle and precedes mitosis. Condensation of the chromosomes occurs during prophase of mitosis. Fragmentation of the nuclear envelope occurs during prometaphase of mitosis. The chromatids align at the equatorial plate during metaphase and separate into two complete sets of daughter chromosomes during anaphase.
    TMP11 37

16. (C) An individual's genome is represented in its entirety in every nucleated cell in the body. The differences among a neuron and an epithelial cell and a leukocyte reflect differences in their proteomes, or the proteins expressed by each cell type. Differential cell-specific protein expression results from programmed activation and repression of certain genes during cell differentiation.
    TMP11 40

17. (C) The cholesterol content of a membrane determines the packing density of phospholipids. The higher the cholesterol content, the more fluid the membrane and the greater the lateral mobility of membrane components, including proteins and phospholipid molecules themselves. To a lesser extent, cholesterol content also affects the "leakiness" of a membrane to water-soluble molecules.
    TMP11 13

18. (E) Nucleic acids and proteins, together, constitute the fundamental replicable unit of life, exemplified by viruses. Membranes and even organelles appear in prokaryotic cells, but only eukaryotic cells possess a nucleus.
    TMP11 18

Membrane Physiology, Nerve, and Muscle

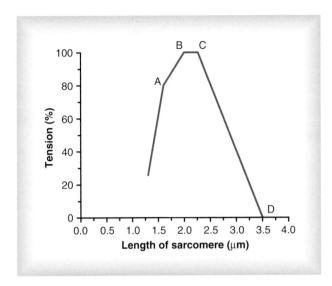

1. The diagram above shows the length-tension relationship for a single sarcomere. Why is the tension development maximal between points B and C?
   (A) There is maximal overlap between the actin and myosin filaments
   (B) There is minimal overlap between the actin and myosin filaments
   (C) The Z discs of the sarcomere abut the ends of the myosin filament
   (D) The myosin filament is at its minimal length
   (E) Actin filaments are overlapping each other

2. Both simple and facilitated diffusion have which characteristic?
   (A) Display saturation kinetics
   (B) Require some type of carrier mechanism for transport
   (C) Can work in the absence of adenosine triphosphate (ATP)
   (D) Can transport material against a concentration gradient
   (E) Can be blocked by specific inhibitors

3. Excitation-contraction coupling in skeletal muscle involves all of the following events except one. Which one is not involved?
   (A) Increase in the permeability of the muscle fiber to Na^+
   (B) Binding of Ca^{++} to calmodulin
   (C) Conformational change in the dihydropyridine receptor
   (D) Depolarization of the transverse tubule (T tubule) membrane
   (E) ATP hydrolysis

4. Skeletal muscle contraction is terminated by which action?
   (A) Removal of acetylcholine from the neuromuscular junction
   (B) Removal of Ca^{++} from the terminal of the motor neuron
   (C) Closure of the postsynaptic nicotinic acetylcholine receptor
   (D) Removal of sarcoplasmic Ca^{++}
   (E) Return of the dihydropyridine receptor to its resting conformation

5. Which of the following statements about smooth muscle contraction is most accurate?
   (A) It requires more energy than skeletal muscle contraction
   (B) It can occur without the generation of an action potential
   (C) It is increased under conditions that stimulate adenylate cyclase
   (D) It is shorter in duration than skeletal muscle contraction
   (E) It is Ca^{++} independent

6. In what way does visceral smooth muscle differ from skeletal muscle?
   (A) Visceral smooth muscle can contract in response to stretch
   (B) Visceral smooth muscle does not contain actin filaments
   (C) Visceral smooth muscle is capable of generating only about half the maximal force of contraction
   (D) Contraction of visceral smooth muscle is ATP dependent
   (E) The rate of cross-bridge cycling in visceral smooth muscle is approximately 100 times faster than that in skeletal muscle

Questions 7-10

Intracellular (mM)	Extracellular (mM)
140 K^+	14 K^+
10 Na^+	100 Na^+
11 Cl^-	110 Cl^-
10^{-4} Ca^{++}	2 Ca^{++}

The table above shows the relative concentrations of four ions across the plasma membrane of a model cell. Refer to this table when answering the following four questions.

7. What is the equilibrium potential for Cl^- across the plasma membrane of this cell?
   (A) –120 millivolts
   (B) –60 millivolts
   (C) 0 millivolts
   (D) 60 millivolts
   (E) 120 millivolts

8. What is the equilibrium potential for K^+ across the plasma membrane of this cell?
   (A) –120 millivolts
   (B) –60 millivolts
   (C) 0 millivolts
   (D) 60 millivolts
   (E) 120 millivolts

9. If the membrane potential of this cell is –80 millivolts, the driving force is greatest for which ion?
   (A) K^+
   (B) Na^+
   (C) Cl^-
   (D) Ca^{++}
   (E) Both Cl^- and Na^+

10. If this cell were permeable only to K$^+$, what would be the effect of reducing the extracellular K$^+$ concentration from 14 to 1.4 millimolar?
   (A) 10 millivolts hyperpolarization
   (B) 60 millivolts hyperpolarization
   (C) 10 millivolts depolarization
   (D) 60 millivolts depolarization
   (E) 12.6 millivolts depolarization

11. In a normal, healthy muscle, what occurs as a result of propagation of an action potential to the terminal membrane of a motor neuron?
   (A) Opening of voltage-gated Ca^{++} channels in the presynaptic membrane
   (B) Depolarization of the T tubule membrane follows
   (C) Always results in muscle contraction
   (D) Increase in intracellular Ca^{++} concentration in the motor neuron terminal
   (E) All of the above are correct

12. Which of the following best describes the change in cell volume that will occur if red blood cells are placed in a solution of 140 millimolar NaCl containing 20 millimolar urea, a relatively large but permeant molecule?
   (A) Cells will swell and lyse
   (B) Cells will swell transiently and return to their original volume over time
   (C) Cells will shrink transiently and return to their original volume over time
   (D) Cells will initially shrink, then swell and lyse
   (E) No change in cell volume will occur

13. Which of the following decreases in length during the contraction of a skeletal muscle fiber?
   (A) Thin filaments
   (B) Thick filaments
   (C) Z discs of the sarcomere
   (D) A band of the sarcomere
   (E) I band of the sarcomere

14. A cross-sectional view of a skeletal muscle fiber through the H zone would reveal the presence of what?
   (A) Actin, but no myosin
   (B) Actin and myosin
   (C) Myosin, but no actin
   (D) Actin and titin
   (E) Actin, myosin, and titin

15. Calmodulin is most closely related, both structurally and functionally, to which of the following proteins?
   (A) G-actin
   (B) Troponin I
   (C) Troponin C
   (D) Tropomyosin
   (E) Myosin light chain

16. The resting potential of a myelinated nerve fiber is primarily dependent on the concentration gradient of which ion?
   (A) K$^+$
   (B) Na$^+$
   (C) Ca^{++}
   (D) Cl$^-$
   (E) HCO$_3^-$

17. What is the calculated osmolarity of a solution containing 12 millimolar NaCl, 3 millimolar KCl, and 1 millimolar CaCl$_2$?
   (A) 16 mOsm/L
   (B) 18 mOsm/L
   (C) 32 mOsm/L
   (D) 33 mOsm/L
   (E) 45 mOsm/L

18. Tetanic contraction of a skeletal muscle fiber results from a cumulative increase in the intracellular concentration of which of the following?
   (A) Na$^+$
   (B) K$^+$
   (C) Troponin
   (D) ATP
   (E) Ca^{++}

19. Malignant hyperthermia is a potentially fatal genetic disorder characterized by a hyperresponsiveness to inhaled anesthetics and results in elevated body temperature, skeletal muscle rigidity, and lactic acidosis. Which of the following molecular changes could account for these clinical manifestations?
   (A) Inhibition of the ryanodine receptor
   (B) Reduction in the density of voltage-sensitive Na$^+$ channels in the T tubule membrane
   (C) Prolonged opening of the ryanodine receptor channel
   (D) Decreased voltage sensitivity of the dihydropyridine receptor
   (E) Enhanced activity of the sarcoplasmic reticulum Ca^{++}-ATPase

20. Weightlifting can result in a dramatic increase in skeletal muscle mass. This increase in muscle mass is primarily attributable to which of the following?
   (A) Increase in skeletal muscle blood supply
   (B) Increase in the number of neuromuscular junctions
   (C) Hypertrophy of individual muscle fibers
   (D) Fusion of sarcomeres between adjacent myofibrils
   (E) Increase in the number of motor neurons

21. Which of the following transport mechanisms is not rate-limited by an intrinsic V$_{max}$?
   (A) Simple diffusion through protein channels
   (B) Facilitated diffusion via carrier proteins
   (C) Primary active transport via carrier proteins
   (D) Secondary co-transport
   (E) Secondary counter-transport

22. Assuming complete dissociation of all solutes, which of the following solutions would be hyperosmotic relative to 1 millimolar NaCl?
    (A) 1 millimolar glucose
    (B) 1.5 millimolar glucose
    (C) 1 millimolar $CaCl_2$
    (D) 1 millimolar sucrose
    (E) 1 millimolar KCl

Questions 23 and 24

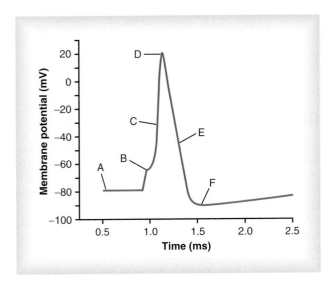

The above figure describes the change in membrane potential during an action potential in a giant squid axon. Refer to it when answering the next two questions.

23. Which of the following is primarily responsible for the change in membrane potential between points B and D?
    (A) Movement of Na^+ into the cell
    (B) Movement of Na^+ out of the cell
    (C) Movement of K^+ into the cell
    (D) Movement of K^+ out of the cell
    (E) Inhibition of the Na^+, K^+-ATPase

24. Which of the following is primarily responsible for the change in membrane potential between points D and E?
    (A) Movement of Na^+ into the cell
    (B) Movement of Na^+ out of the cell
    (C) Movement of K^+ into the cell
    (D) Movement of K^+ out of the cell
    (E) Inhibition of the Na^+, K^+-ATPase

25. The delayed onset and prolonged duration of smooth muscle contraction, as well as the greater force generated by smooth muscle compared with skeletal muscle, are all consequences of which of the following?
    (A) Higher energy requirement of smooth muscle
    (B) Slower cycling rate of the smooth muscle myosin cross-bridges
    (C) Slower uptake of Ca^{++} ions following contraction
    (D) Physical arrangement of actin and myosin filaments
    (E) Greater amount of myosin filaments present in smooth muscle

Questions 26-28

A 60-year-old man visits his physician complaining of double vision, eyelid droop, difficulty chewing and swallowing, and general weakness in his limbs. All these symptoms are made worse with exercise and occur more frequently late in the day. The physician suspects myasthenia gravis and orders a Tensilon test. The test is positive.

26. The increased muscle strength observed during the Tensilon test is due to an increase in which of the following?
    (A) Amount of acetylcholine (ACh) released from the motor nerves
    (B) Levels of ACh at the muscle end plates
    (C) Number of ACh receptors on the muscle end plates
    (D) Amount of norepinephrine released from the motor nerves
    (E) Synthesis of norepinephrine

27. What is the most likely basis for the symptoms described in this patient?
    (A) Autoimmune response
    (B) Overexertion
    (C) Depletion of voltage-gated Ca^{++} channels in certain motor neurons
    (D) Development of macro motor units following recovery from poliomyelitis
    (E) Botulinum toxicity

28. Which of the following drugs would likely alleviate this patient's symptoms?
    (A) Curare
    (B) Atropine
    (C) Neostigmine
    (D) Botulinum toxin antiserum
    (E) Halothane

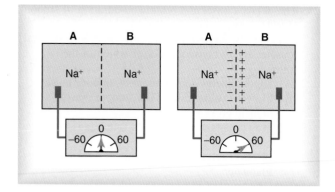

29. The diagrams above depict rigid containers composed of two aqueous chambers, A and B, each containing an Na^+ solution and separated by an Na^+-permeable membrane. The panel on the left represents the distribution of Na^+ ions at rest in the absence of any electrical potential. In this scenario, the concentration of Na^+ ions in chamber A equals the concentration of Na^+ ions in chamber B ($[Na]_A = [Na]_B$). The panel on the right illustrates the effect of a +60-millivolt potential applied across the membrane (chamber B relative to chamber A). Assuming a temperature of 37°C, which of the following expressions best describes the resulting distribution of Na^+ ions between the two chambers?
    (A) $[Na]_A = 2[Na]_B$
    (B) $[Na]_A = 10[Na]_B$
    (C) $[Na]_A = 60[Na]_B$
    (D) $[Na]_B = 10[Na]_A$
    (E) $[Na]_B = 60[Na]_A$

Questions 30-32

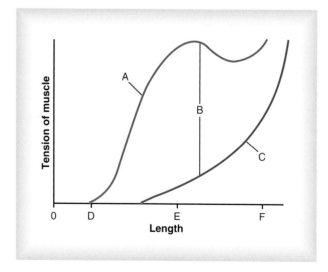

The diagram below illustrates the isometric length-tension relationship in a representative intact skeletal muscle. When answering the following three questions, use the letters in the diagram to identify each of the following.

30. So-called "active" or contraction-dependent tension ( )
31. The muscle length at which active tension is maximal ( )
32. The contribution of noncontractile muscle elements to total tension ( )
33. Smooth muscle contraction is terminated by which of the following?
    (A) Efflux of Ca^{++} ions across the plasma membrane
    (B) Uptake of Ca^{++} ions into the sarcoplasmic reticulum
    (C) Dephosphorylation of myosin kinase
    (D) Dephosphorylation of myosin light chain
    (E) Inhibition of myosin phosphatase

Questions 34-36

A 55-year-old woman sees a neurologist because of weakness in her legs that improves over the course of the day or with exercise. Extracellular electrical recordings from a single skeletal muscle fiber reveal normal miniature end plate potentials. Low-frequency electrical stimulation of the motor neuron, however, elicits an abnormally small depolarization of the muscle fibers. The amplitude of the depolarization is increased after exercise.

34. Based on these findings, which of the following is the most likely cause of this patient's leg weakness?
    (A) Blockade of postsynaptic acetylcholine receptors
    (B) Acetylcholinesterase deficiency
    (C) Reduced acetylcholine synthesis
    (D) Impaired presynaptic voltage-sensitive Ca^{++} influx
    (E) Inhibition of Ca^{++} re-uptake into the sarcoplasmic reticulum
35. A preliminary diagnosis is confirmed by the presence of which of the following?
    (A) Antibodies against the voltage-sensitive Ca^{++} channel
    (B) Antibodies against the acetylcholine receptor
    (C) Mutation in the gene that codes for the ryanodine receptor
    (D) Residual acetylcholine in the neuromuscular junction
    (E) Relatively few vesicles in the presynaptic terminal

36. The molecular mechanism underlying these symptoms is most similar to which of the following?
 (A) Botulinum toxin
 (B) Curare
 (C) Neostigmine
 (D) Acetylcholine
 (E) Tetrodotoxin

Questions 37-39

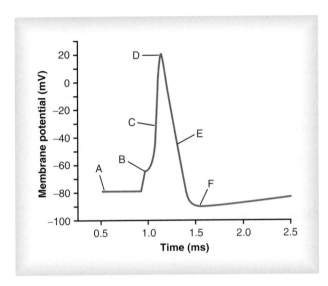

Match each of the descriptions below to one of the points on the diagram of the nerve action potential shown above.

37. Point at which the membrane potential ($_m$V) is closest to the Na$^+$ equilibrium potential ( )

38. Point at which the driving force for Na$^+$ is the greatest ( )

39. Point at which the ratio of K$^+$ permeability to Na$^+$ permeability (P_K/P_{Na}) is the greatest ( )

40. An experimental drug is being tested as a potential therapeutic treatment for asthma. Preclinical studies have shown that this drug induces the relaxation of cultured porcine tracheal smooth muscle cells pre-contracted with acetylcholine. Which of the following mechanisms of action is most likely to induce this effect?
 (A) Decreased plasma membrane K$^+$ permeability
 (B) Inhibition of the sarcoplasmic reticulum Ca^{++}-ATPase
 (C) Increased plasma membrane Na$^+$ permeability
 (D) Decreased affinity of troponin C for Ca^{++}
 (E) Stimulation of adenylate cyclase

41. ATP is used directly for each of the following processes except one. Which one does not use ATP?
 (A) Accumulation of Ca^{++} by the sarcoplasmic reticulum
 (B) Transport of Na$^+$ from the intracellular to extracellular fluid
 (C) Transport of K$^+$ from the extracellular to intracellular fluid
 (D) Transport of H$^+$ from the parietal cells into the lumen of the stomach
 (E) Transport of glucose into muscle cells

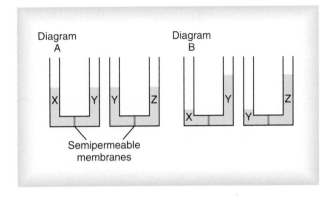

42. In the experiment illustrated in diagram A, equal volumes of solutions X, Y, and Z are placed into the compartments of two U-shaped vessels, as shown. The two compartments of each vessel are separated by semipermeable membranes (i.e., impermeable to ions and large polar molecules). Diagram B illustrates the fluid distribution across the membranes at equilibration. Assuming complete dissociation, identify each of the solutions shown above.

	Solution X	Solution Y	Solution Z
(A)	1 M CaCl$_2$	1 M NaCl	1 M glucose
(B)	1 M NaCl	2 M glucose	3 M CaCl$_2$
(C)	1 M glucose	1 M NaCl	1 M CaCl$_2$
(D)	Pure water	1 M CaCl$_2$	2 M glucose
(E)	2 M NaCl	1 M NaCl	Pure water

43. The force produced by a single skeletal muscle fiber can be increased by what means?
 (A) Increasing the frequency of stimulation of the fiber
 (B) Increasing the amplitude of the depolarizing stimulus
 (C) Decreasing extracellular K$^+$ concentration
 (D) Increasing the permeability of the sarcolemma to K$^+$
 (E) Increasing the number of voltage-gated Na$^+$ channels in the sarcolemma

Questions 44 and 45

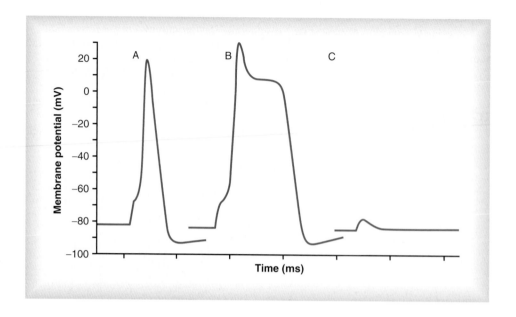

44. Trace A represents a typical action potential recorded under control conditions from a "normal" nerve cell in response to a depolarizing stimulus. Which of the following perturbations would explain the conversion of the response shown in trace A to the action potential shown in trace B?
    (A) Blockade of voltage-sensitive Na^+ channels
    (B) Blockade of voltage-sensitive K^+ channels
    (C) Blockade of Na-K "leak" channels
    (D) Replacement of the voltage-sensitive K^+ channels with "slow" Ca^{++} channels
    (E) Replacement of the voltage-sensitive Na^+ channels with "slow" Ca^{++} channels

45. Which of the following perturbations would account for the failure of the same stimulus to elicit an action potential in trace C?
    (A) Blockade of voltage-sensitive Na^+ channels
    (B) Blockade of voltage-sensitive K^+ channels
    (C) Blockade of Na-K "leak" channels
    (D) Replacement of the voltage-sensitive K^+ channels with "slow" Ca^{++} channels
    (E) Replacement of the voltage-sensitive Na^+ channels with "slow" Ca^{++} channels

Questions 46 and 47

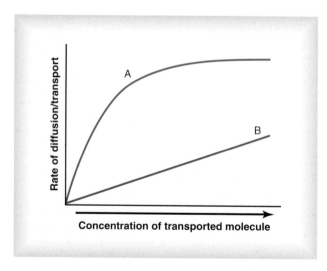

46. Trace A best describes the kinetics of which of the following events?
    (A) Movement of CO_2 across the plasma membrane
    (B) Transport of K^+ into a muscle cell
    (C) Voltage-dependent movement of Ca^{++} into the terminal of a motor neuron
    (D) Na^+ flux through an open nicotinic acetylcholine receptor channel
    (E) Movement of O_2 across a lipid bilayer

47. Trace B best describes which of the following events?
    (A) Transport of Ca^{++} into the sarcoplasmic reticulum of a smooth muscle cell
    (B) Transport of O_2 across an artificial lipid bilayer
    (C) Na^+-dependent transport of glucose into an epithelial cell
    (D) Transport of Na^+ out of a nerve cell
    (E) Transport of K^+ into a muscle cell

48. A 16-year-old high school football player suffered a fracture to the right tibia. After his lower leg has been in a cast for 8 weeks, he is surprised to find that the right gastrocnemius muscle is significantly smaller in circumference than it was before the fracture. What is the most likely explanation?
    (A) Decrease in the number of individual muscle fibers in the right gastrocnemius
    (B) Decrease in blood flow to the muscle caused by constriction from the cast
    (C) Temporary reduction in actin and myosin protein synthesis
    (D) Increase in glycolytic activity in the affected muscle
    (E) Progressive denervation

49. Smooth muscle that exhibits rhythmical contraction in the absence of external stimuli also necessarily exhibits which of the following?
    (A) "Slow" voltage-sensitive Ca^{++} channels
    (B) Intrinsic pacemaker wave activity
    (C) Higher resting cytosolic Ca^{++} concentration
    (D) Hyperpolarized membrane potential
    (E) Action potentials with "plateaus"

Questions 50-54

    (A) Simple diffusion
    (B) Facilitated diffusion
    (C) Primary active transport
    (D) Co-transport
    (E) Counter-transport

Match each of the processes described below with the correct type of transport listed above (each answer may be used more than once).

50. Ouabain-sensitive transport of Na^+ ions from the cytosol to the extracellular fluid ( )

51. Glucose uptake into skeletal muscle ( )

52. Na^+-dependent transport of Ca^{++} from the cytosol to the extracellular fluid ( )

53. Transport of glucose from the intestinal lumen to an intestinal epithelial cell ( )

54. Movement of Na^+ ions into a nerve cell during the upstroke of an action potential ( )

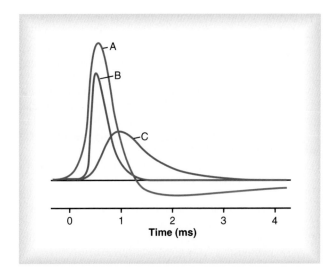

55. Traces A, B, and C in the above diagram summarize the changes in membrane potential ($_mV$) and the underlying membrane permeabilities (P) that occur in a nerve cell over the course of an action potential. Choose the combination of labels below that accurately identifies each of the traces.

	Trace A	Trace B	Trace C
(A)	P_K:P_{Na}	$_mV$	P_K
(B)	P_{Na}	$_mV$	P_K
(C)	$_mV$	P_{Na}	P_K
(D)	$_mV$	P_K	P_{Na}
(E)	P_K	$_mV$	P_{Na}

56. Which of the following is a consequence of myelination in large nerve fibers?
    (A) Increase in the nonselective diffusion of ions across the axon membrane
    (B) Decrease in the velocity of nerve impulses along the axon
    (C) Increase in the energy required to maintain ion gradients across the membrane
    (D) Generation of action potentials only at the nodes of Ranvier
    (E) Increase in the membrane capacitance of the axon

57. During a demonstration for first-year medical students, a neurologist uses magnetic cortical stimulation to trigger firing of the ulnar nerve in a volunteer. At relatively low-amplitude stimulation, action potentials are recorded only from muscle fibers in the index finger. As the amplitude of the stimulation is increased, action potentials are recorded from muscle fibers in both the index finger and the biceps muscle. What is the fundamental principle underlying this amplitude-dependent response?
    (A) Large motor neurons that innervate large motor units require a larger depolarizing stimulus
    (B) Recruitment of multiple motor units requires a larger depolarizing stimulus
    (C) The biceps muscle is innervated by more motor neurons
    (D) The motor units in the biceps are smaller than those in the muscles of the fingers
    (E) The muscles in the fingers are innervated only by the ulnar nerve
58. Similarities between smooth and cardiac muscle include which of the following?
    (A) Striated arrangement of the actin and myosin filaments
    (B) Role of myosin kinase in muscle contraction
    (C) Dependence of contraction on extracellular Ca^{++} ions
    (D) Presence of a T tubule network
    (E) Ability to contract in the absence of an action potential
59. If the intracellular concentration of a membrane-permeant substance doubles from 10 to 20 millimolar and the extracellular concentration remains at 5 millimolar, the rate of diffusion of that substance across the plasma membrane will increase by a factor of how much?
    (A) 2
    (B) 3
    (C) 4
    (D) 5
    (E) 6

Questions 60 and 61

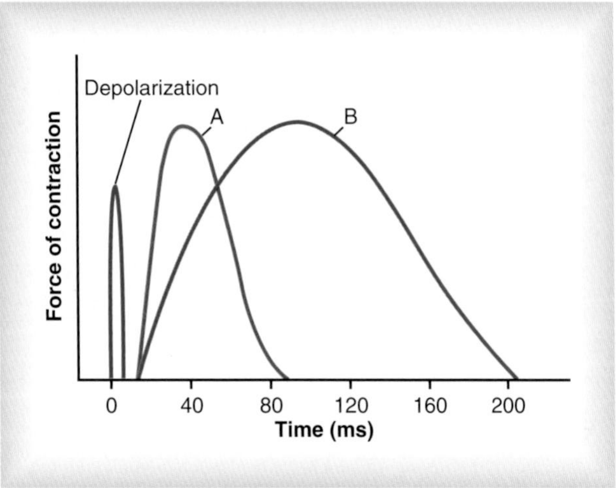

The diagram above illustrates the single isometric twitch characteristics of two skeletal muscles, A and B, in response to a depolarizing stimulus. Refer to it when answering the next two questions.

60. When comparing muscle A to muscle B, which statement is true?
    (A) Muscle B is composed of larger muscle fibers
    (B) Muscle B is innervated by smaller nerve fibers
    (C) Muscle B has fewer mitochondria
    (D) Muscle B has a less extensive blood supply
    (E) Muscle B is adapted for rapid contraction
61. The delay between the termination of the transient depolarization of the muscle membrane and the onset of muscle contraction observed in both muscles A and B reflects the time necessary for what event to occur?
    (A) ATP to be synthesized
    (B) G-actin to polymerize into F-actin
    (C) Ca^{++} to accumulate in the sarcoplasm
    (D) ADP to be released from the myosin head
    (E) Myosin head to complete one cross-bridge cycle

Answers

1. (A) Tension development in a single sarcomere is directly proportional to the number of active myosin cross-bridges attached to actin filaments. At sarcomere lengths of 2.0 to 2.5 micrometers, there is an optimal overlap between the myosin and actin filaments, allowing maximal contact between the myosin heads and the actin filaments. At lengths less than 2.0 micrometers, the actin filaments protrude into the H band, where no myosin heads exist. At lengths greater than 2.5 micrometers, the actin filaments are pulled toward the ends of the myosin filaments, again reducing the number of possible cross-bridges.
   TMP11 77, 78

2. (C) In contrast to primary and secondary transport, diffusion does not require the input of additional energy and, therefore, can work in the absence of ATP. Only facilitated diffusion displays saturation kinetics and involves a carrier protein. By definition, neither simple nor facilitated diffusion can move molecules from low to high concentration. The concept of specific inhibitors is not applicable to simple diffusion that occurs through a lipid bilayer without the aid of protein.
   TMP11 46

3. (B) Excitation-contraction coupling in skeletal muscle begins with an excitatory depolarization of the muscle membrane. This depolarization triggers the all-or-none opening of voltage-sensitive Na^{+} channels and an action potential that travels deep into the muscle via the T tubule network. At the T tubule–sarcoplasmic reticulum "triad," the depolarization of the T tubule causes a conformational change in the dihydropyridine receptor and subse-

quently in the ryanodine receptor on the sarcoplasmic reticulum. The latter causes the release of Ca^{++} into the sarcoplasm and the binding of Ca^{++} to troponin C (not to calmodulin) on the actin filament.
   TMP11 89-91

4. (D) Skeletal muscle contraction is tightly regulated by the concentration of Ca^{++} in the sarcoplasm. As long as sarcoplasmic Ca^{++} is sufficiently high, none of the remaining events—removal of acetylcholine from the neuromuscular junction, removal of Ca^{++} from the presynaptic terminal, closure of the acetylcholine receptor channel, and return of the dihydropyridine receptor to its resting conformation—would have any effect on the contractile state of the muscle.
   TMP11 90, 91

5. (B) In contrast to skeletal muscle, smooth muscle can be stimulated to contract without the generation of an action potential. For example, smooth muscle contracts in response to any stimulus that increases the cytosolic Ca^{++} concentration. This includes Ca^{++} channel openers, subthreshold depolarization, and a variety of tissue factors and circulating hormones that stimulate the release of intracellular Ca^{++} stores. Smooth muscle contraction uses less energy and lasts longer than skeletal muscle contraction does. Smooth muscle contraction is heavily Ca^{++} dependent and is inhibited by any stimulus that activates either adenylate or guanylate cyclase and increases cytosolic cyclic nucleotide concentrations.
   TMP11 95

6. (A) An important characteristic of visceral smooth muscle is its ability to contract in response to stretch. Stretch results in depolarization and potentially the generation of action potentials. These action potentials, coupled with normal slow-wave potentials, stimulate rhythmical contractions. Like skeletal muscle, smooth muscle contraction is both actin and ATP dependent. However, the cross-bridge cycle in smooth muscle is considerably slower than in skeletal muscle, which allows for a higher maximal force of contraction.
   TMP11 97

7. (B) The equilibrium potential for a monovalent ion can be calculated using the Nernst equation. For a monovalent anion such as Cl^-, $E = 60 \log (C_i/C_o)$. In this case, $E_{Cl^-} = 60 \log (11/110)$, or –60 millivolts. The chemical gradient for Cl^-, 110 millimolar extracellular and 11 millimolar intracellular, is balanced by a membrane potential of –60 millivolts.
   TMP11 58

8. (B) The equilibrium potential for a monovalent cation is $E = -60 \log (C_i/C_o)$. Here, $E_{K^+} = -60 \log (140/14)$, or –60 millivolts. It takes a membrane potential of –60 millivolts to counter a 10-fold K^+ concentration gradient, 140 millimolar intracellular and 14 millimolar extracellular.
   TMP11 58

9. (D) Quantitatively, the driving force on any given ion is the difference in millivolts between the membrane potential ($_mV$) and the equilibrium potential for that ion (E_{ion}). In this cell, $E_K = -60$ millivolts, $E_{Cl} = -60$ millivolts, $E_{Na} = 60$ millivolts, and $E_{Ca} = >125$ millivolts. Therefore, the ion with the equilibrium potential farthest from $_mV$ is Ca^{++}. Qualitatively, this means that under these conditions, Ca^{++}, a divalent cation with a 20,000-fold concentration gradient outside to inside, would have the highest tendency to cross the membrane, given an open channel.
   TMP11 58

10. (B) If a membrane is permeable to only a single ion, $_mV$ equals the equilibrium potential for that ion. In this cell, $E_K = -60$ millivolts. If the extracellular K^+ concentration is reduced 10-fold, $E_K = 60 \log (1.4/140)$, or –120 millivolts. This is a hyperpolarization of 60 millivolts.
   TMP11 58

11. (E) The neuromuscular junction is equipped with a so-called safety factor that ensures that every nerve impulse that travels to the terminal of a motor neuron results in an action potential in the sarcolemma. Given a normal, healthy muscle, contraction is also ensured. The voltage sensitivity of the Ca^{++} channels in the presynaptic membrane and the high concentration of extracellular Ca^{++} ensure an influx of Ca^{++} sufficient to stimulate the fusion of synaptic vesicles to the presynaptic membrane and the release of acetylcholine. The overabundance of acetylcholine released guarantees a depolarization of the postsynaptic membrane and the firing of an action potential.
   TMP11 88

12. (C) A solution of 140 millimolar NaCl has an osmolarity of 280 milliosmoles, which is iso-osmotic relative to "normal" intracellular osmolarity. If red blood cells were placed in 140 millimolar NaCl alone, there would be no change in cell volume because intracellular and extracellular osmolarities are equal. The presence of 20 millimolar urea, however, increases the solution's osmolarity and makes it hypertonic relative to the intracellular solution. Water will initially move out of the cell, but because the plasma membrane is permeable to urea, urea will diffuse into the cell and equilibrate across the plasma membrane. As a result, water will re-enter the cell, and the cell will return to its normal volume.
   TMP11 51; SEE ALSO CHAPTER 25

13. (E) The physical lengths of the actin and myosin filaments do not change during contraction. Therefore, the A band, which is composed of myosin filaments, does not change either. The distance between Z discs decreases, but the Z discs themselves do not change. Only the I band decreases in length as the muscle contracts.
   TMP11 74, 75

14. (C) The H zone is the region in the center of the sarcomere composed of the lighter bands on either side of and including the M line. In this region, the myosin filaments are centered on the M line, and there are no overlapping actin filaments. Therefore, a cross section through this region would reveal only myosin.

TMP11 74, 75

15. (C) In smooth muscle, the binding of four Ca^{++} ions to the protein calmodulin permits the interaction of the Ca^{++}-calmodulin complex with myosin light chain kinase. This interaction activates myosin light chain kinase, resulting in the phosphorylation of the myosin light chains and, ultimately, muscle contraction. In skeletal muscle, the activating Ca^{++} signal is received by the protein troponin C. Like calmodulin, each molecule of troponin C can bind with up to four Ca^{++} ions. Binding results in a conformational change in the troponin C protein that dislodges the tropomyosin molecule and exposes the active sites on the actin filament.

TMP11 95

16. (A) The resting potential of any cell is dependent on the concentration gradients of the permeant ions and their relative permeabilities (Goldman equation). In the myelinated nerve fiber, as in most cells, the membrane is predominantly permeable to K^+ at rest. The highly negative $_mV$ observed in cells such as nerve cells is primarily due to the greater than 10-fold higher concentration of K^+ in the cytosol compared with the extracellular fluid.

TMP11 60

17. (D) One osmole equals 1 g MW/L dissociated solute. Therefore, a solution of 12 millimolar NaCl contributes 0.012 g MW/L × 2, or 0.024 osmol/L. Likewise, 3 millimolar KCl contributes 0.003 g MW/L × 2, or 0.006 osmol/L, and 1 millimolar $CaCl_2$ contributes 0.001 g MW/L × 3, or 0.003 osmol/L. The overall osmolarity of this solution is 0.033 osmol/L, or 33 mOsm/L.

TMP11 52

18. (E) Contraction is dependent on an elevation of intracellular Ca^{++} concentration. At relatively low twitch frequency, the increase in intracellular Ca^{++} is transient. As the twitch frequency increases, the initiation of a subsequent twitch can occur before the previous twitch has subsided. As a result, the amplitude of the individual twitches is summed. This results from the prolonged increase in intracellular Ca^{++} concentration. At very high twitch frequencies, the muscle exhibits tetanic contraction. Under these conditions, intracellular Ca^{++} accumulates and supports sustained maximal contraction.

TMP11 81

19. (C) As long as the ryanodine receptor channel on the sarcoplasmic reticulum remains open, Ca^{++} will continue to flood the sarcoplasm and stimulate contraction. This prolonged contraction results in heat production, muscle rigidity, and lactic acidosis. In contrast, factors that either inhibit Ca^{++} release or stimulate Ca^{++} uptake into the sarcoplasmic reticulum, or that prevent either the depolarization of the T tubule membrane or the transduction of the depolarization into Ca^{++} release, would favor muscle relaxation.

TMP11 90

20. (C) Prolonged or repeated maximal contraction results in a concomitant increase in the synthesis of contractile proteins and an increase in muscle mass. This increase in mass, or hypertrophy, is observed at the level of individual muscle fibers.

TMP11 83

21. (A) Facilitated diffusion and both primary and secondary active transport all involve protein transporters or carriers that must undergo some rate-limited conformational change. The rate of simple diffusion is linear with solute concentration.

TMP11 46, 47

22. (C) The term "hyperosmotic" refers to a solution that has a higher osmolarity relative to another solution. The osmolarity of a 1-millimolar NaCl solution is 2 mOsm/L. The osmolarity of a 1-millimolar solution of either glucose or sucrose is only 1 mOsm/L. The osmolarity of a 1.5-millimolar glucose solution is 1.5 mOsm/L. These solutions are all "hypoosmotic" relative to 1 millimolar NaCl. The osmolarity of a 1-millimolar KCl solution is 2 mOsm/L. It is "iso-osmotic" relative to 1 millimolar NaCl. Only 1 millimolar $CaCl_2$, with an osmolarity of 3 mOsm/L, is hyperosmotic relative to 1 millimolar NaCl.

TMP11 51, 52

23. (A) At point B in this action potential, $_mV$ has reached threshold potential and has triggered the opening of voltage-gated Na^+ channels. The resulting Na^+ influx is responsible for the rapid, self-perpetuating depolarization phase of the action potential.

TMP11 61, 62

24. (D) The rapid depolarization phase is terminated at point D by the inactivation of the voltage-gated Na^+ channels and the opening of the voltage-gated K^+ channels. The latter results in the efflux of K^+ from the cytosol into the extracellular fluid and hyperpolarization or repolarization of the cell membrane.

TMP11 62

25. (B) The slower cycling rate of the cross-bridges in smooth muscle means that a higher percentage of possible cross-bridges is active at any point in time. The more active cross-bridges there are, the greater the force that is generated. Although the relatively slow cycling rate means that it takes longer for the myosin head to attach to the actin filament, it also means that the myosin head remains attached longer, prolonging muscle contraction. Because of the slow cross-bridge cycling rate, smooth muscle actually

requires *less* energy to maintain a contraction compared with skeletal muscle.
TMP11 94

26. (B) Myasthenia gravis is a neuromuscular junction disorder. Its symptoms result from the partial blockade of postsynaptic nicotinic acetylcholine receptors by antibodies against the receptor channel. This blockade prevents the firing of an action potential in the postsynaptic membrane. A positive Tensilon test reflects the ability of acetylcholine, when increased in the synapse, to compete with these antibodies and reverse the muscle weakness.
TMP11 89

27. (A) Myasthenia gravis is an autoimmune disease characterized by the presence of anti–acetylcholine receptor antibodies in the plasma. Overexertion can cause junction fatigue, and both a decrease in the density of voltage-sensitive Ca^{++} channels in the presynaptic membrane and botulinum toxicity can cause muscle weakness. However, these effects are presynaptic and therefore would not be reversed by acetylcholinesterase inhibition. Although the macro motor units formed during reinnervation following poliomyelitis compromise the patient's fine motor control, they do not affect muscle strength.
TMP11 89

28. (C) Neostigmine is an acetylcholinesterase inhibitor. Administration of this drug would increase the amount of acetylcholine (ACh) present in the synapse and its ability to sufficiently depolarize the postsynaptic membrane and trigger an action potential. Botulinum toxin antiserum is effective only against botulinum toxicity. Curare blocks the nicotinic ACh receptor and causes muscle weakness. Atropine is a muscarinic ACh receptor antagonist, and halothane is an anesthetic gas. Neither atropine nor halothane has any effect on the neuromuscular junction.
TMP11 89

29. (B) When a positive electrical charge of 60 millivolts is applied to chamber B, the positively charged Na^+ ions are repelled from chamber B into chamber A until the diffusional force from the concentration gradient is sufficient to counter the electromotive force. Using the Nernst equation, a 60-millivolt electromotive force would be offset by a 10-fold Na^+ concentration gradient. Therefore, at the new steady state, the $[Na]_A$ would be 10 times the $[Na]_B$.
TMP11 50

30. (B) In this diagram, "active" or contraction-dependent tension is the difference between total tension (trace A) and the tension contributed by noncontractile elements (trace C). The length-tension relationship in intact muscle resembles the biphasic relationship observed in individual sarcomeres and reflects the same physical interactions between actin and myosin filaments.
TMP11 78

31. (E) "Active" tension is maximal at normal physiological muscle lengths. At this point, there is optimal overlap between actin and myosin filaments to support maximal cross-bridge formation and tension development.
TMP11 78

32. (C) Trace C represents the passive tension contributed by noncontractile elements, including fascia, tendons, and ligaments. This passive tension accounts for an increasingly large portion of the total tension recorded in intact muscle as it is stretched beyond its normal length.
TMP11 78

33. (D) Smooth muscle contraction is regulated by both Ca^{++} and myosin light chain phosphorylation. When the cytosolic Ca^{++} concentration decreases following the initiation of contraction, myosin kinase becomes inactivated. However, cross-bridge formation continues, even in the absence of Ca^{++}, until the myosin light chains are dephosphorylated through the action of myosin light chain phosphatase.
TMP11 95

34. (D) The normal miniature end plate potentials indicate sufficient synthesis and packaging of ACh and the presence and normal function of ACh receptor channels. The most likely explanation for this patient's symptoms is a presynaptic deficiency—in this case, an impairment of the voltage-sensitive Ca^{++} channels responsible for the increase in cytosolic Ca^{++} that triggers the release of ACh into the synapse. The increase in postsynaptic depolarization observed after exercise is indicative of an accumulation of Ca^{++} in the presynaptic terminal after multiple action potentials have reached the nerve terminal.
TMP11 86

35. (A) Inhibition of the presynaptic voltage-sensitive Ca^{++} channels is most consistent with the presence of antibodies against this channel. Antibodies against the ACh receptor, a mutation in the ryanodine receptor, and residual ACh in the junction are all indicative of postsynaptic defects. Although it is a presynaptic defect, a deficit of ACh vesicles is unlikely in this scenario, given the normal miniature end plate potentials recorded in the postsynaptic membrane.
TMP11 86

36. (A) Botulinum toxin inhibits muscle contraction presynaptically by decreasing the amount of ACh released into the neuromuscular junction. In contrast, curare acts postsynaptically, blocking the nicotinic ACh receptors and preventing the excitation of the muscle cell membrane. Tetrodotoxin blocks voltage-sensitive Na^+ channels, impacting both the initiation and the propagation of action potentials in the motor neuron. Both ACh and neostigmine stimulate muscle contraction.
TMP11 86

37. (D) During an action potential in a nerve cell, $_mV$ approaches E_{Na} during the rapid depolarization phase when the permeability of the membrane to Na^+ (P_{Na}) increases relative to its permeability to K^+ (P_K). In a "typical" cell, E_{Na} is close to 60 millivolts. $_mV$ is closest to E_{Na} at point D in this diagram. At this point, the ratio of P_{Na} to P_K is the greatest.
    TMP11 61

38. (F) The driving force for Na^+ is greatest at the point at which $_mV$ is the farthest from E_{Na}. If E_{Na} is very positive (approximately 60 millivolts), $_mV$ is farthest from E_{Na} at point F, or when the cell is the most hyperpolarized.
    TMP11 61

39. (F) Generally, $_mV$ is closest to the equilibrium potential of the most permeant ion. In nerve cells, $P_K \gg P_{Na}$ at rest. As a result, $_mV$ is relatively close to E_K. During the afterpotential or the hyperpolarization phase of the action potential, the ratio of P_K to P_{Na} is even greater than it is at rest. This is due to the residual opening of voltage-gated K^+ channels and the inactivation of the voltage-gated Na^+ channels. $P_K:P_{Na}$ is greatest at point F, at which point $_mV$ comes closest to E_K.
    TMP11 61-63

40. (E) The stimulation of either adenylate or guanylate cyclase induces smooth muscle contraction. The cyclic nucleotides produced by these enzymes stimulate cAMP- and cGMP-dependent kinases, respectively. These kinases phosphorylate, among other things, enzymes that remove Ca^{++} from the cytosol, and in doing so they inhibit contraction. In contrast, either a decrease in K^+ permeability or an increase in Na^+ permeability results in membrane depolarization and contraction. Likewise, inhibition of the sarcoplasmic reticulum Ca^{++}-ATPase, one of the enzymes activated by cyclic nucleotide-dependent kinases, would also favor muscle contraction. Smooth muscle does not express troponin.
    TMP11 98

41. (E) The accumulation of Ca^{++} by the sarcoplasmic reticulum, the transport of Na^+ into and K^+ out of a cell, and the transport of H^+ from parietal cells all occur through primary active transport mechanisms involving ATPase enzymes. In this case, only glucose transport, which occurs via facilitated diffusion in muscle, does not directly utilize ATP.
    TMP11 49-50

42. (C) The redistribution of fluid volume shown in diagram B reflects the net diffusion of water, or osmosis, due to differences in the osmolarity of the solutions on either side of the semipermeable membrane. Osmosis occurs from solutions of high water concentration to low water concentration or from low osmolarity to high osmolarity. In diagram B, osmosis has occurred from X to Y and from Y to Z. Therefore, the osmolarity of solution Z is higher than that of solution Y, and the osmolarity of solution Y is higher than that of solution X.
    TMP11 51-52

43. (A) Increasing the sarcoplasmic Ca^{++} concentration can increase force generation in a single muscle fiber. This can be accomplished by increasing the frequency of stimulation of the fiber. Neither increasing the amplitude of the depolarization at the postsynaptic membrane of the neuromuscular junction nor increasing the number of voltage-gated Na^+ channels is likely to affect the release of Ca^{++} from the sarcoplasmic reticulum. In contrast, both a decrease in the extracellular K^+ concentration and an increase in the permeability of the muscle membrane to K^+ would decrease excitability of the muscle cell.
    TMP11 81

44. (E) The "plateau" exhibited by the action potential in trace B is characteristic of cells that use voltage-gated Ca^{++} channels rather than voltage-gated Na^+ channels to generate the rapid depolarization phase of the action potential. These so-called slow Ca^{++} channels have a slower inactivation rate, thereby lengthening the time during which they are open. This, in turn, delays the repolarization phase of the action potential, creating a "plateau" before the channels inactivate.
    TMP11 64; SEE ALSO CHAPTER 9

45. (A) In the absence of hyperpolarization, the inability of an otherwise excitatory stimulus to initiate an action potential is most likely the result of the blockade of the voltage-gated channels responsible for the generation of the all-or-none depolarization. In nerve cells, these are the voltage-gated Na^+ channels.
    TMP11 61

46. (B) Trace A reflects the kinetics of a process that is limited by an intrinsic V_{max}. Of the choices provided, only the transport of K^+, which occurs through the activity of the Na^+, K^+-ATPase, is the result of an active transport or facilitated diffusion event. The movement of CO_2 and O_2 through a biological membrane and the movement of Ca^{++} and Na^+ through ion channels are all examples of simple diffusion.
    TMP11 53

47. (B) Trace B is indicative of a process not limited by an intrinsic V_{max}. This excludes active transport and facilitated diffusion. Therefore, of the choices provided, only the rate of transport of O_2 across an artificial lipid bilayer via simple diffusion would be accurately reflected by trace B.
    TMP11 46

48. (C) Skeletal muscle continuously remodels in response to its level of use. When a muscle is inactive for an extended period, the rate of synthesis of the contractile proteins in individual muscle fibers decreases, resulting in an overall reduction in muscle

mass. This reversible reduction in muscle mass is called atrophy.
TMP11 82, 83

49. (B) For a muscle to contract spontaneously and rhythmically, there must be an intrinsic rhythmical "pacemaker." Intestinal smooth muscle, for example, exhibits a rhythmical slow-wave potential that transiently depolarizes and repolarizes the muscle membrane. This slow wave does not stimulate contraction itself, but if the amplitude is sufficient, it can trigger one or more action potentials that result in Ca^{++} influx and contraction. Although they are typical of smooth muscle, neither "slow" voltage-sensitive Ca^{++} channels nor action potentials with "plateaus" play a necessary role in rhythmical contraction. A high resting cytosolic Ca^{++} concentration would support a sustained contraction, and hyperpolarization would favor relaxation.
TPM11 97

50. (C) Ouabain inhibits Na^+, K^+-ATPase. This ATP-dependent enzyme transports three Na^+ ions out of the cell for every two K^+ ions it transports into the cell. It is a classic example of primary active transport.
TMP11 53

51. (B) Glucose is transported into skeletal muscle cells via insulin-dependent facilitated diffusion.
TMP11 49, 50; SEE ALSO CHAPTER 78

52. (E) The activity of Na^+, K^+-ATPase maintains the relatively high K^+ concentration inside the cell and the relatively high Na^+ concentration in the extracellular solution. This large concentration gradient for Na^+ across the plasma membrane, together with the net negative charge on the inside of the cell, continuously drives Na^+ ions from the extracellular solution into the cytosol. This energy is used to transport other molecules, such as Ca^{++}, against their concentration gradients. Because ATP is required to maintain the Na^+ gradient that drives this counter-transport, this type of transport is called secondary active transport.
TMP11 54, 55

53. (D) Much like Na^+-Ca^{++} counter-transport, the strong tendency for Na^+ to move across the plasma membrane into the cytosol can be harnessed by transport proteins and used to co-transport molecules against their concentration gradients into the cytosol. An example of this type of secondary co-transport is the transport of glucose into intestinal epithelial cells.
TMP11 55

54. (A) During the rapid depolarization phase of a nerve action potential, voltage-sensitive Na^+ channels open and allow the influx of Na^+ ions into the cytosol. Transport through membrane channels is an example of simple diffusion.
TMP11 47; SEE ALSO CHAPTER 5

55. (C) Trace A exhibits the characteristic shape of an action potential, including the rapid depolarization followed by a rapid repolarization that temporarily overshoots the resting potential. Trace B best illustrates the change in P_{Na} that occurs during an action potential. The rapid increase in P_{Na} closely parallels the rapid depolarization phase of the action potential. Trace C best illustrates the slow onset of the increase in P_K that reflects the opening of the voltage-gated K^+ channels.
TMP11 64

56. (D) Myelination of the axons of large nerve fibers has several consequences. It provides insulation to the axon membrane, decreasing membrane capacitance and thereby decreasing the "leakage" of ions across the cell membrane. Action potentials in myelinated axons occur only at the periodic breaks in the myelin sheath, called nodes of Ranvier. Voltage-gated Na^+ channels are concentrated at these nodes. This arrangement both increases the velocity of the nerve impulses along the axon and minimizes the number of charges that cross the membrane during an impulse, thereby minimizing the energy required by Na^+, K^+-ATPase to re-establish the relative concentration gradients for Na^+ and K^+.
TMP11 68

57. (A) Muscle fibers involved in fine motor control are generally innervated by small motor neurons with relatively small motor units, including those that innervate single fibers. These neurons fire in response to a smaller depolarizing stimulus compared with motor neurons with larger motor units. As a result, during weak contractions, increases in muscle contraction can occur in small steps, allowing for fine motor control. This concept is called the size principle.
TMP11 81

58. (C) The strongest common denominator among smooth, skeletal, and cardiac muscle contraction is their shared dependence on Ca^{++} for the initiation of contraction. Cardiac and skeletal muscles exhibit several characteristics not shared by smooth muscle. For example, the contractile proteins in both cardiac and skeletal muscles are organized into discrete sarcomeres. Both muscle types also possess some semblance of a T tubule system and are dependent on the generation of action potentials for their contraction. Smooth muscle, in contrast, is relatively less organized, is uniquely regulated by myosin light chain phosphorylation, and can contract in vivo in the absence of action potentials.
TMP11 95; SEE ALSO CHAPTER 9

59. (B) Net diffusion of a substance across a permeable membrane is proportional to the concentration difference of the substance on either side of the membrane. Initially, the concentration difference is 5 millimolar (10 millimolar – 5 millimolar). When the intracellular concentration doubles to 20

millimolar, the concentration difference becomes 15
millimolar (20 millimolar − 5 millimolar). The concentration difference has tripled; therefore, the rate
of diffusion would also increase by a factor of 3.
  TMP11 50

60. (B) Muscle B is characteristic of a "slow" muscle;
that is, it is made up of predominantly "slow"
muscle fibers. These fibers are smaller in size and
are innervated by smaller nerve fibers. They typically have a more extensive blood supply, a greater
number of mitochondria, and large amounts of myoglobin, all of which support the high levels of oxidative phosphorylation.
  TMP11 80, 81

61. (C) Muscle contraction is triggered by an increase in
sarcoplasmic Ca^{++} concentration. The delay between
the termination of the depolarizing pulse and the
onset of muscle contraction, also called the "lag,"
reflects the time necessary for the depolarizing pulse
to be translated into an increase in sarcoplasmic Ca^{++}
concentration. This process involves a conformational change in the voltage-sensing, or dihydropyridine, receptor located on the T tubule membrane; the
subsequent conformational change in the ryanodine
receptor on the sarcoplasmic reticulum; and the
release of Ca^{++} from the sarcoplasmic reticulum.
  TMP11 74; SEE ALSO CHAPTER 7

The Heart

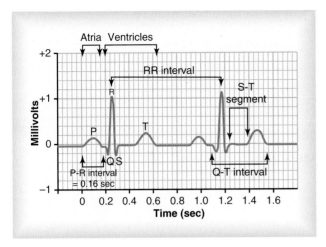

Questions 5-8

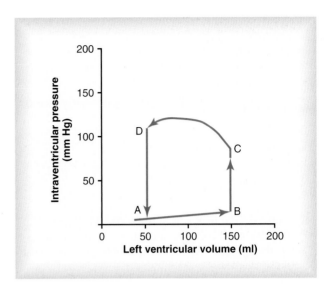

1. A 50-year-old man was admitted to the emergency department because of nausea. The electrocardiogram above was taken, showing standard lead II. What is his Q-T interval?
   (A) 0.12 second
   (B) 0.16 second
   (C) 0.22 second
   (D) 0.30 second
   (E) 0.35 second

2. Which of the following best explains how sympathetic stimulation affects the heart?
   (A) The permeability of the sinoatrial (S-A) node to sodium decreases
   (B) The permeability of the atrioventricular (A-V) node to sodium decreases
   (C) The permeability of the S-A node to potassium increases
   (D) The rate of upward drift of the resting membrane potential of the S-A node increases
   (E) The permeability of the cardiac muscle to calcium decreases

3. Which of the following structures has the slowest rate of conduction of the cardiac action potential?
   (A) Atrial muscle
   (B) Anterior internodal pathway
   (C) Atrioventricular bundle fibers
   (D) Purkinje fibers
   (E) Ventricular muscle

4. A 75-year-old man comes into the emergency department and faints. Five minutes later, he is alert. An electrocardiogram shows 75 P waves per minute and 35 QRS waves per minute, with a normal QRS width. Which of the following is the most likely diagnosis?
   (A) First degree atrioventricular block
   (B) Stokes-Adams syndrome
   (C) Atrial paroxysmal tachycardia
   (D) Electrical alternans
   (E) Atrial premature contractions

A 54-year-old woman has a resting cardiac output of 7000 ml/min. Her arterial pressure is 125/85 mm Hg, and her body temperature is normal. A diagram of the pressure-volume of the left ventricle is shown above.

5. What is her heart rate?
   (A) 46.7 beats/min
   (B) 50 beats/min
   (C) 70 beats/min
   (D) 100 beats/min
   (E) 140 beats/min

6. What is her ejection fraction?
   (A) 33.3 per cent
   (B) 50 per cent
   (C) 66.7 per cent
   (D) 80 per cent
   (E) 100 per cent

7. Which of the following events occurs at point D in her pressure-volume relationship?
   (A) A-V valves close
   (B) Aortic valve opens
   (C) Aortic valve closes
   (D) A-V valves open
   (E) Third heart sound

8. Which phase of her cardiac cycle occurs between points D and A?
   (A) Isovolumic contraction
   (B) Ventricular ejection
   (C) Isovolumic relaxation
   (D) Ventricular filling
   (E) Atrial contraction

9. When traveling −60 degrees in the frontal plane, a ventricular depolarization wave causes a large negative deflection in which lead?
   (A) aVR
   (B) aVL
   (C) Lead II
   (D) Lead III
   (E) aVF

10. If the sinoatrial node discharges at 0.00 seconds, when will the action potential normally arrive at the epicardial surface at the base of the left ventricle?
    (A) 0.22 second
    (B) 0.18 second
    (C) 0.16 second
    (D) 0.12 second
    (E) 0.09 second

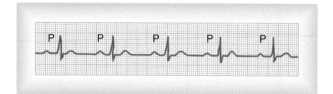

11. A 60-year-old man who weighs 100 kilograms (220 pounds) had the electrocardiogram above, showing standard lead II. Which of the following is the most likely diagnosis?
    (A) A-V nodal rhythm
    (B) First degree A-V heart block
    (C) Second degree A-V heart block
    (D) Third degree A-V heart block
    (E) Atrial flutter

12. Which of the following events occurs at the end of isovolumic contraction?
    (A) A-V valves close
    (B) Aortic valve opens
    (C) Aortic valve closes
    (D) A-V valves open
    (E) Pulmonary valve closes

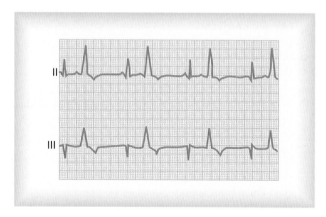

13. A 35-year-old woman felt unusual sensations in her chest after she smoked a cigarette. She was taken to the emergency department, where the electrocardiogram shown above was recorded. Which of the following is the most likely diagnosis?
    (A) Premature contraction originating in the atrium
    (B) Premature contraction originating high in the A-V node
    (C) Premature contraction originating low in the A-V node
    (D) Premature contraction originating in the apex of the ventricle
    (E) Premature contraction originating in the base of the ventricle

14. If the sinoatrial node discharges at 0.00 seconds, when will the action potential normally arrive at the atrioventricular bundle (bundle of His)?
    (A) 0.22 second
    (B) 0.18 second
    (C) 0.16 second
    (D) 0.12 second
    (E) 0.09 second

Questions 15 and 16

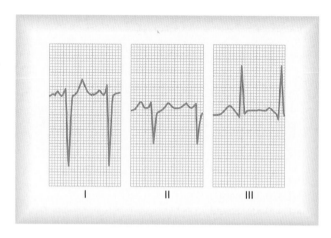

A 55-year-old man reports to his physician that he becomes easily fatigued while doing routine work around the house. The electrocardiogram shown above was recorded at his physician's office.

15. What is the mean electrical axis calculated from standard leads I, II, and III shown in the electrocardiogram above?
    (A) −170 degrees
    (B) −20 degrees
    (C) 0 degrees
    (D) +60 degrees
    (E) +170 degrees

16. Which of the following is the most likely diagnosis?
    (A) Right ventricular hypertrophy
    (B) Complete left bundle branch block
    (C) Pulmonary valve stenosis
    (D) Right bundle branch block
    (E) Left ventricular hypertrophy

17. According to Einthoven's law, if the QRS voltage is 1.0 millivolt in lead I and 2.0 millivolts in lead II, what is the QRS voltage in lead III?
    (A) 0.05 millivolt
    (B) 0.5 millivolt
    (C) 1.0 millivolt
    (D) 1.2 millivolts
    (E) 2.05 millivolts

Questions 18 and 19

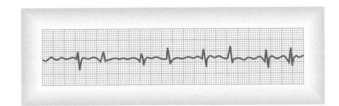

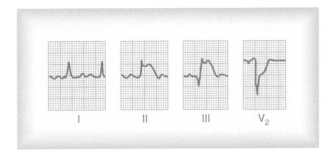

A 55-year-old man had the above electrocardiogram recorded at his physician's office during a routine examination.

18. Which of the following is the most likely diagnosis?
    (A) Normal electrocardiogram
    (B) Atrial flutter
    (C) High A-V junctional pacemaker
    (D) Middle A-V junctional pacemaker
    (E) Low A-V junctional pacemaker

19. What is his ventricular heart rate?
    (A) 37.5 beats/min
    (B) 60 beats/min
    (C) 75 beats/min
    (D) 100 beats/min
    (E) 120 beats/min

20. The electrocardiogram of a 60-year-old man shows that he has an R-R interval of 0.55 second. Which of the following best explains his condition?
    (A) He has a fever
    (B) He has a normal heart rate
    (C) He has excess parasympathetic stimulation of the sinoatrial (S-A) node
    (D) He is a trained athlete at rest
    (E) He has hyperpolarization of the S-A node

21. Which of the following is most likely to cause the heart to go into spastic contraction?
    (A) Increased body temperature
    (B) Increased sympathetic activity
    (C) Decreased extracellular fluid potassium ions
    (D) Excess extracellular fluid potassium ions
    (E) Excess extracellular fluid calcium ions

22. Which of the following conditions at the sinoatrial node causes the heart rate to decrease?
    (A) Increased norepinephrine levels
    (B) Increased sodium permeability
    (C) Increased calcium permeability
    (D) Increased potassium permeability
    (E) Decreased acetylcholine levels

23. A 60-year-old woman is brought to the emergency department because of chest pain. Based on the electrocardiogram tracing shown above, which of the following is the most likely diagnosis?
    (A) Acute anterior infarction in the base of the heart
    (B) Acute anterior infarction in the apex of the heart
    (C) Acute posterior infarction in the base of the heart
    (D) Acute posterior infarction in the apex of the heart
    (E) Right ventricular hypertrophy

24. Increased sympathetic stimulation of the heart causes which of the following?
    (A) Decreased heart rate
    (B) Hyperpolarization of the atrioventricular node
    (C) Decreased atrial contractility
    (D) Decreased ventricular contractility
    (E) Increased norepinephrine release at the ventricular sympathetic nerve endings

25. Which of the following conditions usually results in right axis deviation in an electrocardiogram?
    (A) Systemic hypertension
    (B) Aortic valve stenosis
    (C) Aortic valve regurgitation
    (D) Excess abdominal fat
    (E) Pulmonary hypertension

26. A 60-year-old woman has been diagnosed with atrial fibrillation. Which of the following statements best describes this condition?
    (A) The ventricular rate of contraction is 140 beats/min
    (B) The P waves of the electrocardiogram are pronounced
    (C) Ventricular contractions occur at regular intervals
    (D) The QRS waves are more pronounced than normal
    (E) The atria are smaller than normal

27. Which of the following is most characteristic of atrial fibrillation?
    (A) It occurs less frequently in patients with atrial enlargement
    (B) The ventricular heart rate is about 40 beats/min
    (C) The efficiency of ventricular pumping is decreased 20 to 30 per cent
    (D) The ventricular beat is regular
    (E) The atrial P wave is easily seen

28. When traveling –30 degrees in the frontal plane, a ventricular depolarization wave causes a large positive deflection in which of the following leads?
    (A) aVR
    (B) aVL
    (C) Lead I
    (D) Lead II
    (E) aVF

29. In a resting adult, the typical ventricular ejection fraction has what value?
    (A) 20 per cent
    (B) 30 per cent
    (C) 40 per cent
    (D) 60 per cent
    (E) 80 per cent

30. If the sinoatrial node discharges at 0.00 seconds, when will the action potential normally arrive at the atrioventricular node?
    (A) 0.80 second
    (B) 0.16 second
    (C) 0.12 second
    (D) 0.09 second
    (E) 0.03 second

31. Which of the following responses is caused by acetylcholine?
    (A) Depolarization of the sinoatrial node
    (B) Depolarization of the atrioventricular node
    (C) Increased permeability of the sinoatrial node to potassium ions
    (D) Increased heart rate
    (E) Increased permeability of the cardiac muscle to calcium ions

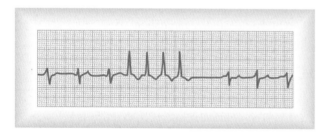

32. A 65-year-old woman who had a myocardial infarction 10 days ago returns to her physician's office for a checkup. She reports that her pulse rate seems rapid. Based on the electrocardiogram shown above, which of the following is the most likely diagnosis?
    (A) Stokes-Adams syndrome
    (B) Atrial fibrillation
    (C) A-V nodal tachycardia
    (D) Atrial paroxysmal tachycardia
    (E) Ventricular paroxysmal tachycardia

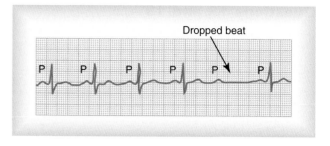

Dropped beat

33. A 65-year-old man had the above electrocardiogram recorded during his annual physical examination. Which of the following is the most likely diagnosis?
    (A) Atrial paroxysmal tachycardia
    (B) First degree A-V block
    (C) Second degree A-V block
    (D) Third degree A-V block
    (E) Atrial flutter

34. What is the membrane potential (threshold level) at which the sinoatrial node discharges?
    (A) –40 millivolts
    (B) –55 millivolts
    (C) –65 millivolts
    (D) –85 millivolts
    (E) –105 millivolts

Questions 35 and 36

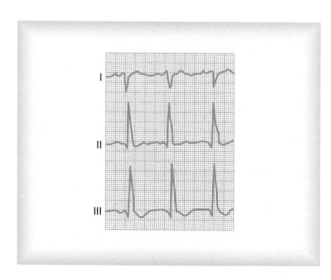

I

II

III

A 62-year-old man has smoked cigarettes for 30 years and weighs about 114 kilograms (250 pounds). His electrocardiogram recorded at the hospital is shown above.

35. Which of the following is the mean electrical axis calculated from standard leads I, II, and III in this patient's electrocardiogram?
    (A) –110 degrees
    (B) –20 degrees
    (C) +90 degrees
    (D) +105 degrees
    (E) +180 degrees

36. Which of the following is the most likely diagnosis?
    (A) Left ventricular hypertrophy
    (B) Left bundle branch block
    (C) Tricuspid stenosis
    (D) Right bundle branch block
    (E) Right ventricular hypertrophy

37. A 30-year-old man has an ejection fraction of 0.25 and an end-systolic volume of 150 milliliters. What is his end-diastolic volume?
    (A) 50 milliliters
    (B) 100 milliliters
    (C) 125 milliliters
    (D) 200 milliliters
    (E) 250 milliliters

38. Which of the following usually results in an inverted P wave that occurs after the QRS complex?
    (A) Premature contraction originating in the atrium
    (B) Premature contraction originating high in the A-V junction
    (C) Premature contraction originating in the middle of the A-V junction
    (D) Premature contraction originating low in the A-V junction
    (E) Atrial fibrillation

39. Which of the following decreases the risk of ventricular fibrillation?
    (A) Dilated heart
    (B) Increased ventricular refractory period
    (C) Decreased electrical conduction velocity
    (D) Exposure of the heart to 60-cycle alternating current
    (E) Administration of epinephrine

40. A 60-year-old woman has lost some of her ability to perform normal household tasks and is not feeling well. An electrocardiogram shows a QRS complex with a width of 0.20 second; the T wave is inverted in lead I, and the R wave has a large negative deflection in lead III. Which of the following is the most likely diagnosis?
    (A) Right ventricular hypertrophy
    (B) Left bundle branch block
    (C) Pulmonary valve stenosis
    (D) Right bundle branch block
    (E) Left ventricular hypertrophy

41. Which of the following conditions at the A-V node causes a decrease in heart rate?
    (A) Increased sodium permeability
    (B) Decreased acetylcholine levels
    (C) Increased norepinephrine levels
    (D) Increased potassium permeability
    (E) Increased calcium permeability

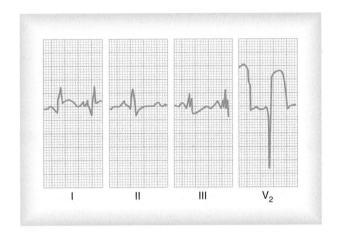

I   II   III   V$_2$

42. A 70-year-old woman is brought to the emergency department because she is experiencing chest pain. Based on the electrocardiogram tracing shown above, which of the following is the most likely diagnosis?
    (A) Acute anterior infarction in the left ventricle of the heart
    (B) Acute anterior infarction in the right ventricle of the heart
    (C) Acute posterior infarction in the left ventricle of the heart
    (D) Acute posterior infarction in the right ventricle of the heart
    (E) Right ventricular hypertrophy

43. Which of the following statements about cardiac muscle is most accurate?
    (A) The T tubules of cardiac muscle can store much less calcium than the T tubules of skeletal muscle can
    (B) The strength and contraction of cardiac muscle depend on the amount of calcium surrounding cardiac myocytes
    (C) In cardiac muscle, the initiation of the action potential causes an immediate opening of slow calcium channels
    (D) Cardiac muscle repolarization is caused by the opening of sodium channels
    (E) Mucopolysaccharides inside the T tubules bind chloride ions

44. Which of the following events occurs at the end of the period of ventricular ejection?
    (A) A-V valves close
    (B) Aortic valve opens
    (C) Aortic valve remains open
    (D) A-V valves open
    (E) Pulmonary valve closes

45. Which of the following occurs after the heart is stimulated with a 60-cycle alternating current?
    (A) Velocity of conduction through the heart muscle decreases
    (B) Longer ventricular refractory period
    (C) Decreased tendency for circus movements
    (D) Decreased tendency for ventricular fibrillation

46. Which of the following statements best describes a patient with premature atrial contractions?
    (A) The pulse taken from the radial artery immediately following the premature contraction is weak
    (B) The stroke volume immediately following the premature contraction is increased
    (C) The P wave is never seen
    (D) The probability of these premature contractions occurring is decreased in a patient with a high caffeine intake
    (E) The QRS interval is lengthened

47. A 30-year-old man had an electrocardiogram at his physician's office, but his records were lost. The technician remembered that the QRS deflection was large and positive in lead aVF and 0 in lead I. What is the mean electrical axis in the frontal plane?
    (A) 90 degrees
    (B) 60 degrees
    (C) 0 degrees
    (D) –60 degrees
    (E) –90 degrees

Questions 48 and 49

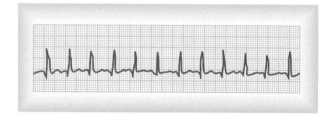

A 63-year-old man had a myocardial infarction at age 55. The standard limb lead I is shown above.

48. What is this patient's heart rate?
    (A) 40 beats/min
    (B) 50 beats/min
    (C) 75 beats/min
    (D) 100 beats/min
    (E) 150 beats/min

49. Which of the following is the current diagnosis?
    (A) Sinus tachycardia
    (B) First degree heart block
    (C) Second degree heart block
    (D) S-T segment depression
    (E) Third degree heart block

50. If the atrioventricular node becomes the pacemaker of the heart, what is the expected heart rate?
    (A) 30 beats/min
    (B) 50 beats/min
    (C) 65 beats/min
    (D) 75 beats/min
    (E) 85 beats/min

51. A 25-year-old well-conditioned athlete weighs 80 kilograms (176 pounds). During maximal sympathetic stimulation, what is the plateau level of his cardiac output function curve?
    (A) 3 L/min
    (B) 5 L/min
    (C) 10 L/min
    (D) 13 L/min
    (E) 25 L/min

52. A 55-year-old man has been diagnosed with Stokes-Adams syndrome. Two minutes after the syndrome starts to cause active blockade of the cardiac impulse, which of the following is the pacemaker of the heart?
    (A) Sinus node
    (B) A-V node
    (C) Purkinje fibers
    (D) Cardiac septum
    (E) Left atrium

53. What is the normal total delay of the cardiac impulse in the A-V node and the A-V bundle system?
    (A) 0.03 second
    (B) 0.06 second
    (C) 0.09 second
    (D) 0.13 second
    (E) 0.17 second

54. If the origin of the stimulus that causes atrial paroxysmal tachycardia is near the atrioventricular node, which of the following statements about the P wave in standard limb lead I is most accurate?
    (A) The P wave originates in the sinus node
    (B) The P wave is upright
    (C) The P wave is inverted
    (D) The P wave is missing

55. A 35-year-old man has dyspnea. His electrocardiogram shows no P waves, and he has a heart rate of 42 beats/min. Which of the following is the most likely diagnosis?
    (A) First degree heart block
    (B) Second degree heart block
    (C) Third degree heart block
    (D) Sinoatrial heart block
    (E) Sinus bradycardia

56. Which of the following events is associated with the first heart sound?
    (A) Closing of the aortic valve
    (B) Inrushing of blood into the ventricles during diastole
    (C) Beginning of diastole
    (D) Opening of the A-V valves
    (E) Closing of the A-V valves

Questions 57 and 58

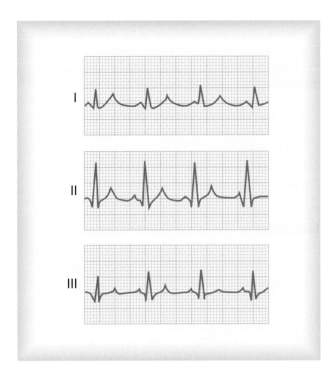

A 65-year-old man was injured in a motor vehicle accident and was taken to the emergency department. Physical examination showed a blood pressure of 160/80 mm Hg, and the electrocardiogram above was taken.

57. What is this patient's heart rate?
 (A) 64 beats/min
 (B) 74 beats/min
 (C) 88 beats/min
 (D) 94 beats/min
 (E) 104 beats/min

58. What is this patient's P-Q interval?
 (A) 0.07 second
 (B) 0.10 second
 (C) 0.14 second
 (D) 0.20 second
 (E) 0.24 second

59. What is the resting membrane potential of the sinus nodal fibers?
 (A) –100 millivolts
 (B) –90 millivolts
 (C) –80 millivolts
 (D) –55 millivolts
 (E) –20 millivolts

60. Which of the following conditions in ventricular muscle decreases the tendency for circus movement?
 (A) Longer refractory period
 (B) Dilated heart
 (C) Decreased conduction velocity
 (D) Repetitive electrical stimulation
 (E) Administration of epinephrine

61. Which of the following phases of the cardiac cycle follows immediately after the beginning of the QRS wave?
 (A) Isovolumic relaxation
 (B) Ventricular ejection
 (C) Atrial systole
 (D) Diastasis
 (E) Isovolumic contraction

62. Which of the following is most likely to occur at the J point in an electrocardiogram of a patient with a damaged cardiac muscle?
 (A) The entire heart is depolarized
 (B) All the heart is depolarized except for the damaged cardiac muscle
 (C) About half the heart is depolarized
 (D) All the heart is repolarized
 (E) All the heart is repolarized except for the damaged cardiac muscle

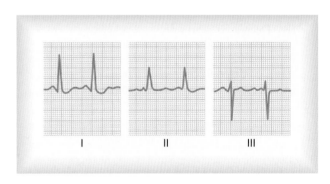

63. A 50-year-old man undergoes a routine physical examination as a new employee at ABC Software. The electrocardiogram above is recorded during the examination. Which of the following is the most likely diagnosis?
 (A) Chronic systemic hypertension
 (B) Chronic pulmonary hypertension
 (C) Second degree heart block
 (D) Paroxysmal tachycardia
 (E) Tricuspid valve stenosis

64. If the Purkinje fibers, situated distal to the atrioventricular junction, become the pacemaker of the heart, what is the expected heart rate?
 (A) 30 beats/min
 (B) 50 beats/min
 (C) 60 beats/min
 (D) 70 beats/min
 (E) 80 beats/min

65. Which of the following conditions results in a dilated, flaccid heart?
 (A) Excess calcium ions in the blood
 (B) Excess potassium ions in the blood
 (C) Excess sodium ions in the blood
 (D) Increased sympathetic stimulation
 (E) Increased norepinephrine concentration in the blood

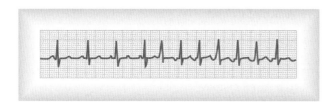

66. A 45-year-old man has the above electrocardiogram recorded during his annual physical examination. Which of the following is the most likely diagnosis?
    (A) Atrial paroxysmal tachycardia
    (B) First degree A-V block
    (C) Second degree A-V block
    (D) Ventricular paroxysmal tachycardia
    (E) Atrial flutter

67. Which of the following conditions is normally caused by sympathetic stimulation of the heart?
    (A) Acetylcholine release at the sympathetic endings
    (B) Decreased heart rate
    (C) Decreased rate of conduction of the cardiac impulse
    (D) Decreased force of contraction of the atria
    (E) Increased force of contraction of the ventricles

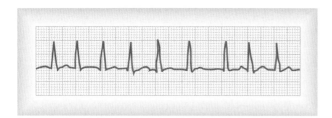

68. A 60-year-old woman sees her physician for an annual physical examination. The physician orders an electrocardiogram, which is shown above. Which of the following is the most likely diagnosis?
    (A) First degree A-V block
    (B) Second degree A-V block
    (C) Third degree A-V block
    (D) Atrial paroxysmal tachycardia
    (E) Atrial fibrillation

69. A 55-year-old man has an electrocardiogram as part of his annual physical examination. The net deflection (R wave – Q or S wave) in standard limb lead I is –1.2 millivolts, and standard limb lead II has a net deflection of +1.2 millivolts. What is the mean electrical axis of his QRS?
    (A) –30 degrees
    (B) +30 degrees
    (C) +60 degrees
    (D) +120 degrees
    (E) –120 degrees

70. Which of the following conditions at the atrioventricular node causes a decrease in heart rate?
    (A) Increased sodium permeability
    (B) Decreased acetylcholine levels
    (C) Increased norepinephrine levels
    (D) Increased potassium permeability
    (E) Increased calcium permeability

71. A 65-year-old patient with a heart murmur has a mean QRS axis of 120 degrees, and the duration of the QRS complex is 0.18 second. Which of the following is the most likely diagnosis?
    (A) Aortic valve stenosis
    (B) Aortic valve regurgitation
    (C) Pulmonary valve stenosis
    (D) Right bundle branch block
    (E) Left bundle branch block

Questions 72 and 73

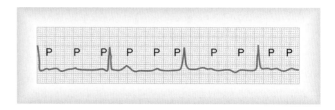

An 80-year-old man went to his family physician for an annual checkup. His electrocardiogram tracing is shown above.

72. What is this patient's heart rate?
    (A) 105 beats/min
    (B) 95 beats/min
    (C) 85 beats/min
    (D) 75 beats/min
    (E) 40 beats/min

73. Which of the following is the most likely diagnosis?
    (A) Left bundle branch block
    (B) First degree A-V block
    (C) Second degree A-V block
    (D) Electrical alternans
    (E) Complete A-V block

74. What is the normal P-R interval?
    (A) 0.03 second
    (B) 0.13 second
    (C) 0.16 second
    (D) 0.20 second
    (E) 0.35 second

75. A 60-year-old woman is easily fatigued. Her electrocardiogram shows a QRS complex that is positive in the aVF lead and negative in standard limb lead I. Which of the following is the most likely cause of her condition?
    (A) Chronic systemic hypertension
    (B) Pulmonary hypertension
    (C) Aortic valve stenosis
    (D) Aortic valve regurgitation

Answers

1. (D) The contraction of the ventricles lasts almost from the beginning of the Q wave and continues to the end of the T wave. This interval is called the Q-T interval, and it ordinarily lasts about 0.35 second. This patient's Q-T interval is somewhat shorter than average and equals 0.30 second.
   TMP11 124

2. (D) During sympathetic stimulation, the permeability of the sinoatrial (S-A) node and the atrioventricular node increases. Also, the permeability of cardiac muscle to calcium increases, resulting in an increased contractile strength. In addition, there is an upward drift of the resting membrane potential of the S-A node. Increased permeability of the S-A node to potassium does not occur during sympathetic stimulation.
   TMP11 121, 122

3. (C) The atrial and ventricular muscles conduct the cardiac action potential at a relatively rapid rate, and the anterior internodal pathway also conducts the impulse fairly rapidly. However, the atrioventricular bundle myofibrils have a slow rate of conduction because they are considerably smaller than the normal atrial and ventricular muscles. Also, their slow conduction is partly caused by a diminished number of gap junctions between successive muscle cells in the conducting pathway, causing a great resistance to conduction of the excitatory ions from cell to cell.
   TMP11 118, 119

4. (B) A sudden onset of A-V block that comes and goes is called the Stokes-Adams syndrome. The patient depicted here has about 75 P waves per minute, which means that the atria are contracting normally. However, the A-V block that occurs allows only 35 QRS waves to occur each minute.
   TMP11 149, 150

5. (C) Heart rate can be determined by using the following formula: Cardiac output = Heart rate × Stroke volume. This patient has a cardiac output of 7000 ml/min. The stroke volume can be determined from the figure, which is the volume change during the C-D segment, or 100 milliliters. Thus, the heart rate is 70 beats/min.
   TMP11 110

6. (C) The ejection fraction is the stroke volume divided by the end-diastolic volume. Thus, stroke volume is 100 milliliters, and the end-diastolic volume at point D is 150 milliliters. The ejection fraction is thus 0.667, or 66.7 per cent.
   TMP11 108

7. (C) During the ejection phase, the aortic valve opens and blood flows into the aorta. The ejection phase is between points C and D, so the aortic valve opens at C and closes at D.
   TMP11 111

8. (C) The period of ventricular filling is between points A and B. The period of isovolumic contraction is between points B and C, and the period of ejection is between points C and D. The period of isovolumic relaxation is between points D and A. The word "isovolumic" means the same volume. Therefore, notice that the volume remains the same between points D and A.
   TMP11 111

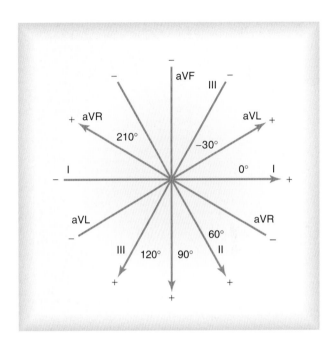

9. (D) As can be seen in the figure above, the positive portion of lead III has an axis of 120 degrees, and the negative part of this lead has an axis of –60 degrees. Notice that the difference between the positive and negative ends of this vector is 180 degrees.
   TMP11 132

10. (A) After the sinoatrial node discharges, the action potential travels through the atria, through the atrioventricular bundle system, and finally to the ventricular septum and throughout the ventricle. The last site where the impulse arrives is the epicardial surface at the base of the left ventricle, which requires a transit time of 0.22 second.
    TMP11 119, 120

11. (B) By definition, first degree A-V heart block occurs when the P-R interval exceeds a value of 0.20 second but without any dropped QRS waves. In this patient, the P-R interval is about 0.30 second, which is considerably prolonged. However, there are no dropped QRS waves. During second degree or third degree A-V block, QRS waves are dropped.
    TMP11 148, 149

12. (B) During the period of isovolumic contraction, the pressure inside the left ventricle increases until the ventricular pressure is greater than the pressure in

the aorta. At this time, the ventricular pressure opens
the aortic valve, which allows the period of ejection
to begin.
   TMP11 111

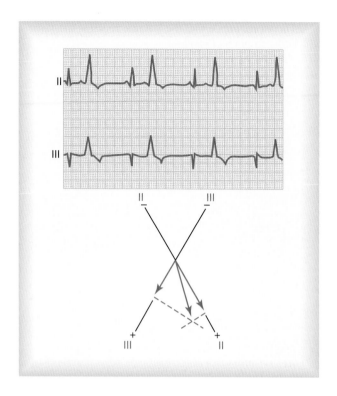

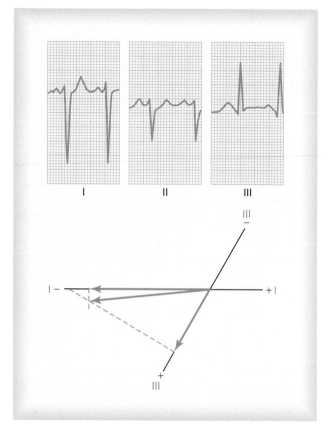

13. (E) Notice that the premature ventricular contrac-
    tions (PVCs) have wide and tall QRS waves in the
    electrocardiogram. The mean electrical axis of the
    premature contraction can be determined by plotting
    these large QRS complexes on the standard limb
    leads (see the figure above). The PVC originates at
    the negative end of the resultant mean electrical axis,
    which is at the base of the ventricle. Notice also that
    the QRS of the PVC is wider and much taller than
    the normal QRS waves in this electrocardiogram.
       TMP11 151

14. (D) The action potential arrives at the A-V bundle at
    0.12 second. It arrives at the A-V node at 0.03
    second and is delayed 0.09 second in the A-V node,
    which results in an arrival time at the bundle of His
    of 0.12 second.
       TMP11 118

15. (E) The mean electrical axis can be determined by
    plotting the resultant voltage of the QRS for leads I,
    II, and III. The result is shown in the figure above.
       TMP11 133

16. (A) Because of the large right axis deviation and the
    slightly prolonged QRS complex, this patient has
    right ventricular hypertrophy. If the patient had right
    bundle branch block, the QRS complex would be
    much more prolonged.
       TMP11 139

17. (C) Einthoven's law states that the voltage in lead I
    plus the voltage in lead III is equal to the voltage in
    lead II.
       TMP11 128

18. (B) This patient has atrial flutter, which is character-
    ized by several P waves for each QRS complex. The
    electrocardiogram shows some areas with two P
    waves for each QRS complex and other areas with
    three P waves for each QRS complex. Notice the
    rapid heart rate, which is characteristic of atrial
    flutter, and the irregular R-R intervals.
       TMP11 156

19. (E) The average ventricular rate is 120 beats/min,
    which is typical of atrial flutter. Notice that the heart
    rate is irregular because of the impulses' inability to
    pass quickly through the atrioventricular node,
    owing to its refractory period.
       TMP11 156

20. (A) Heart rate is determined by dividing 60 by the R-R interval; thus, this patient's heart rate is 109 beats/min. This is a fast rate, which would occur during fever. A trained athlete has a slow heart rate. Excess parasympathetic stimulation and hyperpolarization of the sinoatrial node both decrease heart rate.
TMP11 121, 126

21. (E) If the calcium ion concentration surrounding the cardiac myofibrils increases excessively, the heart goes into spastic contraction. An excess potassium concentration in extracellular fluid causes the heart to become dilated because of the decrease in resting membrane potential of the cardiac muscle fibers.
TMP11 114

22. (D) Increases in sodium and calcium permeability at the sinoatrial (S-A) node result in an increase in heart rate. Increased potassium permeability causes hyperpolarization of the S-A node, which causes the heart rate to decrease.
TMP11 121, 122

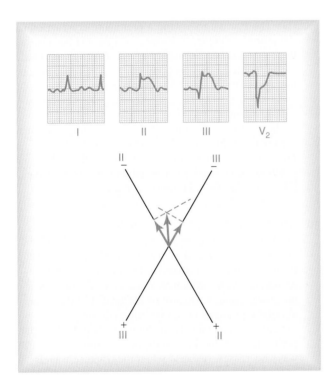

23. (D) In the figure above, the current of injury is plotted on a graph. This is not a plot of the QRS voltages but of the current-of-injury voltages. These voltages are plotted for leads II and III, which are both negative, and the resultant vector is nearly vertical. The negative end of the vector points to the area where the current of injury originated, which is in the apex of the heart.
TMP11 141-143

24. (E) Increased sympathetic stimulation increases heart rate, atrial contractility, and ventricular contractility and also increases norepinephrine release at the ventricular sympathetic nerve endings. It does not cause hyperpolarization of the A-V node. In fact, it causes an increased sodium permeability of the A-V node, which increases the rate of upward drift of the membrane potential to the threshold level for self-excitation.
TMP11 121, 122

25. (E) Systemic hypertension results in a left axis deviation because of enlargement of the left ventricle. Aortic valve stenosis and aortic valve regurgitation also result in a large left ventricle and left axis deviation. When there is excessive abdominal fat, the mechanical pressure of the fat causes a rotation of the heart to the left, resulting in a leftward shift of the mean electrical axis. Pulmonary hypertension causes enlargement of the right heart and thus causes right axis deviation.
TMP11 138, 139

26. (A) Atrial fibrillation has a rapid, irregular heart rate. The P waves are missing or are very weak. The atria exhibit circus movements and often are very enlarged, causing the atrial fibrillation.
TMP11 155

27. (C) Atrial fibrillation often occurs in patients with atrial enlargement, causing an increased tendency for circus movements. The ventricular beat is irregular because impulses arrive rapidly at the A-V node; however, because the A-V node is often in a refractory period, it does not pass a second impulse until about 0.35 second after the previous impulse. There is also a variable interval between atrial impulses reaching the A-V node. This results in a very irregular, rapid heartbeat with a rate of 125 to 150 beats/min.
TMP11 155

28. (B) The aVL lead has a positive vector at the −30-degree angle. The positive end of the aVR lead is at +210 degrees.
TMP11 132

29. (D) The typical ejection fraction is 60 per cent, and lower values are indicative of a weakened heart.
TMP11 108

30. (E) The impulse from the sinoatrial (S-A) node travels rapidly through the internodal pathways and arrives at the atrioventricular node at 0.03 second.
TMP11 119-122

31. (C) Acetylcholine does not increase the permeability of cardiac muscle to calcium ions, but it causes hyperpolarization of the sinoatrial and atrioventricular nodes by increasing permeability to potassium ions. This results in a decreased heart rate.
TMP11 121

32. (E) The term "paroxysmal" means that the heart rate becomes rapid in paroxysms that begin suddenly and can last for a few seconds, a few minutes, a few hours, or much longer. The paroxysm usually ends as suddenly as it began, and the pacemaker shifts

back to the sinoatrial node. The mechanism is believed to occur by a re-entrant circus movement feedback pathway that sets up an area of local, repeated self–re-excitation. The electrocardiogram shows ventricular paroxysmal tachycardia. The ventricular origin can be determined because of the changes in the QRS complexes, which have high voltages and look much different from the preceding normal QRS complexes. This is very characteristic of an irritable ventricular locus.
   TMP11 152

33. (C) Notice that in the electrocardiogram a P wave precedes each of the first four QRS complexes. After that, there is a P wave but a dropped QRS wave. This is characteristic of second degree atrioventricular block.
   TMP11 149

34. (A) The normal resting membrane potential of the sinoatrial (S-A) node is –55 millivolts. As sodium leaks into the membrane, an upward drift of the membrane potential occurs until it reaches –40 millivolts. This is the threshold level that initiates the action potential at the S-A node.
   TMP11 117

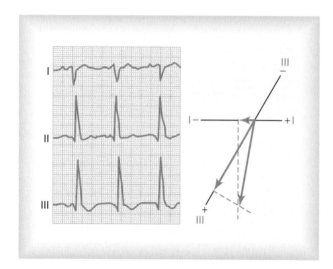

35. (D) Notice in the figure above that lead III has the strongest vector; therefore, the mean electrical axis will be closer to this lead than to lead I or II. The angle of lead III is 120 degrees, and the resultant vector (mean electrical axis) is close to that lead and has a value of +105 degrees.
   TMP11 140

36. (D) This patient has right bundle branch block. The diagnosis can be determined by the rightward shift in the mean electrical axis, as well as by the greatly prolonged QRS complex. In right ventricular hypertrophy, the QRS complex is only moderately prolonged.
   TMP11 140

37. (D) The end-diastolic volume (EDV) is always greater than the end-systolic volume (ESV). Multiply the ejection fraction (EF) by the end-diastolic volume to determine the stroke volume, which is 50 milliliters in this case. Therefore, the end-diastolic volume is 50 milliliters greater than the end-systolic volume, or 200 milliliters. Apply the following formula: $\dfrac{EDV - ESV}{EDV} = EF$. Insert all known information and solve for EDV.
   TMP11 108

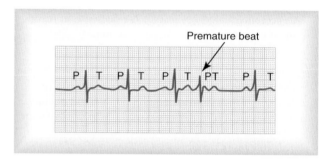

38. (D) The P wave following a premature contraction in the atrioventricular (A-V) node is inverted because the cardiac impulse travels backward into the atria at the same time it travels forward into the ventricles. If the premature contraction is high in the A-V junction, an inverted P wave occurs before the QRS complex. If the premature contraction originates in the middle of the A-V junction, the P wave is superimposed on the QRS complex and thus cannot be seen. If the premature contraction originates low in the A-V junction, the P wave is inverted and occurs after the QRS complex (see the figure above).
   TMP11 151

39. (B) A dilated heart increases the risk of ventricular fibrillation because of an increased likelihood of circus movements. Also, if the conduction velocity decreases, it takes longer for the impulse to travel around the heart, which increases the risk of ventricular fibrillation. Exposure of the heart to 60-cycle alternating current or epinephrine administration increases the irritability of the heart. If the refractory period is long, the likelihood of re-entrant–type pathways decreases, because when the impulse travels around the heart, the ventricles remain in a refractory period.
   TMP11 153, 154

40. (B) This patient has a left axis deviation because of the large negative deflection of the R wave in lead III. Also, her T wave is inverted in lead I, which means that it is in the opposite direction of the QRS complex. This is characteristic of bundle branch block. Also, the QRS complex has a width of 0.20 second, which is very prolonged. A QRS complex with a width greater than 0.12 second is normally caused by a conduction block. All these factors indicate that this patient has left bundle branch block.
   TMP11 139

41. (D) An increase in potassium permeability causes a decrease in the membrane potential of the atrioventricular node. Thus, it will be extremely hyperpolarized, making it much more difficult for the membrane potential to reach its threshold level for conduction. This results in a decrease in heart rate. Increases in sodium and calcium permeability and norepinephrine levels increase the membrane potential, which tends to increase the heart rate.
TMP11 117, 121, 122

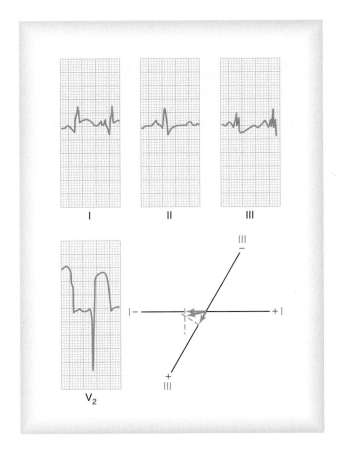

42. (A) This patient has an acute anterior infarction in the left ventricle of the heart. This can be determined by plotting the currents of injury from the different leads (see the figure above). The limb leads are used to determine whether the infarction is coming from the left or right side of the heart and from its base or apex. The chest leads are used to determine whether it is an anterior or posterior infarct. When the currents of injury are analyzed, a negative potential, caused by the current of injury, occurs in lead I, and a positive potential, caused by the current of injury, occurs in lead III. This is determined by subtracting the J point from the T-P segment. The negative end of the resultant vector originates in the ischemic area, which is therefore the left side of the heart. In lead V_2, the chest lead, the electrode is in a field of very negative potential, which occurs in patients with anterior lesions.
TMP11 143

43. (B) Cardiac muscle stores much more calcium in its tubular system than skeletal muscle does, and it is much more dependent on extracellular calcium than skeletal muscle is. An abundance of calcium is bound by the mucopolysaccharides inside the T tubule. This calcium is necessary for the contraction of cardiac muscle, and the strength of contraction depends on the calcium concentration surrounding the cardiac myocytes. At the initiation of the action potential, the fast sodium channels open first, followed by the opening of the slow calcium channels.
TMP11 106

44. (E) At the end of ventricular ejection, both the aortic valves and the pulmonary valves close. This is followed by the period of isovolumic relaxation.
TMP11 107, 108

45. (A) The risk of ventricular fibrillation increases in a heart exposed to a 60-cycle alternating current. A shortened ventricular refractory period and decreased conduction through the heart muscle occur, increasing the probability of re-entrant pathways. Therefore, when the electrical stimulus travels around the heart and reaches the ventricular muscle that was initially stimulated, the risk of ventricular fibrillation increases if this muscle has a short refractory period.
TMP11 153, 154

46. (A) The heartbeat immediately following a premature atrial contraction is weakened because the diastolic period is very short in this condition. Therefore, the ventricular filling time is very short, and the stroke volume decreases. The P wave is usually visible in this type of arrhythmia unless it coincides with the QRS complex. The probability of these premature contractions increases in patients with toxic irritation of the heart and local ischemic areas.
TMP11 150

47. (A) Because the deflection is 0 in lead I, the axis must be 90 degrees away from this lead. Therefore, the mean electrical axis must be +90 degrees or –90 degrees. Because the aVF lead has a positive deflection, the mean electrical axis must be +90 degrees.
TMP11 132, 133

48. (E) The heart rate can be determined as follows: 60 divided by the R-R interval. In this case, the result is 150 beats/min. This patient has tachycardia, which is defined as a heart rate greater than 100 beats/min.
TMP11 110

49. (A) The relationship between the P waves and the QRS complexes appears to be normal, and there are no missing beats. Therefore, this patient has a sinus rhythm, and there is no heart block. Nor is there any S-T segment depression in this patient. Because there are normal P waves, QRS complexes, and T waves, this patient is diagnosed with sinus tachycardia.
TMP11 148

50. (B) If there is a failure in conduction of the sinoatrial (S-A) nodal impulse to the A-V node, or if the

S-A node stops firing, the A-V node will take over as the pacemaker of the heart. The intrinsic rhythmical rate of the A-V node is 40 to 60 times/min. If the Purkinje fibers take over as pacemaker, the heart rate will be between 15 and 40 beats/min.
TMP11 120, 121

51. (E) The normal plateau level of the cardiac output function curve is 13 L/min. This level decreases in any type of cardiac failure and increases markedly during sympathetic stimulation.
TMP11 113

52. (B) During a Stokes-Adams syndrome attack, total A-V block begins suddenly and can persist for a few seconds up to several weeks. The new pacemaker of the heart is distal to the point of blockade, but it is usually the A-V node or the A-V bundle.
TMP11 149

53. (D) The impulse being transmitted from the sinoatrial (S-A) node to the A-V node arrives in 0.03 second. There is then a total delay of 0.13 second in the A-V node and bundle system, allowing the impulse to arrive at the ventricular septum in 0.16 second.
TMP11 118

54. (C) During atrial paroxysmal tachycardia, the impulse is initiated by an ectopic focus somewhere in the atria. If the point of initiation is near the atrioventricular node, the P wave travels backward toward the sinoatrial node and then forward into the ventricles simultaneously. Therefore, the P wave is inverted.
TMP11 152

55. (D) If a patient has no P waves and a very low heart rate, it is likely that the impulse leaving the sinus node is totally blocked before entering the atrial muscle. This is called sinoatrial block. The ventricles pick up the new rhythm, usually initiated in the A-V node at this point. In contrast, during sinus bradycardia, there are still P waves associated with each QRS complex. In first degree, second degree, and third degree heart blocks, there are P waves in each instance, although some are not associated with QRS complexes.
TMP11 146

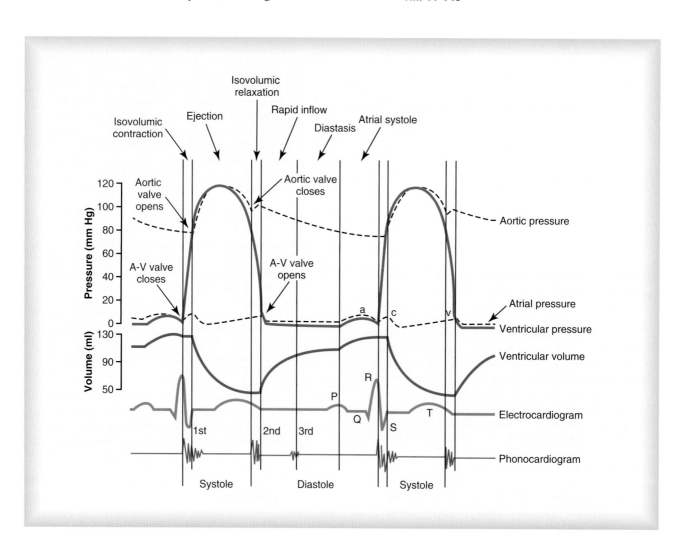

56. (E) By definition, the first heart sound occurs just after the ventricular pressure exceeds the atrial pressure (see the figure on page 38). This causes the atrioventricular valves to mechanically close. The second heart sound occurs when the aortic and pulmonary valves close.
TMP11 107

57. (C) Heart rate can be calculated as follows: 60 divided by the R-R interval, which is 0.68 second. This results in a heart rate of 88 beats/min.
TMP11 110

58. (C) The P-Q interval is 0.14 second. This number is determined by measuring the time between the first deflection of the P wave and the first deflection of the QRS complex. The P-Q interval is also the time required for the cardiac impulse to travel from the sinoatrial node to the ventricular septum.
TMP11 123, 124

59. (D) The resting membrane potential of the sinus nodal fibers is –55 millivolts, in contrast to the –85- to –90-millivolt membrane potential of cardiac muscle. Another major difference between the sinus nodal fibers and the ventricular muscle fibers is that the sinus fibers exhibit self-excitation from inward leaking of sodium ions.
TMP11 117

60. (A) Circus movements occur in ventricular muscle, particularly if the heart is dilated or the conduction velocity is decreased. Other conditions that cause circus movements are repetitive electrical stimulation and the administration of catecholamines, such as epinephrine. A longer refractory period tends to prevent circus movements of the heart, because when the impulses travel around the heart and contact the area of ventricular muscle with a longer refractory period, the action potential stops at that point.
TMP11 153, 154

61. (E) Immediately after the QRS wave, the ventricles begin to contract, and the first phase that occurs is isovolumic contraction. This phase occurs before the ejection phase and increases the ventricular pressure enough to mechanically open the aortic and pulmonary valves.
TMP11 107, 108

62. (A) At the J point, the entire heart is depolarized in a patient with a damaged cardiac muscle—or in a patient with a normal cardiac muscle. The area of the heart that is damaged does not repolarize but remains depolarized at all times.
TMP11 142, 143

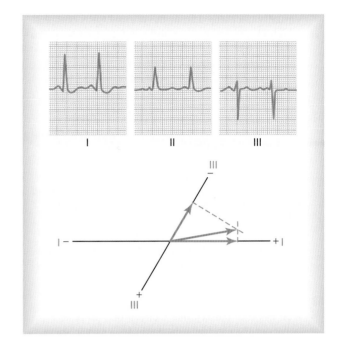

63. (A) Notice in the figure above that the QRS complex has a positive deflection in lead I and a negative deflection in lead III, which indicates a left axis deviation. This occurs in a patient with chronic systemic hypertension. Pulmonary hypertension increases the ventricular mass on the right side of the heart, which produces a right axis deviation.
TMP11 138, 139

64. (A) If the Purkinje fibers are the pacemaker of the heart, the heart rate is between 15 and 40 beats/min. In contrast, the rate of firing of the A-V nodal fibers is 40 to 60 times/min, and the rate of firing of the sinus node is 70 to 80 times/min. If for some reason the sinus node is blocked, the A-V node will take over as the pacemaker; and if the A-V node is blocked, the Purkinje fibers will take over as the pacemaker of the heart.
TMP11 121

65. (B) Excess potassium ions in the blood and extracellular fluid cause the heart to become dilated and flaccid and also slow the heart rate. This effect is important because of the decrease in the resting membrane potential in the cardiac muscle fibers. As the membrane potential decreases, the intensity of the action potential decreases, which causes the contraction of the heart to become progressively weaker. Excess calcium ions, sympathetic stimulation, and increased norepinephrine concentration all cause the heart to contract vigorously.
TMP11 114

66. (A) This electrocardiogram has characteristics of atrial paroxysmal tachycardia, which means that the tachycardia may come and go randomly. The basic shape of the QRS complex and its magnitude are

virtually unchanged from the normal QRS complex, which eliminates the possibility of ventricular paroxysmal tachycardia. This electrocardiogram is not characteristic of atrial flutter because there is only one P wave for each QRS complex.
TMP11 152

67. (E) Sympathetic stimulation of the heart normally causes an increased heart rate, increased rate of conduction of the cardiac impulse, and increased force of contraction in the atria and ventricles. However, it does not cause acetylcholine release at the sympathetic endings, because they contain norepinephrine. Parasympathetic stimulation causes acetylcholine release. The sympathetic nervous system firing increases the permeability of the cardiac muscle fibers, the sinoatrial node, and the atrioventricular node to sodium and calcium.
TMP11 121, 122

68. (E) First, second, and third degree heart blocks, as well as atrial paroxysmal tachycardia, all have P waves in the electrocardiogram. In contrast, there are usually no evident P waves during atrial fibrillation, and the heart rate is irregular. Therefore, this electrocardiogram is characteristic of atrial fibrillation.
TMP11 155

69. (D) Because the plotted QRS wave is –1.2 millivolts on lead I and +1.2 millivolts on lead II, the absolute values of the deflections are the same. Therefore, the mean electrical axis must be exactly halfway between these two leads, which is halfway between the lead II axis of 60 degrees and the lead I negative axis of 180 degrees, which gives a value of 120 degrees.
TMP11 128

70. (D) The increase in potassium permeability causes a hyperpolarization of the atrioventricular (A-V) node, which decreases the heart rate. Increases in sodium permeability partially depolarize the A-V node, and an increase in norepinephrine levels increases the heart rate.
TMP11 121

71. (D) A QRS axis of 120 degrees indicates a rightward shift, and a QRS complex of 0.18 second indicates a conduction block. These characteristics indicate a right bundle branch block.
TMP11 140

72. (E) This patient's heart rate is 40 beats/min, which can be determined by dividing 60 by the R-R interval. This is characteristic of some types of atrioventricular block.
TMP11 110

73. (E) This electrocardiogram is characteristic of complete atrioventricular (A-V) block—also called third degree A-V block. The P waves seem to be totally dissociated from the QRS complexes; sometimes there are three P waves and sometimes there are two P waves between QRS complexes. First degree A-V block causes a lengthened P-R interval, and second degree A-V block has long P-R intervals with dropped beats. However, this does not seem to be occurring in this electrocardiogram, because there is no relationship between the ORS waves and the P waves.
TMP11 149

74. (C) The normal P-R interval is 0.16 second, which is the time that elapses between the initiation of the action potential in the sinoatrial node and the impulse reaching the ventricular septum. It is also the time between the beginning of the P wave and the first deflection of the QRS complex.
TMP11 125

75. (B) This patient's electrocardiogram shows a positive deflection in aVF and a negative deflection in standard limb lead I. Therefore, the mean electrical axis is between 90 and 180 degrees, which is a rightward shift in the mean electrical axis. Systemic hypertension, aortic valve stenosis, and aortic valve regurgitation cause hypertrophy of the left ventricle and thus a leftward shift in the mean electrical axis. Pulmonary hypertension causes a rightward shift in the axis and is therefore the cause of this patient's condition.
TMP11 139

The Circulation

1. A 60-year-old woman has experienced dizziness for the past 6 months when getting out of bed in the morning and when standing up. Her mean arterial pressure is 130/90 mm Hg lying down and 95/60 sitting. Which of the following sets of physiological changes would be expected in response to moving from a supine to an upright position?

	Vagal Tone	Heart Rate	Sympathetic Activity
(A)	↑	↑	↑
(B)	↑	↓	↑
(C)	↑	↓	↓
(D)	↑	↑	↓
(E)	↓	↓	↓
(F)	↓	↑	↓
(G)	↓	↑	↑
(H)	↓	↓	↑

2. If a person has been exercising for 1 hour, which of the following organs experiences the smallest decrease in blood flow?
   (A) Brain
   (B) Intestines
   (C) Kidneys
   (D) Nonexercising skeletal muscle
   (E) Pancreas

3. A healthy 25-year-old male medical student has an exercise stress test at a local health club. Which of the following sets of physiological changes is most likely to occur in this man's skeletal muscles during exercise?

	Arteriolar Diameter	Adenosine Concentration	Vascular Conductance
(A)	↑	↑	↑
(B)	↑	↓	↑
(C)	↑	↓	↓
(D)	↑	↑	↓
(E)	↓	↓	↓
(F)	↓	↑	↓
(G)	↓	↑	↑
(H)	↓	↓	↑

4. A healthy 28-year-old woman stands up from a supine position. Which of the following sets of cardiovascular changes is most likely to occur?

	Plasma Renin Activity	Renal Blood Flow	Total Peripheral Resistance
(A)	↑	↑	↑
(B)	↑	↓	↑
(C)	↑	↓	↓
(D)	↑	↑	↓
(E)	↓	↓	↓
(F)	↓	↑	↓
(G)	↓	↑	↑
(H)	↓	↓	↑

5. Which of the following heart murmurs is heard only during diastole?
   (A) Patent ductus arteriosus
   (B) Mitral regurgitation
   (C) Tricuspid valve stenosis
   (D) Interventricular septal defect
   (E) Aortic stenosis

6. Listed below are the hydrostatic and oncotic pressures across a muscle capillary wall:
   Capillary hydrostatic pressure (Pc) = 25 mm Hg
   Plasma colloid osmotic pressure (Πp) = 25 mm Hg
   Interstitial colloid osmotic pressure (Π_I) = 10 mm Hg
   Interstitial hydrostatic pressure (P$_I$) = −5 mm Hg
   What is the net pressure for fluid movement across the capillary wall?
   (A) 0 mm Hg
   (B) 5 mm Hg
   (C) 10 mm Hg
   (D) 15 mm Hg
   (E) 20 mm Hg

7. Which of the following normally causes either renal sodium or water retention during compensated heart failure?
   (A) Decreased angiotensin II formation
   (B) Decreased aldosterone formation
   (C) Sympathetic vasodilatation of the afferent arterioles
   (D) Increased glomerular filtration rate
   (E) Increased antidiuretic hormone formation

8. Listed below are the hydrostatic and oncotic pressures within a microcirculatory bed:
   Plasma colloid osmotic pressure = 25 mm Hg
   Capillary hydrostatic pressure = 25 mm Hg
   Venous hydrostatic pressure = 5 mm Hg
   Arterial pressure = 80 mm Hg
   Interstitial fluid hydrostatic pressure = −5 mm Hg
   Interstitial colloid osmotic pressure = 10 mm Hg
   Capillary filtration coefficient = 10 ml/min/mm Hg
   What is the rate of net fluid movement across the capillary wall?
   (A) 25 ml/min
   (B) 50 ml/min
   (C) 100 ml/min
   (D) 150 ml/min
   (E) 200 ml/min

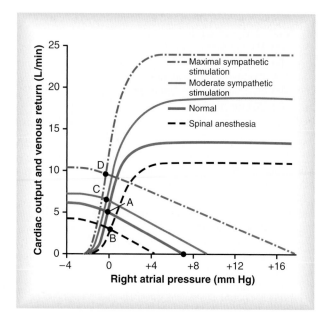

9. For the cardiac output and the venous return curve in the figure above defined by the blue lines, (with equilibrium at point C), what is the resistance to venous return?
   (A) 0.40 mm Hg/L/min
   (B) 0.65 mm Hg/L/min
   (C) 1.40 mm Hg/L/min
   (D) 1.64 mm Hg/L/min
   (E) 1.82 mm Hg/L/min

10. Which of the following often occurs during progressive shock?
    (A) Decreased capillary permeability
    (B) Vasomotor center failure
    (C) Increased mitochondrial activity
    (D) Increased urine output
    (E) Increased pH in the tissues throughout the body

11. Which of the following sets of physiological changes would be expected to occur in response to an increase in atrial natriuretic peptide?

	Angiotensin II	Renal Sodium Transport	Sodium Excretion
(A)	↑	↑	↑
(B)	↑	↓	↑
(C)	↑	↓	↓
(D)	↑	↑	↓
(E)	↓	↓	↓
(F)	↓	↑	↓
(G)	↓	↑	↑
(H)	↓	↓	↑

12. A 30-year-old man is resting and his sympathetic output increases to maximal values because of extreme fright. Which of the following sets of changes would be expected in response to this increased sympathetic output?

	Resistance to Venous Return	Mean Systemic Filling Pressure	Venous Return
(A)	↑	↑	↑
(B)	↑	↓	↑
(C)	↑	↓	↓
(D)	↑	↑	↓
(E)	↓	↓	↓
(F)	↓	↑	↓
(G)	↓	↑	↑
(H)	↓	↓	↑

13. Administration of a drug decreases the diameter of arterioles in the muscle bed of an experimental animal. Which of the following sets of physiological changes would be expected to occur in response to the decrease in diameter?

	Vascular Conductance	Capillary Filtration	Blood Flow
(A)	↑	↑	↑
(B)	↑	↓	↑
(C)	↑	↓	↓
(D)	↑	↑	↓
(E)	↓	↓	↓
(F)	↓	↑	↓
(G)	↓	↑	↑
(H)	↓	↓	↑

14. Which of the following would normally be beneficial to a patient with acute pulmonary edema?
    (A) Infusion of a vasoconstrictor drug
    (B) Infusion of a balanced electrolyte solution
    (C) Administration of furosemide
    (D) Administration of a bronchoconstrictor
    (E) Infusion of whole blood

15. A 35-year-old woman visits her family practitioner for an examination. She has a blood pressure of 160/75 mm Hg and a heart rate of 74 beats/min. Further tests by a cardiologist reveal that the patient has moderate aortic regurgitation. Which of the following sets of changes would be expected in this patient?

	Pulse Pressure	Systolic Pressure	Stroke Volume
(A)	↑	↑	↑
(B)	↑	↓	↑
(C)	↑	↓	↓
(D)	↑	↑	↓
(E)	↓	↓	↓
(F)	↓	↑	↓
(G)	↓	↑	↑
(H)	↓	↓	↑

16. Which of the following conditions is most likely to decrease the risk of coronary artery disease?
    (A) Physical inactivity
    (B) Diabetes mellitus
    (C) Hypertension
    (D) Aging
    (E) Moderately decreased body weight

17. A 65-year-old man with a 5-year history of congestive heart failure is being treated with an angiotensin-converting enzyme (ACE) inhibitor. Which of the following sets of changes would be expected to occur in response to the ACE inhibitor drug therapy?

	Arterial Pressure	Angiotensin II	Total Peripheral Resistance
(A)	↑	↑	↑
(B)	↑	↓	↑
(C)	↑	↓	↓
(D)	↑	↑	↓
(E)	↓	↓	↓
(F)	↓	↑	↓
(G)	↓	↑	↑
(H)	↓	↓	↑

18. Which of the following vasoactive agents is usually the most important controller of coronary blood flow?
    (A) Adenosine
    (B) Bradykinin
    (C) Prostaglandins
    (D) Carbon dioxide
    (E) Potassium ions

19. In which of the following conditions is administration of a sympathomimetic drug the therapy of choice to prevent shock?
    (A) Spinal cord injury
    (B) Shock due to excessive vomiting
    (C) Hemorrhagic shock
    (D) Shock caused by excess diuretics

20. Cognitive stimuli such as reading, problem solving, and talking all result in significant increases in cerebral blood flow. Which of the following changes in cerebral tissue concentrations is the most likely explanation for the increase in cerebral blood flow?

	Carbon Dioxide	pH	Adenosine
(A)	↑	↑	↑
(B)	↑	↓	↑
(C)	↑	↓	↓
(D)	↑	↑	↓
(E)	↓	↓	↓
(F)	↓	↑	↓
(G)	↓	↑	↑
(H)	↓	↓	↑

21. Which of the following is associated with the third heart sound?
    (A) Inrushing of blood into the ventricles due to atrial contraction
    (B) Closing of the atrioventricular (A-V) valves
    (C) Closing of the pulmonary valve
    (D) Opening of the A-V valves
    (E) Inrushing of blood into the ventricles in the early to middle part of diastole

22. A 55-year-old man with a history of normal health visits his physician for a checkup. The physical examination reveals that his blood pressure is 170/98 mm Hg. Further tests indicate that he has renovascular hypertension as a result of stenosis in the left kidney. Which of the following sets of findings would be expected in this man with renovascular hypertension?

	Total Peripheral Resistance	Plasma Renin Activity	Plasma Aldosterone Concentration
(A)	↑	↑	↑
(B)	↑	↓	↑
(C)	↑	↓	↓
(D)	↑	↑	↓
(E)	↓	↓	↓
(F)	↓	↑	↓
(G)	↓	↑	↑
(H)	↓	↓	↑

23. A 40-year-old woman is diagnosed with a heart murmur. During auscultation, a "blowing" murmur of relatively high pitch is heard maximally over the left ventricle. The chest radiograph shows an enlarged heart. Arterial pressure in the aorta is 140/40 mm Hg. Which of the following is the most likely diagnosis?
    (A) Aortic valve stenosis
    (B) Aortic valve regurgitation
    (C) Pulmonary valve stenosis
    (D) Mitral valve stenosis
    (E) Tricuspid valve regurgitation

24. Histamine is infused into the brachial artery. Which of the following sets of microcirculatory changes would be expected in the infused arm?

	Arteriolar Resistance	Capillary Hydrostatic Pressure	Capillary Filtration Rate
(A)	↑	↑	↑
(B)	↑	↑	↓
(C)	↑	↓	↓
(D)	↑	↓	↑
(E)	↓	↓	↓
(F)	↓	↓	↑
(G)	↓	↑	↑
(H)	↓	↑	↓

25. Which of the following conditions often occurs in compensated hemorrhagic shock?
    (A) Decreased heart rate
    (B) Stress relaxation
    (C) Decreased antidiuretic hormone release
    (D) Decreased absorption of interstitial fluid through the capillaries
    (E) Central nervous system ischemic response

26. Bradykinin is infused into the brachial artery of a 22-year-old man. Which of the following sets of microcirculatory changes would be expected in the infused arm?

	Arteriolar Resistance	Interstitial Hydrostatic Pressure	Lymph Flow
(A)	↑	↑	↑
(B)	↑	↑	↓
(C)	↑	↓	↓
(D)	↑	↓	↑
(E)	↓	↓	↓
(F)	↓	↓	↑
(G)	↓	↑	↑
(H)	↓	↑	↓

27. An increase in shear stress in a blood vessel results in which of the following changes?
    (A) Decreased endothelin production
    (B) Decreased cyclic guanosine monophosphate production
    (C) Increased nitric oxide release
    (D) Increased renin production
    (E) Decreased prostacyclin production

28. A 21-year-old man has a cardiac reserve of 300 per cent and a maximum cardiac output of 16 L/min. What is his resting cardiac output?
    (A) 3 L/min
    (B) 4 L/min
    (C) 5.33 L/min
    (D) 6 L/min
    (E) 8 L/min

29. Which of the following increases the heart's tendency to fibrillate following myocardial infarction?
    (A) Decreased irritability of the cardiac muscle
    (B) Decreased potassium ion concentration in the extracellular fluid of the heart
    (C) Current of injury
    (D) Decreased sympathetic stimulation
    (E) Decreased ventricular volume

30. A 72-year-old man had surgery to remove an abdominal tumor. Pathohistological studies reveal that the tumor mass contains a large number of blood vessels. An increase in which of the following is the most likely stimulus for the growth of vessels in a solid tumor?
    (A) Growth hormone
    (B) Plasma glucose concentration
    (C) Angiostatin growth factor
    (D) Tissue oxygen concentration
    (E) Vascular endothelial growth factor

31. If a patient has an oxygen consumption of 240 ml/min, a pulmonary vein oxygen concentration of 180 ml/L of blood, and a pulmonary artery oxygen concentration of 160 ml/L of blood units, what is the cardiac output?
    (A) 8 L/min
    (B) 10 L/min
    (C) 12 L/min
    (D) 16 L/min
    (E) 20 L/min

32. The diameter of a precapillary arteriole is increased in a muscle vascular bed. A decrease in which of the following would be expected?
    (A) Capillary filtration rate
    (B) Vascular conductance
    (C) Capillary blood flow
    (D) Capillary hydrostatic pressure
    (E) Arteriolar resistance

33. If the thorax of a normal, healthy patient is surgically opened, what happens to the cardiac output curve?
    (A) It shifts 2 mm Hg to the left
    (B) It shifts 4 mm Hg to the left
    (C) It shifts 2 mm Hg to the right
    (D) It shifts 4 mm Hg to the right
    (E) It does not shift

34. Under control conditions, flow through a blood vessel is 100 ml/min with a pressure gradient of 50 mm Hg. What would be the approximate flow through the vessel after increasing the vessel diameter by 50 per cent, assuming the pressure gradient is maintained at 100 mm Hg?
    (A) 100 ml/min
    (B) 150 ml/min
    (C) 300 ml/min
    (D) 500 ml/min
    (E) 700 ml/min

35. Left ventricular hypertrophy occurs in which of the following disorders?
    (A) Pulmonary valve regurgitation
    (B) Tricuspid regurgitation
    (C) Mitral stenosis
    (D) Tricuspid stenosis
    (E) Aortic stenosis

36. A 24-year-old woman delivers a 6 pound, 8 ounce female baby. The newborn is diagnosed as having patent ductus arteriosus. Which of the following sets of changes would be expected in this baby?

	Pulse Pressure	Stroke Volume	Systolic Pressure
(A)	↑	↑	↑
(B)	↑	↓	↑
(C)	↑	↓	↓
(D)	↑	↑	↓
(E)	↓	↓	↓
(F)	↓	↑	↓
(G)	↓	↑	↑
(H)	↓	↓	↑

37. Which of the following occurs during heart failure and causes an increase in renal sodium excretion?
    (A) Increased aldosterone release
    (B) Increased atrial natriuretic factor release
    (C) Decreased glomerular filtration rate
    (D) Increased angiotensin II formation
    (E) Decreased mean arterial pressure

38. Which of the following normally causes the cardiac output curve to shift to the left along the right atrial pressure axis?
    (A) Surgically opening the chest
    (B) Severe cardiac tamponade
    (C) Breathing against a negative pressure
    (D) Playing a trumpet
    (E) Positive pressure breathing

39. Which of the following sets of changes would be expected to cause the greatest increase in the net movement of glucose across a muscle capillary wall?

	Wall Permeability to Glucose	Wall Surface Area	Concentration Difference Across Wall
(A)	↑	↑	↑
(B)	↑	↑	↓
(C)	↑	↓	↓
(D)	↑	↓	↑
(E)	↓	↓	↓
(F)	↓	↓	↑
(G)	↓	↑	↑
(H)	↓	↑	↓

40. Which of the following statements about coronary blood flow is most accurate?
    (A) Normal resting coronary blood flow is 500 ml/min
    (B) The majority of flow occurs during systole
    (C) During systole, the percentage decrease in subendocardial flow is greater than the percentage decrease in epicardial flow
    (D) Adenosine release normally decreases coronary flow

41. A 60-year-old man visits his family practitioner for an annual examination. He has a mean blood pressure of 130 mm Hg and a heart rate of 78 beats/min. His plasma cholesterol level is in the upper 25th percentile, and he is diagnosed as having atherosclerosis. Which of the following sets of changes would be expected in this patient?

	Pulse Pressure	Arterial Compliance	Systolic Pressure
(A)	↑	↑	↑
(B)	↑	↓	↑
(C)	↑	↓	↓
(D)	↑	↑	↓
(E)	↓	↓	↓
(F)	↓	↑	↓
(G)	↓	↑	↑
(H)	↓	↓	↑

42. A 65-year-old man enters the emergency department a few minutes after receiving an influenza inoculation. He has pallor, tachycardia, and an arterial pressure of 80/50 mm Hg. He has trouble walking. Which of the following therapies would be recommended to prevent shock?
    (A) Infusion of blood
    (B) Administration of an antihistamine
    (C) Infusion of a balanced electrolyte solution
    (D) Infusion of a sympathomimetic drug
    (E) Administration of a tissue plasminogen activator

43. While participating in a cardiovascular physiology laboratory, a medical student isolates the carotid artery of an animal and partially constricts the artery with a tie around the vessel. Which of the following sets of changes would be expected to occur in response to constriction of the carotid artery?

	Heart Rate	Vagal Tone	Total Peripheral Resistance
(A)	↑	↑	↑
(B)	↑	↓	↑
(C)	↑	↓	↓
(D)	↑	↑	↓
(E)	↓	↓	↓
(F)	↓	↑	↓
(G)	↓	↑	↑
(H)	↓	↓	↑

44. A balloon catheter is advanced from the superior vena cava into the heart and inflated to increase atrial pressure by 5 mm Hg. An increase in which of the following would be expected to occur in response to the elevated atrial pressure?
    (A) Atrial natriuretic peptide
    (B) Angiotensin II
    (C) Aldosterone
    (D) Renal sympathetic nerve activity

45. A 30-year-old patient who took an overdose of furosemide is in shock. Which of the following is the appropriate therapy?
    (A) Infusion of blood
    (B) Infusion of plasma
    (C) Infusion of a balanced electrolyte solution
    (D) Infusion of a sympathomimetic drug
    (E) Administration of a glucocorticoid

46. The diameter of a precapillary arteriole is increased in a muscle vascular bed. Which of the following changes in the microcirculation would be expected?
    (A) Decreased capillary filtration rate
    (B) Decreased interstitial volume
    (C) Increased lymph flow
    (D) Decreased capillary hydrostatic pressure
    (E) Increased arteriolar resistance

47. A 50-year-old man has a 3-year history of hypertension. He complains of fatigue and occasional muscle cramps. There is no family history of hypertension. The patient has not had any other significant medical problems in the past. Examination reveals a blood pressure of 168/104 mm Hg. Additional laboratory tests indicate that the patient has primary hyperaldosteronism. Which of the following sets of findings would be expected in this man with primary hyperaldosteronism hypertension?

	Extracellular Fluid Volume	Plasma Renin Activity	Plasma Potassium Concentration
(A)	↑	↑	↑
(B)	↑	↓	↑
(C)	↑	↓	↓
(D)	↑	↑	↓
(E)	↓	↓	↓
(F)	↓	↑	↓
(G)	↓	↑	↑
(H)	↓	↓	↑

48. Which of the following would be appropriate therapy for a patient in cardiogenic shock?
    (A) Placing tourniquets on the four limbs
    (B) Bleeding the patient moderately
    (C) Administering furosemide
    (D) Infusing a vasoconstrictor drug

49. A 72-year-old man had surgery to remove an abdominal tumor. Pathohistological studies reveal that the tumor mass contains a large number of vessels. A decrease in which of the following is the most likely stimulus for the growth of vessels in a solid tumor?
    (A) Growth hormone
    (B) Plasma glucose concentration
    (C) Angiostatin growth factor
    (D) Vascular endothelial growth factor
    (E) Tissue oxygen concentration

50. Which of the following heart murmurs is heard only during systole?
    (A) Atrial septal defect
    (B) Mitral stenosis
    (C) Tetralogy of Fallot
    (D) Patent ductus arteriosus
    (E) Tricuspid stenosis

51. Under control conditions, flow through a blood vessel is 100 ml/min under a pressure gradient of 50 mm Hg. What would be the approximate flow through the vessel after increasing the vessel diameter to four times normal, assuming the pressure gradient was maintained at 50 mm Hg?
    (A) 300 ml/min
    (B) 1600 ml/min
    (C) 1000 ml/min
    (D) 16,000 ml/min
    (E) 25,600 ml/min

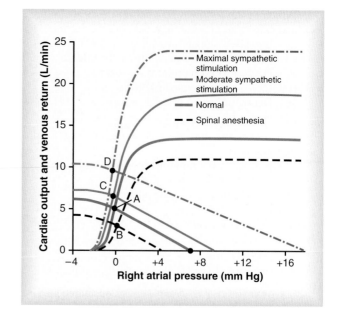

52. In the graph above, for the cardiac output and venous return curves defined by the black dashed lines (with the equilibrium at B), which of the following is accurate?
    (A) Mean systemic filling pressure = approximately 4.3 mm Hg
    (B) Pulmonary arterial blood flow = approximately 5 L/min
    (C) Right atrial pressure = 2 mm Hg
    (D) The plateau of the cardiac output curve is 13 L/min

53. While participating in a cardiovascular physiology laboratory, a medical student isolates an animal's carotid artery proximal to the carotid bifurcation and partially constricts the artery with a tie around the vessel. Which of the following sets of changes would be expected to occur in response to constriction of the carotid artery?

	Mean Carotid Sinus Nerve Impulses	Parasympathetic Nerve Activity	Total Peripheral Resistance
(A)	↑	↑	↑
(B)	↑	↓	↑
(C)	↑	↓	↓
(D)	↑	↑	↓
(E)	↓	↓	↓
(F)	↓	↑	↓
(G)	↓	↑	↑
(H)	↓	↓	↑

54. A 40-year-old man is diagnosed with a heart murmur. A chest radiograph shows an enlarged heart, but there is no fluid on the lungs. The mean QRS axis of his electrocardiogram is 140 degrees. Pulmonary capillary pressure is normal. Which of the following is the most likely diagnosis?
    (A) Aortic stenosis
    (B) Aortic regurgitation
    (C) Pulmonary valve stenosis
    (D) Mitral stenosis
    (E) Mitral regurgitation

55. A 22-year-old man enters the hospital emergency room after severing a major artery in a motorcycle accident. It is estimated that he has lost approximately 700 milliliters of blood. His blood pressure is 90/55 mm Hg. Which of the following sets of changes would be expected in response to hemorrhage in this man?

	Renal Blood Flow	Parasympathetic Nerve Activity	Total Peripheral Resistance
(A)	↑	↑	↑
(B)	↑	↓	↑
(C)	↑	↓	↓
(D)	↑	↑	↓
(E)	↓	↓	↓
(F)	↓	↑	↓
(G)	↓	↑	↑
(H)	↓	↓	↑

56. A 35-year-woman is undergoing spinal anesthesia and experiences a large drop in arterial pressure and goes into shock. Which of the following is the therapy of choice to treat this patient?
    (A) Infusion of plasma
    (B) Infusion of blood
    (C) Infusion of saline
    (D) Infusion of a glucocorticoid
    (E) Infusion of a sympathomimetic drug

57. A 22-year-old man has a muscle blood flow of 250 ml/min and a hematocrit of 50. He has a mean arterial pressure of 130 mm Hg, a muscle venous pressure of 5 mm Hg, and a heart rate of 80 beats/min. Which of the following is the approximate vascular resistance in the muscle of this man?
    (A) 0.10 mm Hg/ml/min
    (B) 0.20 mm Hg/ml/min
    (C) 0.50 mm Hg/ml/min
    (D) 1.00 mm Hg/ml/min
    (E) 2.50 mm Hg/ml/min

58. Which of the following conditions would be expected to decrease mean systemic filling pressure?
    (A) Norepinephrine administration
    (B) Increased blood volume
    (C) Increased sympathetic stimulation
    (D) Increased venous compliance
    (E) Skeletal muscle contraction

59. A healthy 28-year-old woman stands up from a supine position. Moving from a supine to a standing position results in a transient decrease in arterial pressure that is detected by arterial baroreceptors located in the aortic arch and carotid sinuses. Which of the following sets of cardiovascular changes is most likely to occur in response to activation of the baroreceptors?

	Mean Circulatory Filling Pressure	Strength of Cardiac Contraction	Sympathetic Nerve Activity
(A)	↑	↑	↑
(B)	↑	↓	↑
(C)	↑	↓	↓
(D)	↑	↑	↓
(E)	↓	↓	↓
(F)	↓	↑	↓
(G)	↓	↑	↑
(H)	↓	↓	↑

60. Which of the following conditions normally causes arteriolar vasodilatation during exercise?
    (A) Decreased plasma potassium ion concentration
    (B) Increased histamine release
    (C) Decreased plasma nitric oxide concentration
    (D) Increased plasma adenosine concentration
    (E) Decreased plasma osmolality

61. Which of the following vascular beds experiences the most vasoconstriction in a person near the end of a 10-kilometer run?
    (A) Cerebral
    (B) Coronary
    (C) Exercising muscle
    (D) Intestinal
    (E) Skin

62. 35-year-old woman visits her family practice physician for an examination. She has a mean arterial blood pressure of 105 mm Hg and a heart rate of 74 beats/min. Further tests by a cardiologist reveal that the patient has moderate aortic valve stenosis. Which of the following sets of changes would be expected in this patient?

	Pulse Pressure	Stroke Volume	Systolic Pressure
(A)	↑	↑	↑
(B)	↑	↓	↑
(C)	↑	↓	↓
(D)	↑	↑	↓
(E)	↓	↓	↓
(F)	↓	↑	↓
(G)	↓	↑	↑
(H)	↓	↓	↑

63. Which of the following is normally associated with an increased venous return of blood to the heart?
    (A) Decreased mean systemic filling pressure
    (B) Acute large vein dilatation
    (C) Decreased sympathetic tone
    (D) Increased venous compliance
    (E) Increased blood volume

64. A 25-year-old man enters the hospital emergency room after severing a major artery during a farm accident. It is estimated that the patient has lost approximately 800 milliliters of blood. His mean blood pressure is 65 mm Hg, and his heart rate is elevated as a result of activation of the chemoreceptor reflex. Which of the following sets of changes in plasma concentration would be expected to cause the greatest activation of the chemoreceptor reflex?

	Oxygen	Carbon Dioxide	Hydrogen
(A)	↑	↑	↑
(B)	↑	↓	↑
(C)	↑	↓	↓
(D)	↑	↑	↓
(E)	↓	↓	↓
(F)	↓	↑	↓
(G)	↓	↑	↑
(H)	↓	↓	↑

65. Which of the following is associated with the fourth heart sound?
    (A) Inrushing of blood into the ventricles due to atrial contraction
    (B) Closing of the atrioventricular (A-V) valves
    (C) Closing of the pulmonary valve
    (D) Opening of the A-V valves
    (E) Inrushing of blood into the ventricles in the early to middle part of diastole

66. A decrease in which of the following would tend to increase lymph flow?
    (A) Hydraulic conductivity of the capillary wall
    (B) Plasma colloid osmotic pressure
    (C) Capillary hydrostatic pressure
    (D) Interstitial hydrostatic pressure
    (E) Interstitial colloid osmotic pressure

67. A 25-year-old man is involved in a motorcycle accident and is taken to the emergency department. His clothes are covered with blood. His arterial pressure is 70/40 mm Hg, his heart rate is 120 beats/min, and his respiratory rate is 30 breaths/min. Which of the following therapies would the physician recommend?
    (A) Blood infusion
    (B) Plasma infusion
    (C) Balanced electrolyte solution infusion
    (D) Sympathomimetic drug infusion
    (E) Glucocorticoid infusion

68. Under normal physiological conditions, blood flow to the skeletal muscles is determined mainly by which of the following?
    (A) Sympathetic nerves
    (B) Angiotensin II
    (C) Vasopressin
    (D) Metabolic needs
    (E) Capillary osmotic pressure

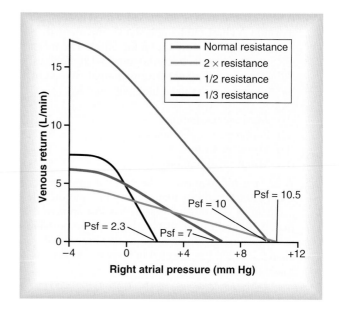

69. Which of the curves in the figure above has the highest resistance to venous return?
    (A) The blue line with mean systemic pressure (Psf) = 10
    (B) The green line with Psf = 10.5
    (C) The black line with Psf = 2.3
    (D) The red line with Psf = 7

70. Which of the following substances in plasma is the major factor that contributes to plasma colloid osmotic pressure?
    (A) Sodium chloride
    (B) Glucose
    (C) Albumin
    (D) Cholesterol
    (E) Potassium

71. A healthy 22-year-old female medical student has an exercise stress test at a local health club. A decrease in which of the following is most likely to occur in this woman's skeletal muscles during exercise?
    (A) Vascular conductance
    (B) Blood flow
    (C) Carbon dioxide concentration
    (D) Arteriolar resistance
    (E) Lactic acid concentration

72. Which of the following blood vessels is responsible for transporting the majority of venous blood flow that leaves the ventricular heart muscle?
    (A) Anterior cardiac veins
    (B) Coronary sinus
    (C) Bronchial veins
    (D) Azygos vein
    (E) Thebesian veins

73. Assuming that vessels A to D are the same length, which one has the greatest flow?

Blood Vessel	Pressure Gradient	Radius	Viscosity
(A)	100	1	10
(B)	50	2	5
(C)	25	4	2
(D)	10	6	1

74. Which of the following conditions normally accompanies acute unilateral right heart failure?
    (A) Increased right atrial pressure
    (B) Increased left atrial pressure
    (C) Increased urinary output
    (D) Increased cardiac output
    (E) Increased arterial pressure

75. Which of the following conditions normally occurs in compensated heart failure?
    (A) Decreased right atrial pressure
    (B) Decreased heart rate
    (C) Decreased aldosterone secretion
    (D) Decreased blood volume
    (E) Increased end-diastolic volume

76. An increase in left atrial pressure is most likely to occur in which of the following heart murmurs?
    (A) Tricuspid stenosis
    (B) Pulmonary valve regurgitation
    (C) Mitral regurgitation
    (D) Tricuspid regurgitation

77. Which blood vessel has the highest vascular resistance?

Blood Vessel (ml/min)	Blood Flow Gradient (mm Hg)	Pressure
(A)	1000	100
(B)	1200	60
(C)	1400	20
(D)	1600	80
(E)	1800	40

78. In which type of shock does cardiac output often increase?
    (A) Hemorrhagic shock
    (B) Anaphylactic shock
    (C) Septic shock
    (D) Neurogenic shock

79. A twofold increase in which of the following would result in the greatest increase in the transport of oxygen across the capillary wall?
    (A) Capillary hydrostatic pressure
    (B) Intercellular clefts in the capillary wall
    (C) Oxygen concentration gradient
    (D) Plasma colloid osmotic pressure
    (E) Capillary wall hydraulic permeability

80. Which of the following vessels has the greatest total cross-sectional area in the circulatory system?
    (A) Aorta
    (B) Small arteries
    (C) Capillaries
    (D) Venules
    (E) Vena cava

81. Which of the following normally occurs in right-sided heart failure?
    (A) Edema of the feet and ankles
    (B) Decrease in cardiac output less than that occurring in acute left-sided heart failure of the same degree
    (C) Increase in urinary output
    (D) Pulmonary edema

82. Which of the following components of the circulatory system contains the largest percentage of the total blood volume?
    (A) Arteries
    (B) Capillaries
    (C) Veins
    (D) Pulmonary circulation
    (E) Heart

83. Which of the following treatments has proved to be beneficial to patients with myocardial ischemia?
    (A) Beta receptor stimulation
    (B) Angiotensin II infusion
    (C) Chelation therapy
    (D) Norepinephrine infusion
    (E) Coronary angioplasty

84. An increase in which of the following would be expected to decrease blood flow in a vessel?
    (A) Pressure gradient across the vessel
    (B) Radius of the vessel
    (C) Plasma colloid osmotic pressure
    (D) Viscosity of the blood
    (E) Plasma sodium concentration

85. A 65-year-old woman is diagnosed with a heart murmur. The mean QRS axis is –60 degrees. Arterial pressure in the aorta is 110/70 mm Hg. Which of the following is the most likely diagnosis?
    (A) Aortic valve stenosis
    (B) Aortic valve regurgitation
    (C) Pulmonary valve stenosis
    (D) Mitral valve stenosis
    (E) Tricuspid valve regurgitation

86. Which of the following is normally beneficial for a patient with cardiogenic shock?
    (A) Placing tourniquets on all four limbs
    (B) Infusing plasma
    (C) Administering furosemide
    (D) Administering a bronchodilator
    (E) Removing blood from the patient

87. Which of the following segments of the circulatory system has the highest velocity of blood flow?
    (A) Aorta
    (B) Arteries
    (C) Capillaries
    (D) Venules
    (E) Veins

88. An increase in which of the following tends to decrease pulse pressure?
    (A) Systolic pressure
    (B) Stroke volume
    (C) Arterial compliance
    (D) Venous return
    (E) Plasma volume

89. An increase in which of the following tends to decrease capillary filtration rate?
    (A) Capillary hydrostatic pressure
    (B) Plasma colloid osmotic pressure
    (C) Interstitial colloid osmotic pressure
    (D) Venous hydrostatic pressure
    (E) Arteriolar diameter

90. Which of the following events normally occurs during exercise?
    (A) Arteriolar dilatation in nonexercising muscle
    (B) Decreased sympathetic output
    (C) Venoconstriction
    (D) Decreased release of epinephrine by the adrenals
    (E) Decreased release of norepinephrine by the adrenals

91. An increase in which of the following tends to increase capillary filtration rate?
    (A) Capillary wall hydraulic conductivity
    (B) Arteriolar resistance
    (C) Plasma colloid osmotic pressure
    (D) Interstitial hydrostatic pressure
    (E) Plasma sodium concentration

92. Which of the following is the most frequent cause of decreased coronary blood flow in patients with ischemic heart disease?
    (A) Increased adenosine release
    (B) Atherosclerosis
    (C) Coronary artery spasm
    (D) Increased sympathetic tone of the coronary arteries
    (E) Occlusion of the coronary sinus

93. A decrease in which of the following tends to increase lymph flow?
    (A) Capillary hydrostatic pressure
    (B) Interstitial hydrostatic pressure
    (C) Plasma colloid osmotic pressure
    (D) Lymphatic pump activity
    (E) Arteriolar diameter

94. A 29-year-old man is diagnosed with a heart murmur. The mean QRS axis of his electrocardiogram is 165 degrees. The arterial blood oxygen content is normal. Which of the following is the most likely diagnosis?
    (A) Aortic stenosis
    (B) Aortic regurgitation
    (C) Pulmonary valve stenosis
    (D) Mitral stenosis
    (E) Tetralogy of Fallot

95. A 20-year-old man arrives at the emergency department hemorrhaging from a gunshot wound. His skin is pale, and he is having trouble walking. He has tachycardia and an arterial pressure of 80/50 mm Hg. The blood bank is out of packed red blood cells. As an alternative, which of the following therapies would the physician recommend to prevent shock?
    (A) Administration of a glucocorticoid
    (B) Administration of an antihistamine
    (C) Infusion of a balanced electrolyte solution
    (D) Infusion of a sympathomimetic drug
    (E) Infusion of plasma

96. Which of the following capillaries has the lowest capillary permeability to plasma molecules?
    (A) Glomerular
    (B) Liver
    (C) Muscle
    (D) Intestinal
    (E) Brain

97. Which of the following is normally associated with an increased cardiac output?
    (A) Increased venous compliance
    (B) Cardiac tamponade
    (C) Surgically opening the chest
    (D) Moderate anemia
    (E) Severe aortic stenosis

98. Which of the following tends to increase the net movement of glucose across a capillary wall?
    (A) Increase in plasma sodium concentration
    (B) Increase in the concentration difference of glucose across the wall
    (C) Decrease in wall permeability to glucose
    (D) Decrease in wall surface area without an increase in the number of pores
    (E) Decrease in plasma potassium concentration

99. In which of the following conditions does right ventricular hypertrophy normally occur?
    (A) Tetralogy of Fallot
    (B) Mild aortic stenosis
    (C) Mild aortic insufficiency
    (D) Mitral stenosis
    (E) Tricuspid stenosis

100. A 65-year-old man is suffering from congestive heart failure. He has a cardiac output of 4 L/min, arterial pressure of 115/85 mm Hg, and a heart rate of 90 beats/min. Further tests by a cardiologist reveal that the patient has a right atrial pressure of 10 mm Hg. An increase in which of the following would be expected in this patient?
    (A) Plasma colloid osmotic pressure
    (B) Interstitial colloid osmotic pressure
    (C) Arterial pressure
    (D) Cardiac output
    (E) Vena cava hydrostatic pressure

101. Which of the following parts of the circulation has the highest compliance?
    (A) Capillaries
    (B) Large arteries
    (C) Veins
    (D) Aorta
    (E) Small arteries

102. Which of the following is normally associated with decompensated heart failure?
    (A) Increased calcium ions in the sarcoplasmic reticulum
    (B) Edema of the heart muscle
    (C) Decreased mean systemic filling pressure
    (D) Increased urinary output of sodium and water

103. Using the following data, calculate the filtration coefficient for the capillary bed:
    Plasma colloid osmotic pressure = 30 mm Hg
    Capillary hydrostatic pressure = 40 mm Hg
    Interstitial hydrostatic pressure = 5 mm Hg
    Interstitial colloid osmotic pressure = 5 mm Hg
    Filtration rate = 150 ml/min
    Venous hydrostatic pressure = 10 mm Hg
    (A) 10 ml/min/mm Hg
    (B) 15 ml/min/mm Hg
    (C) 20 ml/min/mm Hg
    (D) 25 ml/min/mm Hg
    (E) 30 ml/min/mm Hg

104. A 10-year-old girl is hospitalized because of an intestinal obstruction. Her arterial pressure is 70/40 mm Hg, her heart rate is 120 beats/min, and her respiratory rate is 30 breaths/min. Which of the following therapies should the physician recommend?
    (A) Blood infusion
    (B) Plasma infusion
    (C) Infusion of a balanced electrolyte solution
    (D) Infusion of a sympathomimetic drug
    (E) Administration of a glucocorticoid

105. Which of the following sets of physiological changes would be expected to occur in a person who stands up from a supine position?

	Venous Hydrostatic Pressure in Legs	Heart Rate	Renal Blood Flow
(A)	↑	↑	↑
(B)	↑	↑	↓
(C)	↑	↓	↓
(D)	↓	↓	↓
(E)	↓	↓	↑
(F)	↓	↑	↑

106. Which of the following often occurs during progressive shock?
    (A) Patchy areas of necrosis in the liver
    (B) Decreased tendency for blood to clot
    (C) Increased glucose metabolism
    (D) Decreased release of hydrolases by lysosomes
    (E) Decreased capillary permeability

107. Blood flow to a tissue remains relatively constant despite a reduction in arterial pressure (autoregulation). Which of the following would be expected to occur in response to the reduction in arterial pressure?
    (A) Decreased conductance
    (B) Decreased tissue carbon dioxide concentration
    (C) Increased tissue oxygen concentration
    (D) Decreased vascular resistance
    (E) Decreased arteriolar diameter

108. Which of the following is an acceptable treatment for a patient with an acute myocardial infarction?
    (A) Daily exercise
    (B) Beta receptor stimulation
    (C) Discontinue nitroglycerin intake
    (D) Discontinue aspirin intake
    (E) Coronary angioplasty

109. The largest portion of the arterial pressure generated during systole is dissipated at which of the following locations in the vascular tree?
    (A) Aortic arch
    (B) Aortic-arterial juncture
    (C) Arterial-arteriolar juncture
    (D) Arteriolar-capillary juncture
    (E) Capillary-venular juncture

110. Which of the following heart murmurs is heard only during systole?
    (A) Patent ductus arteriosus
    (B) Mitral stenosis
    (C) Tricuspid valve stenosis
    (D) Interventricular septal defect
    (E) Aortic regurgitation

111. The tendency for turbulent flow is greatest in which of the following?
    (A) Arterioles
    (B) Capillaries
    (C) Small arterioles
    (D) Aorta

112. Release of which of the following substances causes vasodilatation and increased capillary permeability during anaphylactic shock?
    (A) Histamine
    (B) Bradykinin
    (C) Nitric oxide
    (D) Atrial natriuretic factor
    (E) Adenosine

113. Autoregulation of tissue blood flow in response to an increase in arterial pressure occurs as a result of which of the following?
    (A) Decrease in vascular resistance
    (B) Initial decrease in vascular wall tension
    (C) Excess delivery of nutrients such as oxygen to the tissues
    (D) Decrease in tissue metabolism

114. Which of the following is normally beneficial for a patient with acute pulmonary edema?
    (A) Placing tourniquets on all four limbs
    (B) Infusing plasma
    (C) Infusing dextran
    (D) Infusing norepinephrine
    (E) Infusing angiotensin II

115. Which of the following is usually associated with compensated heart failure?
    (A) Increased cardiac output
    (B) Increased blood volume
    (C) Decreased mean systemic filling pressure
    (D) Normal right atrial pressure

116. Which of the following is a characteristic of progressive hemorrhagic shock?
    (A) Increased cardiac contractility
    (B) Endotoxin release
    (C) Decreased capillary permeability
    (D) Increased cell membrane active transport of sodium
    (E) Tissue alkalosis

117. Which of the following pressures is normally negative in a muscle capillary bed in the lower extremities?
    (A) Plasma colloid osmotic pressure
    (B) Capillary hydrostatic pressure
    (C) Interstitial hydrostatic pressure
    (D) Interstitial colloid osmotic pressure
    (E) Venous hydrostatic pressure

118. Which of the following would be recommended for a patient with myocardial ischemia?
    (A) Alpha receptor stimulation
    (B) Discontinue medication for hypertension
    (C) Lose excess body weight
    (D) Angiotensin II infusion
    (E) Isometric exercise

119. Which of the following would decrease venous hydrostatic pressure in the legs?
    (A) Increase in right atrial pressure
    (B) Pregnancy
    (C) Movement of leg muscles
    (D) Presence of ascitic fluid in the abdomen

120. Which of the following conditions is normally associated with an increase in mean systemic filling pressure?
    (A) Decreased blood volume
    (B) Congestive heart failure
    (C) Sympathetic inhibition
    (D) Venous dilatation

121. In which of the following conditions is a low arterial oxygen content most likely?
    (A) Tetralogy of Fallot
    (B) Pulmonary artery stenosis
    (C) Tricuspid insufficiency
    (D) Patent ductus arteriosus
    (E) Tricuspid stenosis

122. A 70-year-old man goes to the emergency department because he has been experiencing severe diarrhea. He has pallor, tachycardia, and an arterial pressure of 80/50 mm Hg. He has trouble walking. Which of the following therapies should the physician recommend to prevent shock?
    (A) Blood infusion
    (B) Administration of an antihistamine
    (C) Infusion of a balanced electrolyte solution
    (D) Infusion of a sympathomimetic drug
    (E) Administration of a glucocorticoid

123. Movement of solutes such as Na^+ across the capillary walls occurs primarily by which of the following processes?
    (A) Filtration
    (B) Active transport
    (C) Vesicular transport
    (D) Diffusion

124. Which of the following normally causes the cardiac output curve to shift to the left along the right atrial pressure axis?
    (A) Surgically opening the chest
    (B) Severe cardiac tamponade
    (C) Decreasing intrapleural pressure
    (D) Playing a trumpet
    (E) Placing a patient on a mechanical respirator

125. Which of the following has the fastest rate of movement across the capillary wall?
    (A) Sodium
    (B) Albumin
    (C) Glucose
    (D) Oxygen

126. In which of the following conditions is there normally a decreased cardiac output?
    (A) Hyperthyroidism
    (B) Beriberi
    (C) Atrioventricular fistula
    (D) Anemia
    (E) Acute myocardial infarction

127. A decrease in which of the following would be expected to occur in response to a direct increase in renal arterial pressure?
    (A) Water excretion
    (B) Sodium excretion
    (C) Extracellular fluid volume
    (D) Glomerular filtration rate

128. Which of the following is associated with the second heart sound?
    (A) Inrushing of blood into the ventricles due to atrial contraction
    (B) Closing of the atrioventricular (A-V) valves
    (C) Closing of the pulmonary valve
    (D) Opening of the A-V valves
    (E) Inrushing of blood into the ventricles in the early to middle part of diastole

129. A decrease in which of the following would most likely result in chronic hypertension?
    (A) Renal sympathetic nerve activity
    (B) Aldosterone
    (C) Angiotensin II
    (D) Nitric oxide

130. Which of the following conditions normally occurs during the early stages of compensated heart failure?
    (A) Increased right atrial pressure
    (B) Normal heart rate
    (C) Decreased angiotensin II release
    (D) Decreased aldosterone release
    (E) Increased urinary output of sodium and water

131. Which of the following is one of the major causes of death after myocardial infarction?
(A) Increased cardiac output
(B) Decreased pulmonary interstitial volume
(C) Fibrillation of the heart
(D) Increased cardiac contractility

132. An increase in which of the following would be expected to occur in response to an increase in sodium intake?
(A) Angiotensin II
(B) Aldosterone
(C) Sodium excretion
(D) Renal sympathetic nerve activity

133. At the onset of exercise, which of the following normally occurs?
(A) Decreased cerebral blood flow
(B) Increased venous constriction
(C) Decreased coronary blood flow
(D) Decreased mean systemic filling pressure
(E) Increased parasympathetic impulses to the heart

134. Which of the following would be expected to occur in response to constriction of the renal artery?
(A) Increase in sodium excretion
(B) Decrease in arterial pressure
(C) Increase in renin release
(D) Decrease angiotensin II

135. Which of the following statements about the results of sympathetic stimulation is most accurate?
(A) Epicardial flow increases
(B) Venous resistance decreases
(C) Arteriolar resistance decreases
(D) Heart rate decreases
(E) Venous reservoirs vasoconstrict

136. Which of the following conditions usually increases the plateau level of the cardiac output curve?
(A) Myocarditis
(B) Severe cardiac tamponade
(C) Decreased parasympathetic stimulation of the heart
(D) Myocardial infarction
(E) Mitral stenosis

137. An increase in atrial pressure results in which of the following?
(A) Decrease in plasma atrial natriuretic peptide
(B) Increase in plasma angiotensin II concentration
(C) Increase in plasma aldosterone concentration
(D) Increase in heart rate

138. Which of the following often occurs during decompensated heart failure?
(A) Hypertension
(B) Increased mean pulmonary filling pressure
(C) Decreased pulmonary capillary pressure
(D) Increased cardiac output
(E) Increased norepinephrine in the endings of the cardiac sympathetic nerves

139. Which of the following would be expected to occur during a Cushing reaction caused by brain ischemia?
(A) Increase in parasympathetic activity
(B) Decrease in arterial pressure
(C) Decrease in heart rate
(D) Increase in sympathetic activity

140. Which of the following often occurs in decompensated heart failure?
(A) Increased renal loss of sodium and water
(B) Decreased mean systemic filling pressure
(C) Increased norepinephrine in cardiac sympathetic nerves
(D) Orthopnea
(E) Weight loss

141. An angiotensin-converting enzyme inhibitor is administered to a 65-year-old man with a 20-year history of hypertension. The drug lowers arterial pressure and increases plasma levels of renin and bradykinin. Which of the following would best explain the elevation in plasma bradykinin?
(A) Inhibition of preprobradykinin
(B) Decreased conversion of angiotensin I to angiotensin II
(C) Increased formation of angiotensin II
(D) Increased formation of kallikrein
(E) Inhibition of kininases

142. A 60-year-old woman has been severely burned. Her arterial pressure is 70/40 mm Hg, and her heart rate is 130 beats/min. Which of the following should the physician recommend as initial therapy?
(A) Blood infusion
(B) Plasma infusion
(C) Infusion of a balanced electrolyte solution
(D) Infusion of a sympathomimetic drug
(E) Administration of a glucocorticoid

143. A 60-year-old man has a mean arterial blood pressure of 130 mm Hg, a heart rate of 78 beats/min, a right atrial pressure of 0 mm Hg, and a cardiac output of 3.5 L/min. He also has a pulse pressure of 35 mm Hg and a hematocrit of 40. What is the approximate total peripheral vascular resistance in this man?
(A) 17 mm Hg/L/min
(B) 1.3 mm Hg/L/min
(C) 13 mm Hg/L/min
(D) 27 mm Hg/L/min
(E) 37 mm Hg/L/min

144. The results of an echocardiogram performed on a 50-year-old woman indicate a thickened right ventricle. Other data indicate that the patient has severely decreased arterial oxygen content and equal systolic pressures in both cardiac ventricles. Which of the following conditions is most likely present?
(A) Interventricular septal defect
(B) Tetralogy of Fallot
(C) Pulmonary valve stenosis
(D) Pulmonary valve regurgitation
(E) Patent ductus arteriosus

Answers

1. (G) Moving from a supine to a standing position causes an acute fall in arterial pressure that is sensed by arterial baroreceptors located in the carotid sinuses and aortic arch. Activation of the baroreceptors results in an increase in sympathetic activity and a decrease in parasympathetic activity (or vagal tone), which lead to an increase in heart rate.
   TMP11 209, 210

2. (A) During increases in sympathetic output, the brain and the heart are the two main organs that maintain their blood flow. During 1 hour of exercise, the intestinal flow and the renal and pancreatic blood flow decrease significantly. The skeletal muscle blood flow to nonexercising muscles also decreases at this time. The cerebral blood flow remains close to its control value.
   TMP11 248

3. (A) The increase in local metabolism during exercise causes cells to release vasodilator substances such as adenosine. The increase in tissue adenosine concentration increases arteriolar diameter, vascular conductance, and blood flow to skeletal muscles.
   TMP11 196, 197

4. (B) Moving from a supine to a standing position causes an acute fall in arterial pressure that is sensed by arterial baroreceptors located in the carotid bifurcation and aortic arch. Activation of the arterial baroreceptors leads to an increase in sympathetic outflow to the peripheral vasculature and the kidneys. The increase in sympathetic activity to peripheral vessels results in an increase in total peripheral resistance. The increase in renal sympathetic nerve activity results in an increase in renin release (and plasma renin activity) and a decrease in renal blood flow.
   TMP11 209, 210

5. (C) Mitral regurgitation and aortic stenosis are murmurs heard during the systolic period. A ventricular septal defect murmur is normally heard only during the systolic phase. Tricuspid valve stenosis and patent ductus arteriosus murmurs are heard during diastole, but patent ductus arteriosus is also heard during systole.
   TMP11 271, 272

6. (D) The net pressure (NP) for fluid movement across a capillary wall = capillary hydrostatic pressure – plasma colloid osmotic pressure + interstitial colloid osmotic pressure – interstitial hydrostatic pressure. Thus, the net filtration pressure is 15 mm Hg.
   NP = [Pc – Πp + Π_l – P_l]
   NP = [25 – 25 + 10 – (–5)]
   NP = 15
   TMP11 185, 186

7. (E) In compensated heart failure, the sympathetic output increases. One of the results is a sympathetic vasoconstriction of the afferent arterioles of the kidney. This decreases the glomerular hydrostatic pressure and thus the glomerular filtration rate, resulting in an increase in sodium and water retention in the body. An increased release of angiotensin II also occurs, which causes direct renal sodium retention and stimulates aldosterone secretion, which in turn cause further increases in sodium retention in the kidney. The excess sodium in the body increases osmolality; this increases the release of antidiuretic hormone, which causes renal water retention.
   TMP11 263, 264

8. (D) The rate of net fluid movement across a capillary wall is calculated as capillary filtration coefficient × net filtration pressure. Net filtration pressure = capillary hydrostatic pressure – plasma colloid osmotic pressure + interstitial colloid osmotic pressure – interstitial hydrostatic pressure. Thus, the rate of net fluid movement across the capillary wall is 150 ml/min.
   Filtration rate = Capillary filtration coefficient (K_f) × Net filtration pressure
   Filtration rate = K_f × [Pc – Πc + Πi – P_l]
   Filtration rate = 10 ml/min/mm Hg × [25 – 25 + 10 – (–5)]
   Filtration rate = 10 × 15 = 150 ml/min
   TMP11 185, 186

9. (C) The formula for resistance to venous return is mean systemic filling pressure – right atrial pressure ÷ cardiac output. In this example, the mean systemic filling pressure is 9 mm Hg and the right atrial pressure is –0.5 mm Hg. The cardiac output is 6.8 L/min. Using these values in the previous formula indicates that the resistance to venous return is 1.40 mm Hg/L/min. Note that this formula applies only to the linear portion of the venous return curve.
   TMP11 241, 242

10. (B) Several events occur in progressive shock, including increased capillary permeability, which allows fluid to leak out of the vasculature, thus decreasing the blood volume. Other deteriorating factors include vasomotor center failure, peripheral circulatory failure, decreased cellular mitochondrial activity, and acidosis throughout the body. Usually, urine output decreases strikingly.
    TMP11 281-284

11. (H) Atrial natriuretic peptide (ANP) inhibits renin release (and angiotensin II formation). ANP also inhibits renal tubular sodium reabsorption, which leads to an increase in sodium excretion.
    TMP11 212

12. (A) During increases in sympathetic output to maximal values, several changes occur. First, the mean systemic filling pressure increases markedly and, simultaneously, the resistance to venous return increases. Venous return is determined by the

formula: mean systemic filling pressure – right atrial pressure ÷ resistance to venous return. During maximal sympathetic output, the increase in systemic filling pressure is greater than the increase in resistance to venous return. Therefore, in this formula, the numerator has a much greater increase than the denominator. This results in an increase in the venous return.
TMP11 217, 218

13. (E) Administration of a drug that decreases the diameter of arterioles in a muscle bed increases the vascular resistance. The increased vascular resistance decreases vascular conductance and blood flow. The reduction in arteriolar diameter also leads to a decrease in capillary hydrostatic pressure and capillary filtration rate.
TMP11 167, 168, 189, 190

14. (C) During acute pulmonary edema, the increased fluid in the lungs diminishes the oxygen content in the blood. The decreased oxygen weakens the heart further, causing arteriolar dilatation in the body. This results in increased venous return of blood to the heart, which causes further leakage of the fluid in the lungs and further decreases in oxygen content in the blood. To save a patient's life, it is important to interrupt this vicious circle. This can be done by placing tourniquets on all four limbs, which effectively removes blood volume from the chest. The patient can also breathe oxygen and can be given a bronchodilator. Furosemide can be given to reduce some of the fluid volume in the body, especially in the lungs. This patient should not be infused with whole blood or an electrolyte solution because it may exacerbate the pulmonary edema that is already present.
TMP11 264

15. (A) The difference between systolic pressure and diastolic pressure is the pulse pressure. The two major factors that affect pulse pressure are the stroke volume output of the heart and the compliance of the arterial tree. In patients with moderate aortic regurgitation (due to incomplete closure of aortic valve), the blood that is pumped into the aorta immediately flows back into the left ventricle. The backflow of blood into the left ventricle increases stroke volume and systolic pressure. The rapid backflow of blood also results in a decrease in diastolic pressure. Thus, patients with moderate aortic regurgitation have high systolic pressure, low diastolic pressure, and high pulse pressure.
TMP11 173, 174

16. (E) There are several factors that increase the risk of coronary artery disease, including physical inactivity, diabetes mellitus, hypertension, and aging. Increases in body weight also increase the risk of coronary artery disease. Decreases in body weight reduce the risk of coronary disease.
TMP11 252, 253

17. (E) Angiotensin II is a powerful vasoconstrictor. Angiotensin I is formed by an enzyme (renin) acting on a substrate called angiotensinogen. Angiotensin I is converted to angiotensin II by a converting enzyme. Angiotensin II is a powerful vasoconstrictor and sodium-retaining hormone that increases arterial pressure. Administration of an ACE inhibitor would be expected to decrease angiotensin II formation, total peripheral resistance, and arterial pressure.
TMP11 223, 224

18. (A) Bradykinin, prostaglandins, carbon dioxide, and potassium ions serve as vasodilators for the coronary artery system. However, the major controller of coronary blood flow is adenosine. Adenosine is formed as adenosine triphosphate degrades to adenosine monophosphate. Small portions of the adenosine monophosphate are then further degraded to release adenosine into the tissue fluids of the heart muscle, and this adenosine vasodilates the coronary arteries.
TMP11 250, 251

19. (A) Sympathomimetic drugs are given to counteract hypotension under several circumstances, including spinal cord injury in which the sympathetic output is interrupted. Sympathomimetic drugs are also given during very deep anesthesia, which decreases the sympathetic output, and in anaphylactic shock that results from histamine release and the accompanying vasodilatation. Sympathomimetic drugs such as norepinephrine increase blood pressure by causing vasoconstriction. Shock caused by excess vomiting, hemorrhage, or excess administration of diuretics results in fluid volume depletion that results in decreased blood volume and decreased mean systemic filling pressure. Giving a balanced electrolyte solution best counteracts this condition.
TMP11 287

20. (B) Cognitive stimuli increase cerebral blood flow by decreasing cerebral vascular resistance. The diameter of cerebral vessels is decreased by various metabolic factors in response to cognitive stimuli. Metabolic factors that enhance cerebral blood flow include increases in carbon dioxide, hydrogen ion (decreased pH), and adenosine.
TMP11 196-198

21. (E) The third heart sound is associated with inrushing of blood into the ventricles in the early to middle part of diastole. The next heart sound, the fourth heart sound, is caused by inrushing of blood in the ventricles caused by atrial contraction. The first heart sound is caused by closing of the atrioventricular valves, and the second heart sound is caused by closing of the pulmonary and aortic valves.
TMP11 270

22. (A) Stenosis of one kidney results in the release of renin and the formation of angiotensin II from the

affected kidney. Angiotensin II stimulates aldosterone production and increases total peripheral resistance by constricting most of the blood vessels in the body.
TMP11 226-227

23. (B) "Blowing" murmurs of relatively high pitch are usually associated with valvular insufficiency. The key pieces of data to identify this murmur are the systolic and diastolic pressures. Aortic valve regurgitation typically has a high pulse pressure (systolic pressure minus diastolic pressure), which is 100 mm Hg in this patient. Note also that the diastolic pressure decreases to a very low value of 40 mm Hg as the blood leaks back into the left ventricle.
TMP11 272

24. (G) Histamine is a vasodilator that is typically released by mast cells and basophils. Infusion of histamine into a brachial artery would decrease arteriolar resistance and increase blood flow. The decrease in arteriolar resistance would also increase capillary hydrostatic pressure and capillary filtration rate.
TMP11 164, 202

25. (E) In compensated hemorrhagic shock, several factors prevent the progression of shock, including increased heart rate. Also occurring is reverse stress relaxation, in which the vasculature (particularly the veins) constrict around the available blood volume. Increased amounts of antidiuretic hormone are released, which causes water retention from the kidney and vasoconstriction of the arterioles. A central nervous system ischemic response occurs if blood pressure drops to very low values, which causes an increase in sympathetic output. Increased absorption of interstitial fluid through the capillaries occurs, which increases the volume in the vasculature.
TMP11 280, 281

26. (G) Bradykinin is a vasodilator that is believed to play a role in regulating blood flow and capillary leakage in inflamed tissue. Infusion of bradykinin into the brachial artery would increase arteriolar diameter and decrease arteriolar resistance. The decrease in arteriolar resistance would also result in an increase in capillary hydrostatic pressure and filtration rate. The increase in filtration rate leads to an increase in interstitial hydrostatic pressure and lymph flow.
TMP11 190-192, 202

27. (C) An increase in shear stress in blood vessels is one of the major stimuli for the release of nitric oxide by endothelial cells. Nitric oxide increases blood flow by increasing cyclic guanosine monophosphate.
TMP11 199

28. (B) This patient has a resting cardiac output of 4 L/min, and his cardiac reserve is 300 per cent

of this resting cardiac output, or 12 L/min. The total maximum cardiac output is 16 L/min. Therefore, the cardiac reserve is the percentage increase that the cardiac output can be elevated over the resting cardiac output.
TMP11 264

29. (C) An acute loss of blood supply to cardiac muscle causes depletion of potassium from the cardiac myocytes. This locally increases the extracellular potassium concentration. In turn, this increases the irritability of the cardiac musculature and its likelihood for fibrillating. Therefore, a decreased potassium ion concentration in the extracellular fluid of the heart does not lead to fibrillation. Powerful sympathetic reflexes also increase the irritability of the cardiac muscle and predispose it to fibrillation. Cardiac dilatation increases the likelihood of circus movements, and a current of injury allows electrical current to flow from an ischemic area of the heart to a normal area and can elicit fibrillation.
TMP11 254

30. (E) Solid tumors are metabolically active tissues that need increased quantities of oxygen and other nutrients. When metabolism in a tissue is increased for a prolonged period, the vascularity of the tissue also increases. One of the important factors that increase growth of new blood vessels is vascular endothelial growth factor (VEGF). Presumably, a deficiency of tissue oxygen or other nutrients, or both, leads to the formation of VEGF.
TMP11 200

31. (C) The Fick principle for determining cardiac output can be applied here. The formula for cardiac output is oxygen absorbed per minute by the lungs ÷ atriovenous oxygen difference. In this problem, oxygen consumption of the body is 240 ml/min, and in a steady-state condition, this would exactly equal the oxygen absorbed by the lungs. Therefore, by inserting these values into the equation, the cardiac output equals 12 L/min.
TMP11 244

32. (E) An increase in the diameter of a precapillary arteriole would decrease arteriolar resistance. The decrease in arteriolar resistance would lead to an increase in vascular conductance and capillary blood flow, hydrostatic pressure, and filtration rate.
TMP11 167-168, 189-200

33. (D) The normal intrapleural pressure is –4 mm Hg. When the thorax is surgically opened, the value of all pressures inside the chest immediately become 0 mm Hg, which is the atmospheric pressure. This increased pressure in the chest tends to collapse the atria and decreases the transmural pressure across each atrium. In particular, the right atrial transmural pressure gradient decreases about 4 mm Hg. Therefore, the cardiac output curve shifts 4 mm Hg to the right.
TMP11 238

34. (D) Blood flow in a vessel is directly proportional to the fourth power of the vessel radius. Increasing vessel diameter by 50 per cent (1.5 times control) would increase blood flow 1.5 to the fourth power × normal blood flow (100 ml/min). Thus, blood flow would increase to 100 ml/min × 5.06, or approximately 500 ml/min.
TMP11 168

35. (E) Left ventricular hypertrophy occurs either when the left ventricle has to produce high pressure or when it pumps extra volume with each stroke. In pulmonary valve regurgitation, extra blood leaks back into the ventricle during the diastolic period. This extra volume must be expelled during the next heartbeat but this causes right ventricular hypertrophy. In aortic stenosis, the left ventricle must contract very strongly, producing high wall tension in order to increase the aortic pressure to values that are high enough to expel blood into the aorta. In mitral stenosis and tricuspid stenosis, the ventricles are normal, because the atrium produces extra pressure to move blood through the stenotic valves.
TMP11 276

36. (A) In patent ductus arteriosus, a large quantity of the blood pumped into the aorta by the left ventricle immediately flows backward into the pulmonary artery and then into the lung and left atrium. The shunting of blood from the aorta results in a low diastolic pressure, while the increased inflow of blood into the left atrium and ventricle increases stroke volume and systolic pressure. The combined increase in systolic pressure and decrease in diastolic pressure results in an increase in pulse pressure.
TMP11 173, 174

37. (B) During heart failure, blood volume increases, resulting in an increased cardiac stretch. In particular, the atrial pressure increases, causing a release of atrial natriuretic factor and resulting in an increase in renal sodium excretion. Several factors cause sodium retention during heart failure, including aldosterone release, decreased glomerular filtration rate, and increased angiotensin II release. A decrease in mean arterial pressure results in decreased glomerular hydrostatic pressure and causes a decrease in renal sodium excretion.
TMP11 263, 264

38. (C) Several factors can cause the cardiac output to shift to the right or left. These include surgically opening the chest, which causes the cardiac output curve to shift 4 mm Hg to the right, and severe cardiac tamponade, which increases the pressure inside the pericardium and tends to collapse the heart, particularly the atria. Playing a trumpet or positive pressure breathing tremendously increases the interpleural pressure, thus collapsing the atria and shifting the cardiac output curve to the right.

Breathing against a negative pressure shifts the cardiac output curve to the left.
TMP11 238

39. (A) The net movement of glucose across a capillary wall is directly proportional to the wall permeability to glucose, wall surface area, and concentration gradient across the capillary wall. Thus, increases in glucose permeability, surface area, and glucose concentration gradient wall would all increase the net movement of glucose across the capillary wall.
TMP11 183, 184

40. (C) The normal resting coronary blood flow is approximately 225 ml/min. Infusion of adenosine or local release of adenosine normally increases the coronary blood flow. The contraction of the cardiac muscle around the vasculature, particularly in the subendocardial vessels, causes a decrease in blood flow. Therefore, during the systolic phase of the cardiac cycle, the subendocardial flow clearly decreases, and the decrease in epicardial flow is relatively minor.
TMP11 249-251

41. (B) A person with atherosclerosis would be expected to have decreased arterial compliance. The decrease in arterial compliance would lead to an increase in systolic pressure and pulse pressure.
TMP11 173-174

42. (D) The patient received an influenza inoculation and quickly went into shock. This may be anaphylactic shock, which is a state of extreme vasodilatation because of histamine release. Antihistamines would be somewhat helpful, but they are very slow-acting drugs, and the patient could die in the meantime. Therefore, a very rapid-acting agent must be used, such as a sympathomimetic drug.
TMP11 285, 286

43. (B) Constriction of the carotid artery reduces blood pressure at the carotid bifurcation where the arterial baroreceptors are located. The decrease in arterial pressure activates baroreceptors, which in turn leads to an increase in sympathetic activity and a decrease in parasympathetic activity (or vagal tone). The enhanced sympathetic activity results in constriction of peripheral blood vessels and an increase in total peripheral resistance. The combination of enhanced sympathetic activity and decreased vagal tone also leads to an increase in heart rate.
TMP11 209, 210

44. (A) Atrial natriuretic peptide is released from myocytes in the atria in response to increases in atrial pressure.
TMP11 212

45. (C) An overdose of furosemide causes a tremendous increase in urinary volume. This can cause a

substantial decrease in the plasma volume. There- fore, blood volume decreases, and the arterial pressure reaches very low levels. The appropriate therapy is to replace the volume that was lost by the infusion of a balanced electrolyte solution.
TMP11 285

46. (C) An increase in the diameter of a precapillary arteriole decreases arteriolar resistance while increasing vascular conductance and capillary blood flow, hydrostatic pressure, filtration rate, interstitial volume, and interstitial hydrostatic pressure.
TMP11 167, 168, 189-200

47. (C) Excess secretion of aldosterone results in enhanced tubular reabsorption of sodium and secre- tion of potassium. The increased reabsorption of sodium and water leads to an increase in extracellu- lar fluid volume, which in turn suppresses renin release by the kidney. The increase in potassium secretion leads to a decrease in plasma potassium concentration, or hypokalemia.
TMP11 223

48. (D) A vicious circle of cardiac deterioration occurs in a patient in cardiogenic shock. A weakened heart causes a decreased cardiac output, which decreases arterial pressure. The decreased arterial pressure, particularly the decrease in dias- tolic pressure, decreases the coronary blood flow and further weakens the heart, thus further decreas- ing cardiac output. The therapy of choice for a patient in cardiogenic shock is to increase the arterial pressure with either a vasoconstrictor drug or a volume-expanding drug. Placing tourni- quets on the four limbs, bleeding the patient moderately, or giving furosemide decreases the thoracic blood volume and thus worsens the patient's condition.
TMP11 262, 263

49. (E) A decrease in tissue oxygen tension is thought to be an important stimulus for vascular endothelial growth factor and the growth of blood vessels in solid tumors.
TMP11 200, 201

50. (C) There are several systolic murmurs, including interventricular septal defect. Normally, the septal defect opens during systole and can be heard easily. During systole, mitral regurgitation occurs through the insufficient mitral valve, causing the heart murmur. Tetralogy of Fallot is a systolic murmur because of the sounds created by the interventricu- lar septal defect and the stenotic pulmonary vessel. Patent ductus arteriosus can be heard during systole because of extra blood flowing through the ductus arteriosus, but it is also heard during diastole. Tri- cuspid stenosis is a diastolic murmur because blood flows through the restricted tricuspid valve during the diastolic period.
TMP11 271, 272

51. (E) According to Poiseuille's law, flow through a vessel increases in proportion to the fourth power of the radius. A fourfold increase in vessel diameter (or radius) would increase 4 to the fourth power, or 256 times normal. Thus, flow through the vessel after increasing the vessel four times normal would increase from 100 to 25,600 ml/min.
TMP11 168

52. (A) In the figure shown in the question, the mean systemic filling pressure is approximately 4.3 mm Hg. The average pulmonary arterial blood flow is equal to the cardiac output and venous return, which in this case is approximately 3 L/min. The right atrial pressure is about 0 mm Hg. The plateau of the cardiac output curve is about 10.5 L/min.
TMP11 242

53. (H) Constriction of the carotid artery decreases blood pressure at the level of the carotid sinus. A decrease in carotid sinus pressure leads to a decrease in carotid sinus nerve impulses to the vasomotor center, which in turn leads to enhanced sympathetic nervous activity and decreased parasympathetic nerve activity. The increase in sympathetic nerve activity results in peripheral vasoconstriction and an increase in total peripheral resistance.
TMP11 209, 210

54. (C) In this patient, the mean electrical axis of the QRS is shifted rightward to 140 degrees, indicating that the right side of the heart is involved. Aortic stenosis, aortic regurgitation, and mitral regurgita- tion all cause a leftward shift of the QRS axis. Mitral stenosis does not affect the left ventricle, but when severe enough, it could cause an increase in pulmonary artery pressure. This would cause an increase in pulmonary capillary pressure at the same time. Therefore, pulmonary valve stenosis is the only condition that fits this set of symptoms.
TMP11 271, 272

55. (H) The arterial baroreceptors are activated in response to a fall in arterial pressure. During hem- orrhage, the fall in arterial pressure at the level of the baroreceptors results in enhanced sympathetic outflow from the vasomotor center and a decrease in parasympathetic nerve activity. The increase in sympathetic nerve activity leads to constriction of peripheral blood vessels, increased total peripheral resistance, and a return of blood pressure toward normal. The constriction of renal vessels results in decreased renal blood flow.
TMP11 209, 210

56. (E) Spinal anesthesia, especially when the anesthe- sia extends all the way up the spinal cord, can block the sympathetic nervous outflow from the spinal cord. This can be a very potent cause of neurogenic shock. The therapy of choice is to replace the sympathetic tone that was lost in the body, and the best means of doing this is to

increase the sympathetic tone by infusing a sympathomimetic drug.
TMP11 287

57. (C) Vascular resistance = arterial pressure − venous pressure ÷ blood flow. In this example, arterial pressure is 130 mm Hg, venous pressure is 5 mm Hg, and blood flow is 250 ml/min. Thus, vascular resistance = 125 ÷ 250, or 0.50 mm Hg/ml/min.
TMP11 167

58. (D) Mean systemic filling pressure is a measure of the tightness of fit of the blood in the circulation. Mean systemic filling pressure is increased by factors that increase blood volume and by factors that decrease vascular compliance. Therefore, decreased venous compliance would cause an increase in mean systemic filling pressure, and vice versa. Administering norepinephrine and sympathetic stimulation cause arteriolar vasoconstriction and decreased vascular compliance, resulting in an increase in mean systemic filling pressure. Increased blood volume and skeletal muscle contraction, which causes a contraction of the vasculature, also increase this filling pressure.
TMP11 239

59. (A) Activation of the baroreceptors leads to an increase in sympathetic activity, which in turn increases heart rate, strength of cardiac contraction, and constriction of arterioles and veins. The increase in venous constriction results in an increase in mean circulatory filling pressure, venous return, and cardiac output.
TMP11 209, 210

60. (D) There are several factors that cause arteriolar vasodilatation during exercise, including increases in potassium ion concentration, plasma nitric oxide concentration, plasma adenosine concentration, and plasma osmolality. Although histamine causes arteriolar vasodilatation, histamine release does not normally occur during exercise.
TMP11 247

61. (D) The vascular beds that are spared from vasoconstriction due to increased sympathetic output during exercise include the cerebral and coronary vascular beds. In exercising muscle, the metabolic vasodilatory response overcomes the sympathetic nervous system, resulting in vasodilatation. In the skin vasculature, vasoconstriction occurs only at the beginning of exercise, and when the body temperature rises, the skin arterioles dilate. The intestinal vasculature significantly constricts during long-term exercise.
TMP11 247, 248

62. (E) Pulse pressure is the difference between systolic pressure and diastolic pressure. The two major factors that affect pulse pressure are the stroke volume output of the heart and the compliance of the arterial tree. An increase in stroke volume increases systolic and pulse pressure, while an increase in compliance of the arterial tree decreases pulse pressure. Moderate aortic valve stenosis results in a decrease in stroke volume, which leads to a decrease in systolic pressure and pulse pressure.
TMP11 173, 174

63. (E) Venous return of the heart = mean systemic filling pressure − right atrial pressure ÷ resistance to venous return. Therefore, decreased mean systemic filling pressure decreases the venous return to the heart. Factors that decrease the systemic filling pressure include large vein dilatation, decreased sympathetic tone, increased venous compliance, and decreased blood volume. Increased blood volume increases mean systemic filling pressure and venous return.
TMP11 239, 240

64. (G) When blood pressure falls below 80 mm Hg, carotid and aortic chemoreceptors are activated to elicit a neural reflex to minimize the fall in blood pressure. The chemoreceptors are chemosensitive cells that are sensitive to oxygen lack, carbon dioxide excess, or hydrogen ion excess (or fall in pH). The signals transmitted from the chemoreceptors into the vasomotor center excite the vasomotor center to increase arterial pressure.
TMP11 211, 212

65. (A) The fourth heart sound is caused by the inrushing of blood into the ventricles following atrial contraction. This initiates a vibration similar to those of the third heart sound, but it occurs at the end of the diastolic period. This fourth heart sound is also called the atrial "kick" and increases cardiac output by 25 to 30 per cent.
TMP11 271

66. (B) The two main factors that increase lymph flow are an increase in capillary filtration rate and an increase in lymphatic pump activity. A decrease in plasma colloid osmotic pressure increases capillary filtration rate, interstitial volume and hydrostatic pressure, and lymph flow. In contrast, a decrease in hydraulic conductivity of the capillary wall, capillary hydrostatic pressure, and interstitial colloid osmotic pressure all decrease capillary filtration rate, interstitial volume and pressure, and lymph flow.
TMP11 192, 194

67. (A) This patient has obviously lost a lot of blood, so the most advantageous therapy is to replace the blood lost. An infusion of blood is much better than a plasma infusion. Red blood cells are being replaced, which have a superior oxygen carrying capacity compared with the plasma component of blood. Sympathetic nerves are firing very rapidly in this condition, and an infusion of a sympathomimetic agent would be of little advantage.
TMP11 286, 287

68. (D) Although sympathetic nerves, angiotensin II, and vasopressin are powerful vasoconstrictors, blood flow to skeletal muscles under normal

physiological conditions is mainly determined by local metabolic needs.
TMP11 195

69. (B) The resistance to venous return is the inverse of the slope of the linear portion of the venous return curve. Therefore, the curve with the lowest slope will have the highest resistance to venous return.
TMP11 241

70. (C) Those molecules or ions that fail to pass through the pores of the capillary wall exert osmotic pressure. The capillary wall is highly permeable to sodium chloride, glucose, cholesterol, and potassium but relatively impermeable to albumin. Thus, albumin in the plasma is the major contributor to plasma colloid osmotic pressure.
TMP11 188

71. (D) During exercise, tissue levels of carbon dioxide and lactic acid increase. These metabolites dilate blood vessels, decrease arteriolar resistance, and enhance vascular conductance and blood flow. Thus, a decrease in arteriolar resistance is most likely to occur in skeletal muscle during exercise.
TMP11 197, 198

72. (B) The anterior cardiac veins and the thebesian veins both drain venous blood from the heart. However, 75 per cent of the total coronary flow drains from the heart by the coronary sinus.
TMP11 249

73. (D) The flow in a vessel is directly proportional to the pressure gradient across the vessel and to the fourth power of the radius of the vessel. In contrast, blood flow is inversely proportional to the viscosity of the blood. Because blood flow is proportional to the fourth power of the vessel radius, the vessel with the largest radius (vessel D) would have the greatest flow.
TMP11 168

74. (A) In unilateral right heart failure, the right atrial pressure increases and the overall cardiac output decreases. This results in a decrease in arterial pressure and urinary output. However, left atrial pressure does not increase, but in fact decreases.
TMP11 262

75. (E) During compensated heart failure, several conditions change to stabilize the circulatory system. Because of increased sympathetic output, the heart rate increases. The kidneys retain sodium and water, which increases blood volume and thus increases right atrial pressure. The resulting increased blood volume causes an increase in end-diastolic volume in the ventricles, which helps to increase the cardiac output. This renal retention of sodium is promoted by increases in aldosterone secretion.
TMP11 260

76. (C) Mitral stenosis, aortic regurgitation, and mitral regurgitation all cause large increases in left atrial pressure. Tricuspid stenosis and regurgitation increase only the right atrial pressure and should not affect pressure in the left atrium.
TMP11 273, 274

77. (A) Resistance of a vessel = pressure gradient ÷ blood flow of the vessel. In this example, vessel A has the highest vascular resistance (100 mm Hg/ 1000 ml/min, or 0.1 mm Hg/ml/min).
TMP11 164

78. (C) In hemorrhagic shock, anaphylactic shock, and neurogenic shock, the venous return of blood to the heart markedly decreases. However, in septic shock, the cardiac output increases in many patients because of vasodilatation in affected tissues and a high metabolic rate causing vasodilatation in other parts of the body.
TMP11 284-286

79. (C) The transport of oxygen across a capillary wall is proportional to the capillary surface area, capillary wall permeability to oxygen, and oxygen gradient across the capillary wall. Thus, a twofold increase in the oxygen concentration gradient would result in the greatest increase in the transport of oxygen across the capillary wall. A twofold increase in intercellular clefts in the capillary wall would not significantly impact oxygen transport, because oxygen can permeate the endothelial cell wall.
TMP11 183, 184

80. (C) The capillaries have the largest total cross-sectional area of all vessels of the circulatory system. The venules also have a relatively large total cross-sectional area, but not as great as the capillaries, which explains the large storage of blood in the venous system compared with that in the arterial system.
TMP11 163

81. (A) In acute right-sided heart failure, the kidneys retain sodium and water, and the systemic (not pulmonary) veins become congested. This results in edema of the lower extremities, including the feet and ankles. Cardiac output decreases more compared with the decrease in a patient with an equal amount of left-sided heart damage. This occurs because the right atrial pressure increases only a small amount during right-sided heart failure, whereas in left-sided heart failure, the left atrial pressure increases much more.
TMP11 262

82. (C) The percentage of the total blood volume in the veins is approximately 64 per cent.
TMP11 162

83. (E) Several drugs have proved helpful to patients with myocardial ischemia. Beta receptor blockers inhibit the sympathetic effects on the heart.

Angiotensin-converting enzyme inhibitors prevent the production of angiotensin II, thus decreasing the afterload effect on the heart. Norepinephrine increases the cardiac afterload which increases the myocardial O_2 consumption. Coronary angioplasty opens up the coronary vessels, thus reducing coronary vascular resistance. Chelation therapy has not proved to be of any benefit in patients with myocardial ischemia.
TMP11 261

84. (D) The rate of blood flow is directly proportional to the fourth power of the vessel radius and to the pressure gradient across the vessel. In contrast, the rate of blood flow is inversely proportional to the viscosity of the blood. Thus, an increase in blood viscosity would decrease blood flow in a vessel.
TMP11 168

85. (A) This patient has a QRS axis of –60 degrees, indicating a leftward axis shift. In other words, the left side of the heart is enlarged. In both aortic valve stenosis and aortic valve regurgitation, the left side of the heart is enlarged. However, in aortic valve regurgitation, the pulse pressure is very large, which is not the case in this patient. Therefore, these symptoms are diagnostic of aortic stenosis. In pulmonary valve stenosis, the right side of the heart hypertrophies, and in mitral valve stenosis, there is no left ventricular hypertrophy. In tricuspid valve regurgitation, the right side of the heart enlarges.
TMP11 272-274

86. (B) Cardiogenic shock results from a weakening of the cardiac muscle, often following coronary thrombosis. This can result in a vicious circle when low cardiac output results in low diastolic pressure; this causes a decrease in coronary flow, which decreases the cardiac strength even more. Therefore, in patients with cardiogenic shock, arterial pressure, particularly diastolic pressure, must be increased by administering either vasoconstrictors or volume expanders. In this patient, the best choice is to infuse plasma. Placing tourniquets on all four limbs would decrease the central blood volume, which would worsen the patient's condition.
TMP11 262, 263

87. (A) The velocity of blood flow within each segment of the circulatory system is inversely proportional to the total cross-sectional area of the segment. Because the aorta has the smallest total cross-sectional area of all circulatory segments, it has the highest velocity of blood flow.
TMP11 162

88. (C) The difference between systolic pressure and diastolic pressure is called the pulse pressure. The two main factors that affect pulse pressure are stroke volume and arterial compliance. Pulse pressure is directly proportional to the stroke volume and inversely proportional to the arterial compliance. Thus, an increase in arterial compliance would tend to decrease pulse pressure.
TMP11 173-174

89. (B) An increase in plasma colloid osmotic pressure would reduce net filtration pressure and capillary filtration rate. Increases in capillary hydrostatic pressure and interstitial colloid osmotic pressure would also favor capillary filtration. An increase in venous hydrostatic pressure and arteriolar diameter would tend to increase capillary hydrostatic pressure and capillary filtration rate.
TMP11 189-200

90. (C) During exercise, the sympathetic output increases markedly, which causes arteriolar constriction in many parts of the body, including nonexercising muscle. The increased sympathetic output also causes venoconstriction throughout the body. During exercise, there is an increased release of norepinephrine and epinephrine by the adrenal glands.
TMP11 247, 248

91. (A) An increase in capillary wall permeability to water would increase capillary filtration rate, whereas increases in arteriolar resistance, plasma colloid osmotic pressure, and interstitial hydrostatic pressure would all decrease filtration rate. Plasma sodium concentration would have no effect on filtration.
TMP11 189-200

92. (B) Several factors contribute to decreased coronary flow in patients with ischemic heart disease. Some patients have spasm of the coronary arteries, which acutely decreases coronary flow. However, the major cause of decreased coronary flow is an atherosclerotic narrowing of the lumen of the coronary arteries.
TMP11 250-252

93. (C) The rate of lymph flow increases in proportion to the interstitial hydrostatic pressure and the lymphatic pump activity. A decrease in plasma colloid osmotic pressure would increase filtration rate, interstitial volume, interstitial hydrostatic pressure, and lymph flow. A decrease in arteriolar diameter would decrease capillary hydrostatic pressure, capillary filtration, and lymph flow.
TMP11 192-193

94. (C) This patient has a rightward axis shift, which indicates that the right side of the heart has hypertrophied. Pulmonary value stenosis and tetralogy of Fallot have a rightward axis shift, but in tetralogy of Fallot, the arterial blood oxygen content is low, which is not the case in this patient. Therefore, pulmonary valve stenosis is the correct answer.
TMP11 272-276

95. (E) In this patient, the optimal therapy would be to replace the blood lost. Unfortunately, there is no blood available, so the next best therapy is plasma

infusion. Plasma's high colloid osmotic pressure will help the infused fluid remain in the circulation much longer than a balanced electrolyte solution.
TMP11 286, 287

96. (E) The brain has tight junctions between capillary endothelial cells that allow only extremely small molecules such as water, oxygen, and carbon dioxide to pass in or out of the brain tissues.
TMP11 182

97. (D) Decreased cardiac output can result from a weakened heart or from a decrease in venous return. Increased venous compliance decreases the venous return of blood to the heart. Cardiac tamponade, surgically opening the chest, and severe aortic stenosis effectively weaken the heart, thus decreasing cardiac output. Moderate anemia causes an arteriolar vasodilatation, which increases venous return of blood back to the heart, thus increasing cardiac output.
TMP11 234, 239

98. (B) The factors that determine the net movement of glucose across a capillary wall include the wall permeability to glucose, the glucose concentration gradient across the wall, and the capillary wall surface area. Thus, an increase in the concentration difference of glucose across the wall would enhance the net movement of glucose.
TMP11 183, 184

99. (A) Right ventricular hypertrophy occurs when the right side of the heart must pump a higher volume of blood or pump it against a higher pressure. Tetralogy of Fallot is associated with right ventricular hypertrophy because of the increased pulmonary valvular resistance; this also occurs during pulmonary artery stenosis. Tricuspid insufficiency causes an increased stroke volume by the right heart, which causes hypertrophy. However, tricuspid stenosis does not affect the right ventricle.
TMP11 276

100. (E) An increase in atrial pressure of 10 mm Hg would tend to decrease venous return to the heart and increase vena cava hydrostatic pressure. Plasma colloid osmotic pressure, interstitial colloid osmotic pressure, arterial pressure, and cardiac output would generally be low to normal in this patient.
TMP11 176, 177

101. (C) The vascular compliance is proportional to the vascular distensibility and vascular volume of any given segment of the circulation. The compliance of a systemic vein is 24 times that of its corresponding artery because it is about 8 times as distensible and it has a volume about 3 times as great.
TMP11 171, 172

102. (B) During decompensated heart failure, the kidneys decrease their urinary output of sodium and water in order to increase the blood volume. This increases the mean systemic filling pressure and the venous return of blood back toward the heart. Unfortunately, if the heart is very weak, the end-diastolic volume increases, which overstretches the cardiac sarcomeres, and the heart muscle becomes edematous. At the same time, there is a decreased accumulation of calcium ions in the longitudinal tubules of the sarcoplasmic reticulum. Therefore, there is less calcium available for the cardiac muscle, resulting in a further weakened heart.
TMP11 260, 261

103. (B) Filtration coefficient (K_f) = filtration rate ÷ net filtration pressure. Net filtration pressure = capillary hydrostatic pressure – plasma colloid osmotic pressure + interstitial colloid osmotic pressure – interstitial hydrostatic pressure. The net filtration pressure in this example is 10 mm Hg. Thus, K_f = 150 ml/min ÷ 10 mm Hg, or 15 ml/min/mm Hg.
TMP11 189-200

104. (B) Intestinal obstruction often causes a severe reduction in plasma volume. Obstruction causes distention and partially blocks the venous blood flow in the intestines. This results in an increased intestinal capillary pressure, which causes fluid to leak from the capillary into the intestinal walls and also into the intestinal lumen. The leaking fluid has a high protein content very similar to that of plasma, which reduces the total plasma protein and the plasma volume. Therefore, the therapy of choice is to replace the fluid lost by infusing plasma.
TMP11 284, 285

105. (B) Moving from a supine to a standing position results in pooling of blood in the lower extremities and a fall in blood pressure. The pooling of blood in the legs increases venous hydrostatic pressure. The fall in arterial pressure activates the arterial baroreceptors, which in turn increases sympathetic nerve activity and decreases parasympathetic nerve activity. The increase in sympathetic activity constricts renal vessels and reduces renal blood flow. The heart rate also increases.
TMP11 209, 210

106. (A) Because of the poor blood flow in progressive shock, the pH in the tissues throughout the body decreases. Many vessels are blocked because of local blood agglutination, called sludged blood. Patchy areas of necrosis also occur in the liver. Mitochondrial activity decreases, and capillary permeability increases. There is also an increased release of hydrolases by the lysosomes and a decrease in the cellular metabolism of glucose.
TMP11 281-283

107. (D) Reduction in perfusion pressure to a tissue leads to a decrease in tissue oxygen concentration and an increase in tissue carbon dioxide concentration. Both events lead to an increase in arteriolar

diameter, decreased vascular resistance, and increased vascular conductance.
TMP11 198, 199

108. (E) There are several acceptable treatments for patients with myocardial ischemia. Many patients take a daily dose of aspirin to prevent coronary thrombosis. Angioplasty with placement of stents or coronary bypass surgery effectively increases the coronary blood flow. Blood pressure reduction, administration of angiotensin-converting enzyme inhibitors, and beta receptor blockade are also effective treatments. Beta receptor stimulation or exercise would be detrimental to a patient with ischemia.
TMP11 256

109. (D) The largest portion of the arterial pressure is at the site of greatest vascular resistance, which is the arteriolar-capillary juncture.
TMP11 162, 163

110. (D) During systole, the murmurs from an interventricular septal effect and patent ductus arteriosus are heard clearly. However, patent ductus arteriosus is also heard during diastole. Mitral stenosis, tricuspid valve stenosis, and aortic regurgitation are diastolic murmurs.
TMP11 271

111. (D) The tendency for turbulent flow occurs at vascular sites where the velocity of blood flow is high. The aorta has the highest velocity of blood flow.
TMP11 166

112. (A) Anaphylaxis is an allergic condition that results from an antigen-antibody reaction that takes place after exposure to an antigenic substance. The basophils and mast cells in the pericapillary tissues release histamine or histamine-like substances. The histamine causes venous and arteriolar dilatation and greatly increased capillary permeability, with rapid loss of fluid and protein into the tissue spaces. This reduces venous return and often results in anaphylactic shock.
TMP11 285, 286

113. (C) An increase in perfusion pressure to a tissue results in excessive delivery of nutrients such as oxygen to a tissue. The increase in tissue oxygen concentration constricts arterioles and returns blood flow and nutrient delivery toward normal levels.
TMP11 198, 199

114. (A) Patients with acute pulmonary edema rapidly deteriorate unless the proper therapy is given. The thoracic blood volume must be decreased, and several techniques are available. Tourniquets can be placed on all four limbs and the constriction rotated to increase the blood volume of the limbs and thus decrease the volume of blood in the chest. Patients also can be given rapidly acting diuretics such as furosemide, which reduces plasma volume. Blood can be removed in moderate quantities from the patient to decrease the volume of blood in the chest. Patients should also breathe oxygen to increase the oxygen levels in the blood, but they should never be given a volume expander, such as plasma or dextran, because it could worsen the pulmonary edema.
TMP11 264

115. (B) In compensated heart failure, mean systemic filling pressure increases because of hypervolemia, and cardiac output is often at normal values. There is air hunger, called dyspnea, and excess sweating occurs in the early phases of compensated heart failure. However, right atrial pressure rises to very high values in these patients and is a hallmark of this disease.
TMP11 258, 259

116. (B) During progressive hemorrhagic shock, the cardiac contractility markedly decreases. The vasomotor center becomes depressed, and lack of blood flow throughout the body causes acidosis because of lack of removal of carbon dioxide. During hemorrhagic shock, endotoxin is released from the intestines, and the capillaries fail, causing an increase in capillary permeability. Cell membrane active transport of sodium and potassium also decreases.
TMP11 281, 282

117. (C) Interstitial hydrostatic pressure in a muscle capillary bed is normally negative ($-3\,mm\,Hg$). Pumping by the lymphatic system is the basic cause of the negative pressure.
TMP11 187

118. (C) In a patient with myocardial ischemia, factors that increase stress on the heart must be minimized. This can be done with the use of beta blockers, which inhibit the effects of excess sympathetic output on the heart. It is also important to maintain a normal body weight and a normal arterial pressure, which prevents excess stress on the heart. In conditions of acute myocardial ischemia, nitroglycerin can be taken. Isometric exercise should be avoided because of the large increase in arterial pressure.
TMP11 256

119. (C) Movement of the leg muscles causes blood to flow toward the vena cava, which reduces venous hydrostatic pressure. An increase in right atrial pressure would decrease venous return and increase venous hydrostatic pressure. Pregnancy and the presence of ascitic fluid in the abdomen would tend to compress the vena cava and increase venous hydrostatic pressure in the legs.
TMP11 177, 178

120. (B) Mean systemic pressure is increased by factors that increase blood volume or decrease vascular capacity. Sympathetic inhibition and venous dilatation decrease the mean systemic filling pressure. In congestive heart failure, the kidneys retain great

quantities of sodium and water, which results in an increase in blood volume and causes large increases in mean systemic filling pressure.
TMP11 239

121. (A) In tetralogy of Fallot, there is an interventricular septal defect as well as stenosis of either the pulmonary artery or the pulmonary valve. Therefore, it is very difficult for blood to pass into the pulmonary artery and into the lungs to be oxygenated. Instead, the blood partially shunts to the left side of the heart, thus bypassing the lungs. This results in low arterial oxygen content.
TMP11 274-276

122. (C) In cases of severe diarrhea, there is a large loss of sodium and water from the body, resulting in dehydration and sometimes shock. The best therapy is to replace the electrolytes that were lost by infusing a balanced electrolyte solution.
TMP11 286, 287

123. (D) The primary mechanism whereby solutes move across a capillary wall is simple diffusion.
TMP11 183

124. (C) Several factors cause the cardiac output curve to shift to the right along the right atrial pressure axis. Surgically opening the chest increases intrapleural pressure from a normal value of −4 mm Hg to a value of 0 mm Hg. Severe cardiac tamponade increases the pressure in the intrapleural space, thus tending to collapse the right and left atria. Playing a trumpet or placing a patient on a mechanical respirator distinctly increases the intrapleural pressure and causes the cardiac output curve to shift to the right. Decreasing the intrapleural pressure causes a leftward shift in the cardiac output curve.
TMP11 238

125. (D) Because oxygen is lipid soluble and can cross the capillary wall with ease, it has the fastest rate of movement across the capillary wall.
TMP11 183

126. (E) Cardiac output increases in several medical conditions because of increased venous return. Cardiac output increases in patients with hyperthyroidism because of the increased oxygen use by the peripheral tissues, resulting in arteriolar vasodilatation and thus increased venous return. Beriberi causes increased cardiac output because of a lack of the vitamin thiamine and results in peripheral vasodilatation. Arteriovenous fistula also causes a decreased resistance to venous return, thus increasing cardiac output. Because of the decreased oxygen delivery to the tissues, anemia causes an increase in venous return to the heart and thus an increase in cardiac output. Cardiac output decreases in patients with myocardial infarction.
TMP11 234-236

127. (C) An increase in renal arterial pressure results in pressure natriuresis and diuresis. The loss of

sodium and water tends to decrease extracellular fluid volume. Glomerular filtration rate would be normal or slightly increased in response to an increase in renal artery pressure.
TMP11 216, 217

128. (C) By definition, the second heart sound is always associated with the closing of the pulmonary and aortic valves. The heart sounds are never associated with the opening of any of the valves, but always with the closing of the valves and the associated vibration of blood and the walls of the heart.
TMP11 270

129. (D) Nitric oxide is a potent vasodilator and natriuretic substance. A decrease in nitric oxide production would decrease the ability of the kidney to excrete sodium and water.
TMP11 228

130. (A) During compensated heart failure, the release of angiotensin II and aldosterone increases, causing the kidneys to retain sodium and water, which increases the blood volume in the body and the venous return of blood to the heart. This results in an increase in right atrial pressure. Increased sympathetic output during compensated heart failure would increase the heart rate. Air hunger, called dyspnea, occurs during any type of exertion; orthopnea is the air hunger that occurs when the patient lies in a recumbent position.
TMP11 258-260

131. (C) The major causes of death after myocardial infarction include a decrease in cardiac output, which prevents tissues of the body from receiving adequate nutrition and oxygen delivery and prevents the removal of waste materials. Other causes of death are pulmonary edema, which reduces the oxygenation of the blood; fibrillation of the heart; and rupture of the heart. Cardiac contractility decreases after a myocardial infarction.
TMP11 254

132. (C) An increase in sodium intake would result in an increase in sodium excretion to maintain sodium balance. Angiotensin II, aldosterone, and renal sympathetic nervous system activity decrease in response to a chronic elevation in sodium intake.
TMP11 225-226

133. (B) During exercise, there is very little change in cerebral blood flow, and coronary blood flow increases. Because of the increased sympathetic output, mean systemic filling pressure increases, and the veins constrict. During exercise, there is also a decrease in parasympathetic impulses to the heart.
TMP11 247-249

134. (C) Constriction of the renal artery increases renin release, angiotensin II formation, and arterial pressure. Sodium excretion decreases, but only

transiently, because as arterial pressure increases, sodium excretion returns to normal levels via a pressure natriuresis mechanism.
TMP11 226-227

135. (E) During sympathetic stimulation, venous reservoirs constrict, venous vascular resistance increases, arterioles constrict (which increases their resistance), and heart rate increases. The epicardial coronary vessels have a large number of alpha receptors, but the subendocardial vessels have more beta receptors. Therefore, sympathetic stimulation causes at least a slight constriction of the epicardial vessels, which results in a slight decrease in epicardial flow.
TMP11 248, 250

136. (C) The plateau level of the cardiac output curve, which is one measure of cardiac contractility, decreases in several circumstances, including myocarditis, severe cardiac tamponade that increases the pressure in the pericardial space, myocardial infarction, and various valvular diseases such as mitral stenosis. Decreased parasympathetic stimulation of the heart actually moderately increases the level of the cardiac output curve by increasing the heart rate.
TMP11 238, 242

137. (D) An increase in atrial pressure causes an increase in heart rate by a nervous reflex called the Bainbridge reflex. The stretch receptors of the atria that elicit the Bainbridge reflex transmit their afferent signals through the vagus nerves to the medulla of the brain. The efferent signals are transmitted back via vagal and sympathetic nerves to increase the heart rate. An increase in atrial pressure would also increase plasma levels of atrial natriuretic peptide, which in turn would decrease plasma levels of angiotensin II and aldosterone.
TMP11 212

138. (B) During decompensated heart failure, cardiac output decreases because of weakness of the heart and edema of the cardiac muscle. Pressures in the pulmonary capillary system increase, including the pulmonary capillary pressure and the mean pulmonary filling pressure. Another factor that causes weakness of the heart is depletion of norepinephrine in the endings of the cardiac sympathetic nerves.
TMP11 260-262

139. (D) The Cushing reaction is a special type of central nervous system (CNS) ischemic response that results from increased pressure of the cerebrospinal fluid around the brain in the cranial vault.

When the cerebrospinal fluid pressure rises, it decreases the blood supply to the brain and elicits a CNS ischemic response. The CNS ischemic response includes enhanced sympathetic activity, decreased parasympathetic activity, and increased heart rate, arterial pressure, and total peripheral resistance.
TMP11 213

140. (D) In decompensated heart failure, the kidneys retain sodium and water, which causes weight gain and an increase in blood volume. This increases the mean systemic filling pressure, which stretches the heart. Therefore, a decreased mean systemic filling pressure does not occur in decompensated heart failure. The excess blood volume often overstretches the sarcomeres of the heart, which prevents the sarcomeres from achieving their maximal tension. An excess central fluid volume results in orthopnea, which is the inability to breathe properly except in an upright position.
TMP11 260-262

141. (E) The conversion of angiotensin I to angiotensin II is catalyzed by a converting enzyme that is present in the endothelium of the lung vessels and in the kidneys. The converting enzyme also serves as a kininase that degrades bradykinin. Thus, a converting enzyme inhibitor not only decreases the formation of angiotensin II but also inhibits kininases and the breakdown of bradykinin.
TMP11 223

142. (B) In patients with severe burns, there is a large loss of plasma-like substances from the burned tissues. The plasma protein concentration is thus severely decreased, and the therapy of choice is plasma infusion.
TMP11 284, 285

143. (E) Total peripheral vascular resistance = arterial pressure – right atrial pressure ÷ cardiac output. In this example, total peripheral vascular resistance = 130 mm Hg ÷ 3.5 L/min, or approximately 37 mm Hg/L/min.
TMP11 167

144. (B) In tetralogy of Fallot, there is an interventricular septal defect and increased resistance in the pulmonary valve or pulmonary artery. This causes partial blood shunting toward the left side of the heart without going through the lungs, resulting in a severely decreased arterial oxygen content. The interventricular septal defect causes equal systolic pressures in both cardiac ventricles, causing right ventricular hypertrophy and a wall thickness very similar to that of the left ventricle.
TMP11 275

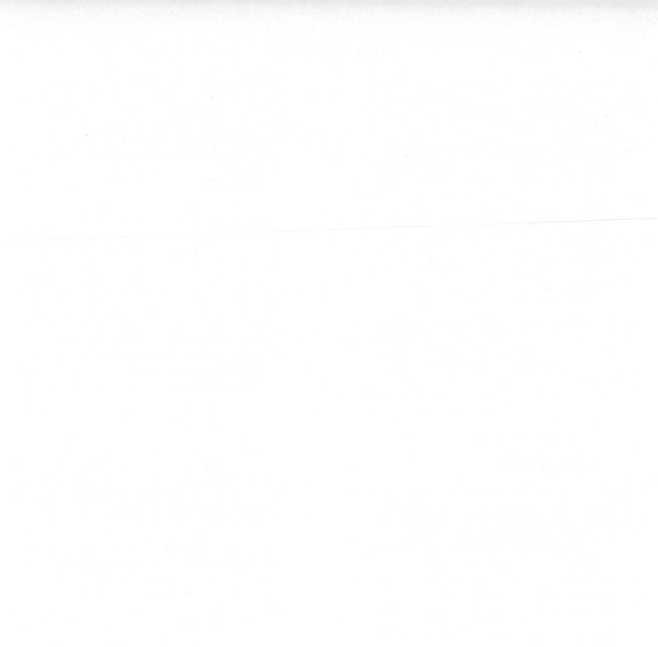

The Body Fluids and Kidneys

Questions 1 and 2

Use the following clinical laboratory test results for questions 1 and 2:

Urine flow rate = 1 ml/min
Urine inulin concentration = 100 mg/ml
Plasma inulin concentration = 2 mg/ml
Urine urea concentration = 50 mg/ml
Plasma urea concentration = 2.5 mg/ml

1. What is the glomerular filtration rate (GFR)?
   (A) 25 ml/min
   (B) 50 ml/min
   (C) 100 ml/min
   (D) 125 ml/min
   (E) None of the above

2. What is the net urea reabsorption rate?
   (A) 0 mg/min
   (B) 25 mg/min
   (C) 50 mg/min
   (D) 75 mg/min
   (E) 100 mg/min

3. Which of the following solutions when infused intravenously would result in an increase in extracellular fluid volume, a decrease in intracellular fluid volume, and an increase in total body water after osmotic equilibrium?
   (A) 1 liter of 0.9 per cent sodium chloride solution
   (B) 1 liter of 0.45 per cent sodium chloride solution
   (C) 1 liter of 3 per cent sodium chloride solution
   (D) 1 liter of 5 per cent dextrose solution
   (E) 1 liter of pure water

4. A 65-year-old man has a heart attack and experiences cardiopulmonary arrest while being transported to the emergency room. The following laboratory values are obtained from arterial blood:
   Plasma pH = 7.12
   Plasma P_{CO_2} = 60 mm Hg
   Plasma HCO_3^- concentration = 19 mEq/L
   Which of the following best describes his acid-base disorder?
   (A) Respiratory acidosis with partial renal compensation
   (B) Metabolic acidosis with partial respiratory compensation
   (C) Mixed acidosis: combined metabolic and respiratory acidosis
   (D) Mixed alkalosis: combined respiratory and metabolic alkalosis

5. In the patient described in question 4, which of the following laboratory results would be expected, compared with normal?
   (A) Increased renal excretion of HCO_3^-
   (B) Decreased urinary titratable acid
   (C) Increased urine pH
   (D) Increased renal excretion of NH_4^+

6. Increases in both renal blood flow and glomerular filtration rate (GFR) are caused by which of the following?
   (A) Dilatation of the efferent arterioles
   (B) Dilatation of the afferent arterioles
   (C) Increased glomerular capillary filtration coefficient
   (D) Increased plasma colloid osmotic pressure
   (E) Increased renal sympathetic nerve activity

7. In normal kidneys, which of the following is true of the osmolarity of renal tubular fluid that flows through the early distal tubule in the region of the macula densa?
   (A) Usually isotonic compared with plasma
   (B) Usually hypotonic compared with plasma
   (C) Usually hypertonic compared with plasma
   (D) Hypertonic, compared with plasma, in antidiuresis

Questions 8-10

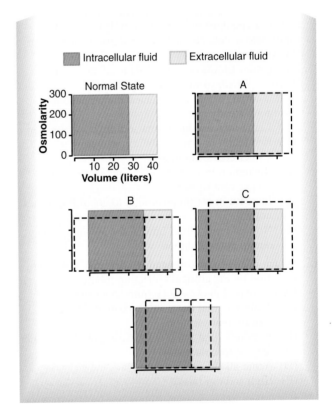

The diagrams above represent various states of abnormal hydration. In each diagram, the normal state (red and yellow) is superimposed on the abnormal state (dashed lines) to illustrate the shifts in the volume (width of rectangles) and total osmolarity (height of rectangles) of the extracellular and intracellular fluid compartments.

8. Which of the diagrams above represents the changes (after osmotic equilibrium) in extracellular and intracellular fluid volumes and osmolarities after the infusion of 1 per cent dextrose? ( )

9. Which of the diagrams above represents the changes (after osmotic equilibrium) in extracellular and intracellular fluid volumes and osmolarities after the infusion of 3 per cent sodium chloride? ( )

10. Which of the diagrams above represents the changes (after osmotic equilibrium) in extracellular and intracellular fluid volumes and osmolarities in a patient with the syndrome of inappropriate antidiuretic hormone (excessive secretion of antidiuretic hormone)? ( )

11. Which of the following changes, compared with normal, would be expected in a patient with chronic renal failure and a decrease in the number of functional nephrons to 25 per cent of normal? Assume steady-state conditions and that the patient has maintained the same diet.
    (A) Decreased maximal urine concentrating ability
    (B) Decreased renal sodium excretion
    (C) Alkalosis
    (D) Decreased filtered load of creatinine
    (E) Increased renal blood flow

12. After receiving a renal transplant, a patient develops severe hypertension (170/110 mm Hg). A renal arteriogram indicates severe renal artery stenosis in his single remaining kidney, with a reduction in glomerular filtration rate (GFR) to 25 per cent of normal. Which of the following changes, compared with normal, would be expected in this patient, assuming steady-state conditions?
    (A) Large increase in plasma sodium concentration
    (B) Reduction in urinary sodium excretion to 25 per cent of normal
    (C) Reduction in urinary creatinine excretion to 25 per cent of normal
    (D) Increase in serum creatinine to about four times normal
    (E) Normal renal blood flow in the stenotic kidney due to autoregulation

13. Which of the following tends to decrease potassium secretion by the cortical collecting tubule?
    (A) Increased plasma potassium concentration
    (B) A diuretic that decreases proximal tubule sodium reabsorption
    (C) A diuretic that inhibits the action of aldosterone (e.g., spironolactone)
    (D) Acute alkalosis
    (E) High sodium intake

14. If a patient has a creatinine clearance of 90 ml/min, a urine flow rate of 1 ml/min, a plasma K^+ concentration of 4 mEq/L, and a urine K^+ concentration of 60 mEq/L, what is the approximate rate of K^+ excretion?
    (A) 0.06 mEq/min
    (B) 0.30 mEq/min
    (C) 0.36 mEq/min
    (D) 3.6 mEq/min
    (E) 60 mEq/min

15. Which of the following changes would be expected in a patient with diabetes insipidus due to a lack of antidiuretic hormone (ADH) secretion?

	Plasma Osmolarity	Plasma Sodium Concentration	Plasma Renin Concentration	Urine Volume
(A)	↔	↔	↓	↑
(B)	↔	↔	↑	↑
(C)	↑	↑	↑	↑
(D)	↑	↑	↔	↔
(E)	↓	↓	↓	↔

16. A patient with severe hypertension (blood pressure 185/110 mm Hg) is referred to you. A renal magnetic resonance imaging scan shows a tumor in the kidney, and laboratory findings include a very high plasma renin activity of 12 ng angiotensin 1/ml/hr (normal = 1). The diagnosis is a renin-secreting tumor. Which of the following changes would you expect to find in this patient, under steady-state conditions, compared with normal?

	Plasma Aldosterone Concentration	Sodium Excretion Rate	Plasma Potassium Concentration	Renal Blood Flow
(A)	↔	↓	↓	↑
(B)	↔	↔	↓	↑
(C)	↑	↔	↓	↓
(D)	↑	↓	↔	↓
(E)	↑	↓	↓	↔

17. Which of the following changes, compared with normal, would you expect to find 3 weeks after a patient ingested a toxin that caused sustained impairment of proximal tubular sodium chloride (NaCl) reabsorption? Assume that there has been no change in diet or ingestion of electrolytes.

	Glomerular Filtration Rate	Afferent Arteriolar Resistance	Sodium Excretion
(A)	↔	↔	↑
(B)	↔	↔	↑
(C)	↓	↑	↑
(D)	↓	↑	↔
(E)	↑	↓	↔

18. Blood pressure in a 55-year-old man with hypertension has been reasonably well controlled by administration of a thiazide diuretic. During his last visit (6 months ago), his blood pressure was 130/75 mm Hg and his serum creatinine was 1 mg/dl. He has been exercising regularly for the past 2 years but recently experienced knee pain and began self-medicating with large amounts of a nonsteroidal anti-inflammatory drug. When he arrives at your office, his blood pressure is 155/85 and his serum creatinine is 2 mg/dl. Which of the following best explains his increased serum creatinine?
    (A) Increased afferent arteriolar resistance that reduced the glomerular filtration rate (GFR)
    (B) Increased efferent arteriolar resistance that reduced the GFR
    (C) Increased glomerular capillary filtration coefficient that reduced the GFR
    (D) Increased angiotensin II formation that decreased the GFR
    (E) Increased muscle mass due to exercise

19. A 26-year-old woman recently decided to adopt a healthier diet and eat more fruits and vegetables. As a result, her potassium intake increased from 80 to 160 mmol/day. Which of the following conditions would you expect to find 2 weeks after she increased her potassium intake, compared with before the increase?

	Potassium Excretion Rate	Sodium Excretion Rate	Plasma Aldosterone Concentration	Plasma Potassium Concentration
(A)	↔	↔	↑	Large increase (>1 mmol/L)
(B)	↔	↓	↑	Small increase (<1 mmol/L)
(C)	↑2×	↔	↑	Small increase (<1 mmol/L)
(D)	↑2×	↑	↓	Large increase (>1 mmol/L)
(E)	↑2×	↑	↔	Large increase (>1 mmol/L)

20. An 8-year-old boy is brought to your office with extreme swelling of the abdomen. His parents indicate that he had a very sore throat a "month or so" ago and that he has been "swelling up" since that time. He appears to be edematous, and when you check his urine, you find large amounts of protein being excreted. Your diagnosis is nephrotic syndrome subsequent to glomerulonephritis. Which of the following changes would you expect to find, compared with normal?

	Thoracic Lymph Flow	Interstitial Fluid Protein Concentration	Interstitial Fluid Hydrostatic Pressure	Plasma Renin Concentration
(A)	↑	↓	↑	↑
(B)	↑	↓	↑	↔
(C)	↑	↓	↔	↑
(D)	↓	↑	↔	↔
(E)	↓	↓	↓	↓

21. Which of the following changes would you expect to find after administering a vasodilator drug that caused a 50 per cent decrease in afferent arteriolar resistance and no change in arterial pressure?
    (A) Decreased renal blood flow, decreased glomerular filtration rate (GFR), and decreased peritubular capillary hydrostatic pressure
    (B) Decreased renal blood flow, decreased GFR, and increased peritubular capillary hydrostatic pressure
    (C) Increased renal blood flow, increased GFR, and increased peritubular capillary hydrostatic pressure
    (D) Increased renal blood flow, increased GFR, and no change in peritubular capillary hydrostatic pressure
    (E) Increased renal blood flow, increased GFR, and decreased peritubular capillary hydrostatic pressure

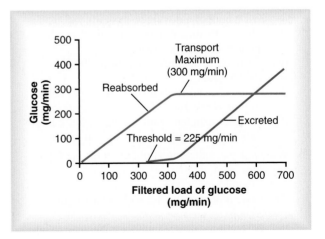

22. A 32-year-old man complains of frequent urination. He is overweight (280 pounds, 5 feet 10 inches tall), and after measuring the 24-hour creatinine clearance, you estimate his glomerular filtration rate (GFR) to be 150 ml/min. His plasma glucose is 300 mg/dl. Assuming that his renal transport maximum for glucose is normal, as shown in the figure above, what would be this patient's approximate rate of urinary glucose excretion?
    (A) 0 mg/min
    (B) 100 mg/min
    (C) 150 mg/min
    (D) 225 mg/min
    (E) 300 mg/min
    (F) Not enough information is given to estimate the glucose excretion rate

23. The clinical laboratory returned the following values for arterial blood taken from a patient:
    Plasma pH = 7.28
    Plasma $HCO_3^- = 32$ mEq/L
    Plasma $PCO_2 = 70$ mm Hg
    What is this patient's acid-base disorder?
    (A) Acute respiratory acidosis without renal compensation
    (B) Respiratory acidosis with partial renal compensation
    (C) Acute metabolic acidosis without respiratory compensation
    (D) Metabolic acidosis with partial respiratory compensation

24. Which of the following changes tends to increase peritubular capillary fluid reabsorption?
    (A) Increased blood pressure
    (B) Decreased filtration fraction
    (C) Increased efferent arteriolar resistance
    (D) Decreased angiotensin II
    (E) Increased renal blood flow

25. Which of the following would cause the greatest degree of hyperkalemia?
    (A) Increase in potassium intake from 60 to 180 mmol/day in a person with normal kidneys and a normal aldosterone system
    (B) Chronic treatment with a diuretic that inhibits the action of aldosterone
    (C) Decrease in sodium intake from 200 to 100 mmol/day
    (D) Chronic treatment with a diuretic that inhibits loop of Henle Na^+-2 Cl^-- K^+ co-transport
    (E) Chronic treatment with a diuretic that inhibits sodium reabsorption in the collecting ducts

26. Which of the following is filtered most readily by the glomerular capillaries?
    (A) Albumin in plasma
    (B) Neutral dextran with a molecular weight of 25,000
    (C) Polycationic dextran with a molecular weight of 25,000
    (D) Polyanionic dextran with a molecular weight of 25,000
    (E) Red blood cells

27. Under conditions of normal renal function, which of the following is true of the concentration of urea in tubular fluid at the end of the proximal tubule?
    (A) It is higher than the concentration of urea in tubular fluid at the tip of the loop of Henle
    (B) It is higher than the concentration of urea in the plasma
    (C) It is higher than the concentration of urea in the final urine in antidiuresis
    (D) It is lower than plasma urea concentration because of active urea reabsorption along the proximal tubule

28. Which of the following changes would be expected in a patient with Liddle's syndrome (excessive activity of amiloride-sensitive sodium channel in the collecting tubule) under steady-state conditions, assuming that intake of electrolytes remained constant?

	Plasma Renin Concentration	Blood Pressure	Sodium Excretion	Plasma Aldosterone Concentration
(A)	↔	↑	↓	↔
(B)	↑	↑	↔	↑
(C)	↑	↑	↓	↓
(D)	↓	↑	↔	↓
(E)	↓	↑	↓	↓
(F)	↓	↓	↑	↑

29. A patient's urine is collected for 2 hours, and the total volume is 600 milliliters during this time. Her urine osmolarity is 150 mOsm/L, and her plasma osmolarity is 300 mOsm/L. What is her "free water clearance"?
    (A) + 5.0 ml/min
    (B) + 2.5 ml/min
    (C) 0.0 ml/min
    (D) −2.5 ml/min
    (E) −5.0 ml/min

30. A patient is referred for treatment of hypertension. After testing, you discover that he has a very high level of plasma aldosterone, and your diagnosis is Conn's syndrome. Assuming no change in electrolyte intake, which of the following changes would you expect to find, compared with normal?

	Plasma pH	Plasma K^+ Concentration	Urine K^+ Excretion	Urine Na^+ Excretion	Plasma Renin Concentration
(A)	↑	↓	↔	↔	↓
(B)	↓	↓	↔	↔	↓
(C)	↑	↓	↑	↓	↓
(D)	↑	↑	↔	↓	↑
(E)	↑	↑	↑	↑	↑

31. A patient with renal disease had a plasma creatinine of 2 mg/dl during an examination 6 months ago. You note that his blood pressure has increased about 30 mm Hg since his previous visit, and the lab tests indicate that his plasma creatinine is now 4 mg/dl. Which of the following changes, compared with his previous visit, would you expect to find, assuming steady-state conditions and no changes in electrolyte intake or metabolism?

	Sodium Excretion Rate	Creatinine Excretion Rate	Creatinine Clearance	Filtered Load of Creatinine
(A)	↔	↔	↓ by 50%	↓
(B)	↔	↔	↓ by 50%	↔
(C)	↔	↔	↓ by 75%	↓
(D)	↓	↓	↔	↔
(E)	↓	↓	↓ by 50%	↓

32. Which of the following changes tends to increase glomerular filtration rate (GFR)?
    (A) Increased afferent arteriolar resistance
    (B) Decreased efferent arteriolar resistance
    (C) Increased glomerular capillary filtration coefficient
    (D) Increased Bowman's capsule hydrostatic pressure
    (E) Decreased glomerular capillary hydrostatic pressure

33. The maximum clearance rate possible for a substance that is totally cleared from the plasma is equal to which of the following?
    (A) Glomerular filtration rate
    (B) Filtered load of that substance
    (C) Urinary excretion rate of that substance
    (D) Renal plasma flow
    (E) Filtration fraction

34. A patient has the following laboratory values:
    Arterial pH = 7.25
    Plasma HCO_3^- = 13 mEq/L
    Plasma chloride concentration = 118 mEq/L
    Arterial P_{CO_2} = 30 mm Hg
    Plasma Na^+ concentration = 141 mEq/L
    What is the most likely cause of his acidosis?
    (A) Salicylic acid poisoning
    (B) Diabetes mellitus
    (C) Diarrhea
    (D) Emphysema

35. A 26-year-old man develops glomerulonephritis, and his glomerular filtration rate (GFR) decreases by 50 per cent and remains at that level. For which of the following substances would you expect to find the greatest increase in plasma concentration?
    (A) Creatinine
    (B) K^+
    (C) Glucose
    (D) Na^+
    (E) Phosphate
    (F) H^+

36. A patient with a history of frequent and severe migraine headaches arrives at your office complaining of stomach pain and breathing rapidly. She informs you that she has had a severe migraine for the past 2 days and has taken eight times the recommended dose of aspirin to relieve her headache during that time. Which of the following changes would you expect to find, compared with normal?

	Plasma HCO_3^- Concentration	Plasma P_{CO_2}	Urine HCO_3^- Excretion	Urine NH_4^+ Excretion	Plasma Anion Gap
(A)	↑	↓	↑	↑	↑
(B)	↑	↑	↑	↓	↑
(C)	↓	↓	↓	↓	↓
(D)	↓	↓	↓	↑	↑
(E)	↓	↓	↓	↑	↓

Questions 37 and 38

Assume the following initial conditions for questions 37 and 38:
Intracellular fluid volume = 40 per cent of body weight before fluid administration
Extracellular fluid volume = 20 per cent of body weight before fluid administration
Molecular weight of NaCl = 58.5 g/mol
No excretion of water or electrolytes

37. A male patient appears to be dehydrated, and after obtaining a plasma sample, you find that he has hyponatremia, with a plasma sodium concentration of 130 mmol/L and a plasma osmolarity of 260 mOsm/L. You decide to administer 2 liters of 3 per cent sodium chloride (NaCl). His body weight was 60 kilograms before giving the fluid. What is his approximate plasma osmolarity after administration of the NaCl solution and after osmotic equilibrium? Assume the initial conditions described above.
    (A) 273 mOsm/L
    (B) 286 mOsm/L
    (C) 300 mOsm/L
    (D) 310 mOsm/L
    (E) 326 mOsm/L

38. What is the approximate extracellular fluid volume in this patient after administration of the NaCl solution and after osmotic equilibrium?
    (A) 15.1 liters
    (B) 17.2 liters
    (C) 19.1 liters
    (D) 19.8 liters
    (E) 21.2 liters

39. If glomerular filtration rate (GFR) suddenly decreases from 100 ml/min to 50 ml/min and tubular fluid reabsorption simultaneously decreases from 99 ml/min to 50 ml/min, which of the following changes will occur (assuming that the changes in GFR and tubular fluid reabsorption are maintained)?
    (A) Urine flow rate will not change
    (B) Urine flow rate will decrease by 50 per cent
    (C) Urine flow rate will decrease to 0
    (D) Urine flow rate will increase by 50 per cent

40. The most serious hypokalemia would occur in which of the following conditions?
    (A) Decrease in potassium intake from 150 to 60 mEq/day
    (B) Increase in sodium intake from 100 to 200 mEq/day
    (C) Fourfold increase in aldosterone secretion plus high sodium intake
    (D) Fourfold increase in aldosterone secretion plus low sodium intake
    (E) Addison's disease

41. If the average hydrostatic pressure in the glomerular capillaries is 50 mm Hg, the hydrostatic pressure in Bowman's space is 12 mm Hg, the average colloid osmotic pressure in the glomerular capillaries is 30 mm Hg, and there is no protein in the glomerular ultrafiltrate, what is the net pressure driving glomerular filtration?
    (A) 8 mm Hg
    (B) 32 mm Hg
    (C) 48 mm Hg
    (D) 60 mm Hg
    (E) 92 mm Hg

42. In a patient who has chronic, uncontrolled diabetes mellitus, which of the following sets of conditions would you expect to find, compared with normal?

	Titratable Acid Excretion	NH^+ Excretion	HCO_3^- Excretion	Plasma P_{CO_2}
(A)	↔	↑	↓	↔
(B)	↓	↑	↔	↓
(C)	↑	↑	↔	↑
(D)	↑	↑	↓	↓
(E)	↓	↓	↓	↓
(F)	↔	↑	↓	↔

43. Intravenous infusion of 1 liter of 0.45 per cent sodium chloride (NaCl) solution (molecular weight of NaCl = 58.5) would cause which of the following changes, after osmotic equilibrium?

	Intracellular Fluid Volume	Intracellular Fluid Osmolarity	Extracellular Fluid Volume	Extracellular Fluid Osmolarity
(A)	↑	↑	↑	↑
(B)	↑	↓	↑	↓
(C)	↔	↑	↑	↑
(D)	↓	↑	↑	↑
(E)	↓	↓	↓	↓

44. The figure above shows the concentration of inulin at different points along the renal tubule, expressed as the tubular fluid/plasma ratio of inulin concentration. If inulin is not reabsorbed, what is the approximate percentage of the filtered water that has been reabsorbed prior to the distal convoluted tubule?
    (A) 25 per cent
    (B) 33 per cent
    (C) 66 per cent
    (D) 75 per cent
    (E) 99 per cent
    (F) 100 per cent

45. Which of the following tends to increase potassium secretion by the cortical collecting tubule?
    (A) A diuretic that inhibits the action of aldosterone (e.g., spironolactone)
    (B) A diuretic that decreases loop of Henle sodium reabsorption (e.g., furosemide)
    (C) Decreased plasma potassium concentration
    (D) Acute metabolic acidosis
    (E) Low sodium intake

46. Which of the following changes would you expect to find in a patient with primary aldosteronism (Conn's syndrome) under steady-state conditions, assuming that electrolyte intake remained constant?

	Sodium Excretion Rate	Potassium Excretion Rate	Plasma Renin Concentration	Plasma Potassium Concentration	Blood Pressure
(A)	↔	↔	↔	↓	↑
(B)	↔	↔	↓	↓	↑
(C)	↔	↑	↓	↓	↑
(D)	↓	↑	↓	↔	↑
(E)	↑	↓	↑	↑	↔

47. A diabetic patient has developed chronic renal disease and is referred to your nephrology clinic. According to his family physician, his creatinine clearance has decreased from 100 ml/min to 40 ml/min over the past 4 years. His glucose has not been well controlled, and his plasma pH is 7.14. Which of the following changes, compared with before the development of renal disease, would you expect to find, assuming steady-state conditions and no change in electrolyte intake?

	Sodium Excretion Rate	Creatinine Excretion Rate	Plasma Creatinine Concentration	Plasma HCO_3^- Concentration	NH_4^+ Excretion Rate
(A)	↓	↓	↑	↑	↑
(B)	↔	↔	↑	↓	↑
(C)	↔	↔	↑	↓	↔
(D)	↔	↓	↑	↓	↔
(E)	↓	↓	↓	↓	↑
(F)	↓	↓	↓	↓	↓

3.0   4.0

100

48. A 20-year-old woman arrives at your office complaining of rapid weight gain and marked fluid retention. Her blood pressure is 105/65 mm Hg, her plasma protein concentration is 3.6 g/dl (normal = 7.0), and she has no detectable protein in her urine. Which of the following changes would you expect to find, compared with normal?

	Thoracic Lymph Flow	Interstitial Fluid Protein Concentration	Capillary Filtration	Interstitial Fluid Pressure
(A)	↓	↓	↓	↓
(B)	↓	↑	↔	↔
(C)	↑	↓	↑	↑
(D)	↑	↓	↑	↔
(E)	↑	↑	↑	↑

49. A 48-year-old woman complains of severe polyuria (producing about 0.5 liter of urine each hour) and polydipsia (drinking two to three glasses of water every hour). Her urine contains no glucose, and she is placed on overnight water restriction for further evaluation. The next morning, she is weak and confused, her sodium concentration is 160 mEq/L, and her urine osmolarity is 80 mOsm/L. Which of the following is the most likely diagnosis?
    (A) Diabetes mellitus
    (B) Diabetes insipidus
    (C) Primary aldosteronism
    (D) Renin-secreting tumor
    (E) Syndrome of inappropriate antidiuretic hormone

50. Furosemide (Lasix) is a diuretic that also produces natriuresis. Which of the following is an undesirable side effect of furosemide due to its site of action on the renal tubule?
    (A) Edema
    (B) Hyperkalemia
    (C) Hypercalcemia
    (D) Decreased ability to concentrate the urine
    (E) Heart failure

51. A patient complains of headaches, and an examination reveals that her blood pressure is 175/112 mm Hg. Laboratory tests give the following results:
    Plasma renin activity = 11.5 ng angiotensin I/ml/hr (normal = 1)
    Plasma Na⁺ = 144 mmol/L
    Plasma K⁺ = 3 .4 mmol/L
    A magnetic resonance imaging procedure suggests that she has a renin-secreting tumor. Which of the following changes would you expect, compared with normal?

	Renal Blood Flow	Filtration Fraction	Glomerular Capillary Hydrostatic Pressure	Peritubular Capillary Hydrostatic Pressure
(A)	↓	↑	↑	↓
(B)	↓	↑	↑	↑
(C)	↓	↓	↑	↓
(D)	↓	↑	↓	↑
(E)	↓	↓	↓	↓

52. When the dietary intake of K⁺ increases, body K⁺ balance is maintained by an increase in K⁺ excretion primarily by which of the following?
    (A) Decreased glomerular filtration of K⁺
    (B) Decreased reabsorption of K⁺ by the proximal tubule
    (C) Decreased reabsorption of K⁺ by the thick ascending limb of the loop of Henle
    (D) Increased K⁺ secretion by the late distal collecting tubules
    (E) Shift of K⁺ into the intracellular compartment

53. A female patient has unexplained severe hypernatremia (plasma Na⁺ = 167 mmol/L) and complains of frequent urination and large urine volumes. A urine specimen reveals that the Na⁺ concentration is 15 mmol/L (very low) and the osmolarity is 155 mOsm/L (very low). Laboratory tests reveal the following:
    Plasma renin activity = 3 ng angiotensin I/ml/hr (normal = 1.0)
    Plasma antidiuretic hormone (ADH) = 30 pg/ml (normal = 3 pg/mL)
    Plasma aldosterone = 20 ng/dl (normal = 6 ng/dl)
    Which of the following is the most likely reason for her hypernatremia?
    (A) Simple dehydration due to decreased water intake
    (B) Nephrogenic diabetes insipidus
    (C) Central diabetes insipidus
    (D) Syndrome of inappropriate ADH
    (E) Primary aldosteronism
    (F) Renin-secreting tumor

54. Juvenile (type I) diabetes mellitus is often diagnosed because of polyuria (high urine flow) and polydipsia (frequent drinking) that occur because of which of the following?
    (A) Increased delivery of glucose to the collecting duct interferes with the action of antidiuretic hormone
    (B) Increased glomerular filtration of glucose increases Na⁺ reabsorption via the sodium-glucose co-transporter
    (C) When the filtered load of glucose exceeds the renal threshold, a rising glucose concentration in the proximal tubule decreases the osmotic driving force for water reabsorption
    (D) High plasma glucose concentration decreases thirst
    (E) High plasma glucose concentration stimulates antidiuretic hormone release from the posterior pituitary

55. You begin treating a hypertensive patient with a powerful loop diuretic (e.g., furosemide). Which of the following changes would you expect to find, compared with pretreatment values, when he returns for a follow-up examination 2 weeks later?

	Urine Sodium Excretion	Extracellular Fluid Volume	Blood Pressure	Plasma Potassium Concentration
(A)	↑	↓	↓	↓
(B)	↑	↓	↔	↔
(C)	↔	↓	↓	↓
(D)	↔	↓	↔	↔
(E)	↑	↔	↓	↑

56. In acidosis, most of the hydrogen ions secreted by the proximal tubule are associated with which of the following processes?
    (A) Excretion of hydrogen ions
    (B) Excretion of NH_4^+
    (C) Reabsorption of bicarbonate ions
    (D) Reabsorption of phosphate ions
    (E) Reabsorption of potassium ions

57. Administration of a thiazide diuretic (e.g., chlorothiazide) would be expected to cause which of the following effects as its primary mechanism of action?
    (A) Inhibition of NaCl co-transport in the early distal tubules
    (B) Inhibition of NaCl co-transport in the proximal tubules
    (C) Inhibition of Na^+-2 Cl^--K^+ co-transport in the loop of Henle
    (D) Inhibition of Na^+-2 Cl^--K^+ co-transport in the collecting tubules
    (E) Inhibition of the renal tubular actions of aldosterone
    (F) Blockade of sodium channels in the collecting tubules

58. Two weeks after constricting the renal artery of a sole remaining kidney to initially reduce renal artery pressure by 20 mm Hg (from 100 to 80 mm Hg), which of the following changes would you expect, compared with before constriction of the artery?
    (A) Large decrease in sodium excretion (>20 per cent)
    (B) Large increase in renin secretion (more than twofold)
    (C) Return of renal artery pressure to nearly 100 mm Hg
    (D) Large decrease in glomerular filtration rate (>20 per cent)
    (E) Large reduction in renal blood flow (>20 per cent)

59. Because the usual rate of phosphate filtration exceeds the transport maximum for phosphate reabsorption, which of the following is true?
    (A) All the phosphate that is filtered is reabsorbed
    (B) More phosphate is reabsorbed than is filtered
    (C) Phosphate in the tubules can contribute significantly to titratable acid in the urine
    (D) The plasma threshold for phosphate is usually not exceeded
    (E) Parathyroid hormone must be secreted for phosphate reabsorption to occur

60. Which of the following changes, compared with normal, would be expected to occur, under steady-state conditions, in a patient whose severe renal disease has reduced the number of functional nephrons to 25 per cent of normal?
    (A) Increased glomerular filtration rate (GFR) of the surviving nephrons
    (B) Decreased urinary creatinine excretion rate
    (C) Decreased urine flow rate in the surviving nephrons
    (D) Decreased urinary excretion of sodium
    (E) Increased urine concentrating ability

61. In a patient with severe syndrome of inappropriate antidiuretic hormone (excessive antidiuretic hormone secretion), which of the following changes, compared with normal, would you expect to find? Assume steady-state conditions and that the intake of water and electrolytes has remained constant.

	Plasma Renin Concentration	Plasma Aldosterone Concentration	Urine Flow Rate	Plasma Sodium Concentration	Plasma Protein Concentration
(A)	↔	↔	↓	↓	↓
(B)	↔	↔	↔	↓	↑
(C)	↓	↓	↔	↓	↓
(D)	↓	↓	↔	↔	↓
(E)	↑	↑	↓	↓	↔

62. Which of the following would likely lead to hyponatremia?
    (A) Excessive antidiuretic hormone secretion
    (B) Restriction of fluid intake
    (C) Excess aldosterone secretion
    (D) Administration of 2 liters of 3 per cent sodium chloride solution
    (E) Administration of 2 liters of 0.9 per cent sodium chloride solution

Questions 63-66

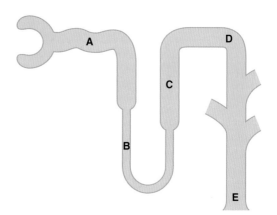

For questions 63 to 66, choose the appropriate nephron site in the diagram above.

63. In a patient with severe central diabetes insipidus caused by a lack of antidiuretic hormone secretion, which part of the tubule would have the lowest tubular fluid osmolarity? ( )

64. In a person on a very low potassium diet, which part of the nephron would be expected to reabsorb the most potassium? ( )

65. Which part of the nephron normally reabsorbs the most water? ( )

66. In a normally functioning kidney, which part of the tubule has the lowest permeability to water during antidiuresis? ( )

67. Which of the following substances are best suited to measure interstitial fluid volume?
    (A) Inulin and heavy water
    (B) Inulin and ^{22}Na
    (C) Heavy water and ^{125}I-albumin
    (D) Inulin and ^{125}I-albumin
    (E) ^{51}Cr red blood cells and ^{125}I-albumin

68. Which of the following changes would you expect to find in a dehydrated person deprived of water for 24 hours?
    (A) Decreased plasma renin activity
    (B) Decreased plasma antidiuretic hormone concentration
    (C) Increased plasma atrial natriuretic peptide concentration
    (D) Increased water permeability of the collecting duct
    (E) Increased water permeability in the ascending loop of Henle

69. Which of the following changes would you expect to find after acute administration of a vasodilator drug that caused a 50 per cent decrease in renal efferent arteriolar resistance and no change in afferent arteriolar resistance or arterial pressure?

	Renal Blood Flow	Glomerular Filtration Rate	Glomerular Capillary Hydrostatic Pressure	Peritubular Capillary Hydrostatic Pressure
(A)	↑	↑	↑	↔
(B)	↑	↑	↑	↑
(C)	↑	↔	↔	↔
(D)	↑	↓	↓	↓
(E)	↑	↓	↓	↑

70. Which of the following would be expected to cause a decrease in extracellular fluid potassium concentration (hypokalemia) at least in part by stimulating potassium uptake into the cells?
    (A) β-Adrenergic blockade
    (B) Insulin deficiency
    (C) Strenuous exercise
    (D) Aldosterone deficiency (Addison's disease)
    (E) Metabolic alkalosis

71. Which of the following is true of the tubular fluid that passes through the lumen of the early distal tubule in the region of the macula densa?
    (A) It is usually isotonic
    (B) It is usually hypotonic
    (C) It is usually hypertonic
    (D) It is hypertonic in antidiuresis
    (E) It is hypertonic when the filtration rate of its own nephron decreases to 50 per cent below normal

72. If a person has a kidney transport maximum for glucose of 350 mg/min, a glomerular filtration rate (GFR) of 100 ml/min, a plasma glucose of 150 mg/dl, a urine flow rate of 2 ml/min, and no detectable glucose in the urine, what would be the approximate rate of glucose reabsorption, assuming normal kidneys?
    (A) Glucose reabsorption cannot be estimated from these data
    (B) 0 mg/min
    (C) 50 mg/min
    (D) 150 mg/min
    (E) 350 mg/min

73. A patient complains that he is always thirsty, and his breath has an acetone smell. You suspect that he has diabetes mellitus, and that diagnosis is confirmed by a urine sample that tests very positive for glucose and a blood sample that shows a fasting blood glucose concentration of 400 mg/dl. Compared with normal, you would expect to find which of the following changes in his urine?

	Urine pH	NH$_4^+$ Excretion	Urine Volume (ml/24 hr)	Renal HCO$_3^-$ Production
(A)	↓	↓	↓	↓
(B)	↓	↑	↓	↓
(C)	↑	↓	↓	↓
(D)	↓	↑	↑	↑
(E)	↑	↑	↑	↑

74. Which of the following statements is correct?
    (A) Urea reabsorption in the medullary collecting tubule is less than in the distal convoluted tubule during antidiuresis
    (B) Urea concentration in the interstitial fluid of the renal cortex is greater than in the interstitial fluid of the renal medulla during antidiuresis
    (C) The thick ascending limb of the loop of Henle reabsorbs more urea than the inner medullary collecting tubule during antidiuresis
    (D) Urea reabsorption in the proximal tubule is greater than in the cortical collecting tubule

75. A healthy 29-year-old man runs a 10-kilometer race on a hot day and becomes very dehydrated. Assuming that his antidiuretic hormone levels are very high, in which part of the renal tubule is the most water reabsorbed?
    (A) Proximal tubule
    (B) Loop of Henle
    (C) Distal tubule
    (D) Cortical collecting tubule
    (E) Medullary collecting duct

Questions 76-78

A person with normal body fluid volumes weighs 60 kilograms and has an extracellular fluid volume of approximately 12.8 liters, a blood volume of 4.3 liters, and a hematocrit of 0.4; 57 per cent of his body weight is water. Answer the following three questions based on this information.

76. What is the approximate intracellular fluid volume?
    (A) 17.1 liters
    (B) 19.6 liters
    (C) 21.4 liters
    (D) 23.5 liters
    (E) 25.6 liters

77. What is the approximate plasma volume?
    (A) 2.0 liters
    (B) 2.3 liters
    (C) 2.6 liters
    (D) 3.0 liters
    (E) 3.3 liters

78. What is the approximate interstitial fluid volume?
    (A) 6.4 liters
    (B) 8.4 liters
    (C) 10.2 liters
    (D) 11.3 liters
    (E) 12.0 liters

79. Which of the following nephron segments is the primary site of magnesium reabsorption under normal conditions?
    (A) Proximal tubule
    (B) Descending limb of the loop of Henle
    (C) Ascending limb of the loop of Henle
    (D) Distal convoluted tubule
    (E) Collecting ducts

80. Autoregulation of the renal blood flow and glomerular filtration rate by tubuloglomerular feedback requires which of the following?
    (A) Increase in the colloid osmotic pressure of the blood in the glomerular capillaries as blood flow increases
    (B) Decrease in the colloid osmotic pressure of the blood in the glomerular capillaries as the filtration fraction increases
    (C) Increased release of renin as blood pressure in the renal artery increases
    (D) Signaling from the macula densa to juxta-glomerular cells
    (E) Relaxation of the renal arteriolar smooth muscle as a direct response to the increased renal artery blood pressure

81. Which of the following changes would you expect to find in a newly diagnosed 10-year-old patient with type I diabetes and uncontrolled hyperglycemia (plasma glucose = 300 mg/dl).

	Thirst (Water Intake)	Urine Volume	Glomerular Filtration Rate	Afferent Arteriolar Resistance
(A)	↑	↓	↑	↓
(B)	↑	↑	↓	↑
(C)	↑	↑	↑	↓
(D)	↓	↑	↑	↑
(E)	↓	↓	↓	↓

Questions 82 and 83

Use the following data for questions 82 and 83.

To evaluate kidney function in a 45-year-old woman with type II diabetes, you ask her to collect her urine over 24 hours. She collects 3600 milliliters of urine in that period. The clinical laboratory returns the following results after analyzing the patient's urine and plasma samples:
Plasma creatinine = 4 mg/dl
Urine creatinine = 32 mg/dl
Plasma potassium = 5 mmol/L
Urine potassium = 10 mmol/L

82. What is this patient's approximate glomerular filtration rate (GFR), assuming that she collected all her urine in the 24-hour period?
    (A) 10 ml/min
    (B) 20 ml/min
    (C) 30 ml/min
    (D) 40 ml/min
    (E) 80 ml/min

83. What is the net renal tubular reabsorption rate of potassium in this patient?
    (A) 1.050 mmol/min
    (B) 0.100 mmol/min
    (C) 0.037 mmol/min
    (D) 0.075 mmol/min
    (E) Potassium is not reabsorbed in this example

Questions 84-88

Match each of the patients described in questions 84 to 88 with the correct set of blood values in the table below (the same values may be used for more than one patient):

	pH	HCO_3^- (mEq/L)	P_{CO_2} (mm Hg)	Na^+ (mEq/L)	Cl^- (mEq/L)
(A)	7.66	22	20	143	111
(B)	7.28	30	65	142	102
(C)	7.24	12	29	144	102
(D)	7.29	14	30	143	117
(E)	7.52	38	48	146	100
(F)	7.07	14	50	144	102

84. A patient with severe diarrhea. ( )

85. A patient with primary aldosteronism. ( )

86. A patient with proximal renal tubular acidosis. ( )

87. A patient with diabetic ketoacidosis and emphysema. ( )

88. A patient treated chronically with a carbonic anhydrase inhibitor. ( )

89. Which of the following changes would you expect to find in a patient who developed acute renal failure after ingesting poisonous mushrooms that caused renal tubular necrosis?
    (A) Increased plasma bicarbonate concentration
    (B) Metabolic acidosis
    (C) Decreased plasma potassium concentration
    (D) Decreased blood urea nitrogen concentration
    (E) Decreased hydrostatic pressure in Bowman's capsule

90. An elderly patient complains of muscle weakness and lethargy. A urine specimen reveals a Na^+ concentration of 600 mmol/L and an osmolarity of 1200 mOsm/L. Additional laboratory tests provide the following information:
Plasma Na^+ concentration = 167 mmol/L
Plasma renin activity = 4 ng angiotensin I/ml/hr (normal = 1)
Plasma antidiuretic hormone (ADH) = 60 pg/ml (normal = 3 pg/ml)
Plasma aldosterone = 15 ng/dl (normal = 6 ng/dl)
Which of the following is the most likely reason for this patient's hypernatremia?
    (A) Dehydration caused by decreased fluid intake
    (B) Syndrome of inappropriate ADH
    (C) Nephrogenic diabetes insipidus
    (D) Primary aldosteronism
    (E) Renin-secreting tumor

91. A patient complains that he is always thirsty, and his breath has an acetone smell. You suspect that he has diabetes mellitus, and that diagnosis is confirmed by a urine sample that tests very positive for glucose and a blood sample that shows a fasting blood glucose concentration of 400 mg/dl. You would expect to find which of the following sets of changes in his plasma, compared with normal?

	Plasma HCO_3^-	Plasma pH	Plasma P_{CO_2}	Plasma Anion Gap
(A)	↓	↓	↓	↓
(B)	↓	↓	↓	↑
(C)	↓	↓	↑	↓
(D)	↑	↓	↑	↑
(E)	↑	↓	↓	↑

92. Which of the following has similar values for both intracellular and interstitial body fluids?
    (A) Potassium ion concentration
    (B) Colloid osmotic pressure
    (C) Sodium ion concentration
    (D) Chloride ion concentration
    (E) Total osmolarity

93. In a patient with very high levels of aldosterone and otherwise normal kidney function, approximately what percentage of the filtered load of sodium would be reabsorbed by the distal convoluted tubule and collecting duct?
    (A) More than 66 per cent
    (B) 40 to 60 per cent
    (C) 20 to 40 per cent
    (D) 10 to 20 per cent
    (E) Less than 10 per cent

94. Which of the following statements is true?
    (A) Antidiuretic hormone (ADH) increases water reabsorption from the ascending loop of Henle
    (B) Water reabsorption from the descending loop of Henle is normally less than that from the ascending loop of Henle
    (C) Sodium reabsorption from the ascending loop of Henle is normally less than that from the descending loop of Henle
    (D) Osmolarity of fluid in the early distal tubule would be less than 300 mOsm/L in a dehydrated person with normal kidneys and increased ADH levels
    (E) ADH decreases the urea permeability in the medullary collecting tubules

95. Which of the following changes tends to increase urinary Ca^{++} excretion?
    (A) Extracellular fluid volume expansion
    (B) Increased plasma parathyroid hormone concentration
    (C) Decreased blood pressure
    (D) Increased plasma phosphate concentration
    (E) Metabolic acidosis

96. A patient's one remaining kidney has moderate renal artery stenosis that reduces renal artery pressure distal to the stenosis to 85 mm Hg, compared with the normal level of 100 mm Hg. Which of the following is most likely decreased in this patient 2 weeks after the stenosis has occurred, assuming that his diet is unchanged?
    (A) Efferent arteriolar resistance
    (B) Afferent arteriolar resistance
    (C) Renin secretion
    (D) Sodium excretion rate
    (E) Plasma aldosterone concentration

97. Which of the following changes would you expect to find in a patient consuming a high-sodium diet (200 mEq/day) compared with the same patient on a normal-sodium diet (100 mEq/day), assuming steady-state conditions?
    (A) Increased plasma aldosterone concentration
    (B) Increased urinary potassium excretion
    (C) Decreased plasma renin activity
    (D) Decreased plasma atrial natriuretic peptide
    (E) An increase in plasma sodium concentration of at least 5 mmol/L

98. A 26-year-old construction worker is brought to the emergency room with a change in mental status after working a 10-hour shift on a hot summer day (average outside temperature was 97°F). The man had been sweating profusely during the day but did not drink fluids. He has a fever of 102°F, heart rate of 140 beats/min, and blood pressure of 100/55 mm Hg in the supine position. On examination, he has no perspiration, appears to have dry mucous membranes, and is poorly oriented to person, place, and time. Assuming that his kidneys were normal yesterday, which of the following sets of hormone levels describes his condition, compared with normal?

   (A) High antidiuretic hormone (ADH), high renin, low angiotensin II, low aldosterone
   (B) Low ADH, low renin, low angiotensin II, low aldosterone
   (C) High ADH, low renin, high angiotensin II, low aldosterone
   (D) High ADH, high renin, high angiotensin II, high aldosterone
   (E) Low ADH, high renin, low angiotensin II, high aldosterone

Answers

1. (B) GFR is equal to inulin clearance, which is calculated as the urine inulin concentration (100 mg/ml) × urine flow rate (1 ml/min) ÷ plasma inulin concentration (2 mg/ml), which is equal to 50 ml/min.
   TMP11 344

2. (D) The net urea reabsorption rate is equal to the filtered load of urea (GFR [50 ml/min] × plasma urea concentration [2.5 mg/ml]) – urinary excretion rate of urea (urine urea concentration [50 mg/ml] × urine flow rate [1 ml/min]). Therefore, net urea reabsorption = (50 ml/min × 2.5 mg/ml) – (50 mg/ml × 1 ml/min) = 75 mg/min.
   TMP11 344

3. (C) A 3 per cent sodium chloride (NaCl) solution is hypertonic and when infused intravenously would increase extracellular fluid volume and osmolarity, thereby causing water to flow out of the cell. This would decrease intracellular fluid volume and further increase extracellular fluid volume. The 0.9 per cent NaCl solution and 5 per cent dextrose solution are isotonic and therefore would not reduce intracellular fluid volume. Pure water and the 0.45 per cent NaCl solution are hypotonic and when infused would increase both intracellular and extracellular fluid volumes.
   TMP11 298-300

4. (C) Because the patient has a low plasma pH (normal = 7.4), he has acidosis. The fact that his plasma bicarbonate concentration is also low (normal = 24 mEq/L) indicates that he has metabolic acidosis. However, he also appears to have respiratory acidosis because his plasma P_{CO_2} is high (normal = 40 mm Hg). The rise in P_{CO_2} is due to his impaired breathing as a result of cardiopulmonary arrest. Therefore, the patient has a mixed acidosis with combined metabolic and respiratory acidosis.
   TMP11 397-400

5. (D) An important compensation for respiratory acidosis is increased renal production of ammonia (NH_4^+) and increased NH_4^+ excretion. In acidosis, urinary excretion of HCO_3^- would be reduced, as would urine pH, and urinary titratable acid would be slightly increased as a compensatory response to the acidosis.
   TMP11 392-394

6. (B) Dilation of afferent arterioles increases glomerular hydrostatic pressure, which in turn increases GFR, decreases total renal vascular resistance, and increases renal blood flow. Dilation of efferent arterioles increases renal blood flow but reduces glomerular hydrostatic pressure and therefore tends to reduce GFR. Increased glomerular capillary filtration coefficient would increase GFR but has no direct effect on renal blood flow. Increases in plasma colloid osmotic pressure or renal sympathetic nerve activity would tend to reduce GFR.
   TMP11 319, 320

7. (B) As water flows up the ascending limb of the loop of Henle, solutes are reabsorbed, but this segment is relatively impermeable to water; progressive dilution of the tubular fluid occurs so that the osmolarity decreases to approximately 100 mOsm/L by the time the fluid reaches the early distal tubule. Even during maximal antidiuresis, this portion of the renal tubule is relatively impermeable to water and is therefore called the diluting segment of the renal tubule.
   TMP11 355, 356

8. (B) A 1 per cent solution of dextrose is hypotonic and when infused would increase both intracellular and extracellular fluid volumes while decreasing osmolarity of these compartments.
   TMP11 298-300

9. (C) A 3 per cent solution of sodium chloride is hypertonic and when infused into the extracellular fluid would raise osmolarity, thereby causing water to flow out of the cells into the extracellular fluid until osmotic equilibrium is achieved. In the steady state, extracellular fluid volume would increase, intracellular fluid volume would decrease, and osmolarity of both compartments would increase.
   TMP11 298-300

10. (B) Excessive secretion of antidiuretic hormone would increase renal tubular reabsorption of water,

thereby increasing extracellular fluid volume and reducing extracellular fluid osmolarity. The reduced osmolarity, in turn, would cause water to flow into the cells and raise intracellular fluid volume. In the steady state, both extracellular and intracellular fluid volumes would increase, and osmolarity of both compartments would decrease.
TMP11 301, 358, 359

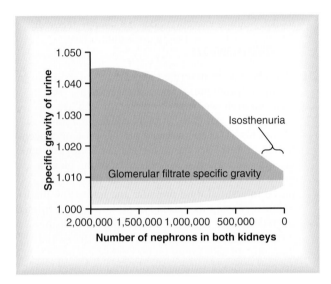

11. (A) With a severe reduction in the number of functional nephrons to 25 per cent of normal, the surviving nephrons must excrete four times as much sodium and four times as much volume as normal to maintain water and electrolyte balance. This rapid flow of urine through the surviving tubules decreases their ability to concentrate the urine. Urinary sodium excretion would be maintained at normal levels, equal to intake, through various compensatory mechanisms (e.g., increased arterial pressure) that reduce renal tubular sodium reabsorption. Although filtered load of creatinine and urinary creatinine excretion transiently decrease with a decreased glomerular filtration rate, this also causes an accumulation of creatinine in the body fluids and raises plasma creatinine concentration until the filtered load of creatinine and the creatinine excretion rate return to normal. Chronic renal failure is associated with a tendency toward acidosis, rather than alkalosis, due to the kidneys' failure to rid the body of normal acid products effectively. With loss of functional nephrons, renal blood flow would also be reduced.
TMP11 409-411

12. (D) A severe renal artery stenosis that reduces GFR to 25 per cent of normal would also decrease renal blood flow but would cause only a transient decrease in urinary creatinine excretion. The transient decrease in creatinine excretion would increase serum creatinine (to about four times normal), which would restore the filtered creatinine load to normal and therefore return urinary creatinine excretion to normal levels under steady-state conditions. Urinary

sodium secretion would also decrease transiently but would also be restored to normal so that intake and excretion of sodium are balanced. Plasma sodium concentration would not change significantly because it is carefully regulated by the antidiuretic hormone–thirst mechanism.
TMP11 323, 345, 409, 410

13. (C) Aldosterone stimulates potassium secretion by the principal cells of the collecting tubules. Therefore, blockade of the action of aldosterone with spironolactone would inhibit potassium secretion. Other factors that stimulate potassium secretion by the cortical collecting tubule include increased potassium concentration, increased cortical collecting tubule flow rate (as would occur with high sodium intake or a diuretic that reduces proximal tubular sodium reabsorption), and acute alkalosis.
TMP11 368-371

14. (A) K^+ excretion rate = urine K^+ concentration (60 mEq/L) × urine flow rate (0.001 L/min) = 0.06 mEq/min.
TMP11 344

15. (C) In the absence of ADH secretion, there is a marked increase in urine volume because the late distal and collecting tubules are relatively impermeable to water. As a result of increased urine volume, there is dehydration and increased plasma osmolarity and high plasma sodium concentration. The resulting decrease in extracellular fluid volume stimulates renin secretion, resulting in an increase in plasma renin concentration.
TMP11 357

16. (C) In a patient with a very high rate of renin secretion, there would also be increased formation of angiotensin II, which in turn would stimulate aldosterone secretion. The increased levels of angiotensin II and aldosterone would cause a transient decrease in sodium excretion, which would cause expansion of the extracellular fluid volume and increased arterial pressure. The increased arterial pressure as well as other compensations would return sodium excretion to normal so that intake and output are balanced. Therefore, under steady-state conditions, sodium excretion would be normal and equal to sodium intake. The increased aldosterone concentration would cause hypokalemia (decreased plasma potassium concentration), whereas the high level of angiotensin II would cause renal vasoconstriction and decreased renal blood flow.
TMP11 322, 373-375

17. (D) Impairment of proximal tubular NaCl reabsorption would increase NaCl delivery to the macula densa, which in turn would cause a tubuloglomerular feedback-mediated increase in afferent arteriolar resistance. The increased afferent arteriolar resistance would decrease the glomerular filtration rate. Initially there would be a transient increase in sodium excretion, but after 3 weeks, steady-state conditions would be achieved. Sodium excretion

would equal sodium intake, and no significant change would occur in urinary sodium excretion.
TMP11 323-325

18. (A) Renal prostaglandins play an important role in preventing excessive vasoconstriction of afferent arterioles and decreased GFR, especially under conditions of volume depletion. Administration of a thiazide diuretic would tend to cause volume depletion, and addition of a nonsteroidal anti-inflammatory drug would inhibit the formation of vasodilator prostaglandins, causing increased afferent arteriolar resistance and decreased GFR. Increased efferent arteriolar resistance or increased glomerular capillary filtration coefficient would actually tend to elevate GFR. Blockade of prostaglandin synthesis would tend to reduce renin secretion and angiotensin II formation. It is unlikely that increased muscle mass due to the exercise could cause a doubling of serum creatinine.
TMP11 322, 323

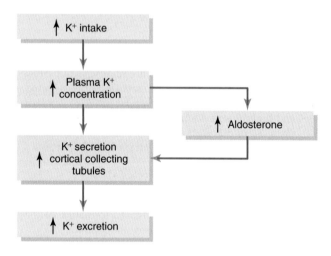

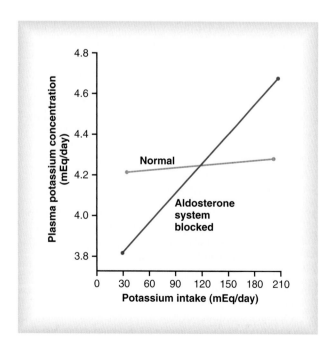

19. (C) When potassium intake is doubled (from 80 to160 mmol/day), potassium excretion also approximately doubles within a few days, and the plasma potassium concentration increases only slightly. Increased potassium excretion is achieved largely by increased secretion of potassium in the cortical collecting tubule. Increased aldosterone concentration plays a significant role in increasing potassium secretion and in maintaining a relatively constant plasma potassium concentration during increases in potassium intake. Sodium excretion does not change markedly during chronic increases in potassium intake.
TMP11 369-371

20. (A) The patient described appears to have protein in the urine (proteinuria) and reduced plasma protein concentration secondary to glomerulonephritis caused by an untreated streptococcal infection ("strep throat"). The reduced plasma protein concentration, in turn, decreased the plasma colloid osmotic pressure and resulted in leakage from the plasma to the interstitium. The extracellular fluid edema raised interstitial fluid pressure and interstitial fluid volume, causing increased lymph flow and decreased interstitial fluid protein concentration. Increasing lymph flow causes a "washout" of the interstitial fluid protein as a safety factor against edema. The decreased blood volume would tend to lower blood pressure and stimulate the secretion of renin by the kidneys, raising the plasma renin concentration.
TMP11 303

21. (C) A 50 per cent reduction in afferent arteriolar resistance with no change in arterial pressure would increase renal blood flow and glomerular hydrostatic pressure, thereby increasing GFR. At the same time, the reduction in afferent arteriolar resistance would raise peritubular capillary hydrostatic pressure.
TMP 11 319, 320

22. (C) The filtered load of glucose in this example is determined as follows: GFR (150 ml/min) × plasma glucose (300 mg/dl) = 450 mg/min. The transport maximum for glucose in this example is 300 mg/min. Therefore, the maximum rate of glucose reabsorption is 300 mg/min. The urinary glucose excretion is equal to the filtered load (450 mg/min) minus the tubular reabsorption of glucose (300 mg/min), or 150 mg/min.
TMP11 327, 331

Characteristics of Primary Acid-Base Disturbances

	pH	H⁺	Pco₂	HCO₃⁻
Normal	7.4	40 mEq/L	40 mm Hg	24 mEq/L
Respiratory acidosis	↓	↑	↑↑	↑
Respiratory alkalosis	↑	↓	↓↓	↓
Metabolic acidosis	↓	↑	↓	↓↓
Metabolic alkalosis	↑	↓	↑	↑↑

The primary event is indicated by the double arrows (↑↑ or ↓↓). Note that respiratory acid-base disorders are initiated by an increase or decrease in Pco₂, whereas metabolic disorders are initiated by an increase or decrease in HCO₃⁻.

23. (B) This patient has respiratory acidosis because the plasma pH is lower than the normal level of 7.4 and the plasma P_{CO_2} is higher than the normal level of 40 mm Hg. The elevation in plasma bicarbonate concentration above normal (~24 mEq/L) is due to partial renal compensation for the respiratory acidosis. Therefore, this patient has respiratory acidosis with partial renal compensation.
TMP11 396

24. (C) Peritubular capillary fluid reabsorption is determined by the balance of hydrostatic and colloid osmotic forces in the peritubular capillaries. Increased efferent arteriolar resistance reduces peritubular capillary hydrostatic pressure and therefore increases the net force favoring fluid reabsorption. Increased blood pressure tends to raise peritubular capillary hydrostatic pressure and reduce fluid reabsorption. Decreased filtration fraction increases the peritubular capillary colloid osmotic pressure and tends to reduce peritubular capillary reabsorption. Decreased angiotensin II causes vasodilatation of efferent arterioles, raising peritubular capillary hydrostatic pressure, decreasing reabsorption, and decreasing tubular transport of water and electrolytes. Increased renal blood flow also tends to raise peritubular capillary hydrostatic pressure and decrease fluid reabsorption.
TMP11 339-341

25. (B) Inhibition of aldosterone causes hyperkalemia by two mechanisms: (1) shifting potassium out of the cells into the extracellular fluid, and (2) decreasing cortical collecting tubular secretion of potassium. Increasing potassium intake from 60 to 180 mmol/day would cause only a very small increase in plasma potassium concentration in a person with normal kidneys and normal aldosterone feedback mechanisms (see TMP11 Figures 29-7 and 29-8). A reduction in sodium intake also has very little effect on plasma potassium concentration. Chronic treatment with a diuretic that inhibits loop of Henle Na^+-2 Cl^--K^+ co-transport would tend to cause potassium loss in the urine and hypokalemia. However, chronic treatment with a diuretic that inhibits sodium reabsorption in the collecting ducts, such as amiloride, would have little effect on plasma potassium concentration.
TMP11 366, 369

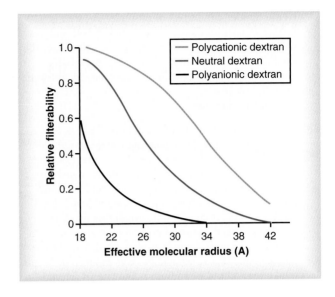

26. (C) The filterability of solutes in the plasma is inversely related to the size of the solute (molecular weight). Also, positively charged molecules are filtered more readily than are neutral molecules or negatively charged molecules of equal molecular weight. Therefore, the positively charged polycationic dextran with a molecular weight of 25,000 would be the most readily filtered substance of the choices provided. Red blood cells are not filtered at all by the glomerular capillaries under normal conditions.
TMP11 317

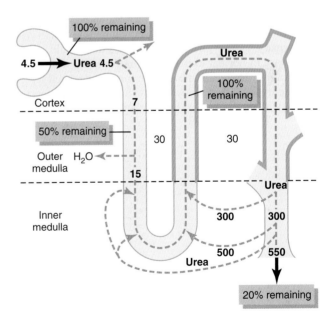

27. (B) Approximately 30 to 40 per cent of the filtered urea is reabsorbed in the proximal tubule. However, the tubular fluid urea concentration increases because urea is not nearly as permeant as water in this nephron segment. Urea concentration increases further in the tip of the loop of Henle because water is reabsorbed in the descending limb of the loop of

Henle. Under conditions of antidiuresis, urea is further concentrated as water is reabsorbed and as fluid flows along the collecting ducts. Therefore, the final urine concentration of urea is substantially greater than the concentration in the proximal tubule or in the plasma.
    TMP11 353-354

28. (D) Excessive activity of the amiloride-sensitive sodium channel in the collecting tubules would cause a transient decrease in sodium excretion and expansion of extracellular fluid volume, which in turn would increase arterial pressure and decrease renin secretion, leading to decreased aldosterone secretion. Under steady-state conditions, sodium excretion would return to normal so that intake and renal excretion of sodium are balanced. One of the mechanisms that re-establishes this balance between intake and output of sodium is the rise in arterial pressure that induces a "pressure natriuresis."
    TMP11 373-375

29. (B) Free water clearance is calculated as urine flow rate (600 ml/2 hr, or 5 ml/min) – osmolar clearance (urine osmolarity × urine flow rate/plasma osmolarity). Therefore, free water clearance is equal to +2.5 ml/min.
    TMP11 357

30. (A) Primary excessive secretion of aldosterone (Conn's syndrome) would be associated with marked hypokalemia and metabolic alkalosis (increased plasma pH). Because aldosterone stimulates sodium reabsorption and potassium secretion by the cortical collecting tubule, there could be a transient decrease in sodium excretion and an increase in potassium excretion, but under steady-state conditions, both urinary sodium and potassium excretion would return to normal to match the intake of these electrolytes. However, the sodium retention as well as the hypertension associated with aldosterone excess would tend to reduce renin secretion.
    TMP11 370, 379

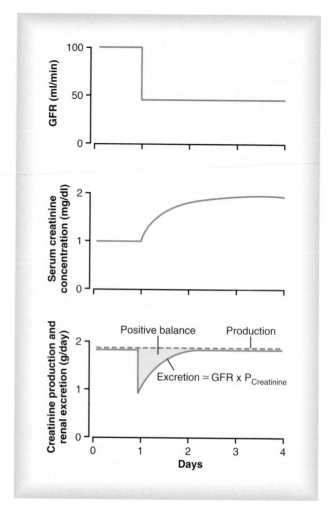

31. (B) A doubling of plasma creatinine implies that the creatinine clearance and glomerular filtration rate have been reduced by approximately 50 per cent. Although the reduction in creatinine clearance would initially cause a transient decrease in filtered load of creatinine, creatinine excretion rate, and sodium excretion rate, the plasma concentration of creatinine would increase until the filtered load of creatinine and the creatinine excretion rate returned to normal. However, creatinine clearance would remain reduced, because creatinine clearance is the urinary excretion rate of creatinine divided by the plasma creatinine concentration. Urinary sodium excretion would also return to normal and would equal the sodium intake, under steady-state conditions, as a result of compensatory mechanisms that reduce renal tubular reabsorption of sodium.
    TMP11 409, 410

32. (C) The glomerular capillary filtration coefficient is the product of the hydraulic conductivity and surface area of the glomerular capillaries. Therefore, increasing the glomerular capillary filtration coefficient tends to increase GFR. Increased afferent arteriolar resistance, decreased efferent arteriolar resistance, increased Bowman's capsule hydrostatic pressure, and decreased glomerular hydrostatic pressure tend to decrease GFR.
    TMP11 317-319

33. (D) If a substance is completely cleared from the plasma, the clearance rate of that substance would equal the total renal plasma flow. In other words, the total amount of substance delivered to the kidneys in the blood (renal plasma flow × concentration of substance in the blood) would equal the amount of that substance excreted in the urine. Complete renal clearance of a substance would require both glomerular filtration and tubular secretion of that substance.
TMP 11 343-347

34. (C) The patient has a lower than normal pH and is therefore acidotic. Because the plasma bicarbonate concentration is also lower than normal, the patient has metabolic acidosis with respiratory compensation (PCO_2 is lower than normal). Plasma anion gap ($Na^+ - Cl^- - HCO_3^- = 10$ mEq/L) is in the normal range, suggesting that the metabolic acidosis is not caused by excess nonvolatile acids such as salicylic acid or ketoacids caused by diabetes mellitus. Therefore, the most likely cause of the metabolic acidosis is diarrhea, which would cause a loss of HCO_3^- in the feces and would be associated with a normal anion gap and a hyperchloremic (increased chloride concentration) metabolic acidosis.
TMP11 397-400

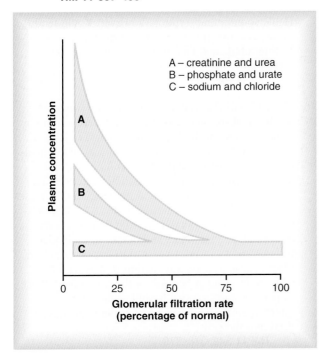

35. (A) A 50 per cent reduction of GFR would approximately double the plasma creatinine concentration, because creatinine is not reabsorbed or secreted and its excretion depends largely on glomerular filtration. Therefore, when GFR decreases, the plasma concentration of creatinine increases until the renal excretion of creatinine returns to normal. Plasma concentrations of glucose, potassium, sodium, and hydrogen ions are closely regulated by multiple mechanisms that keep them relatively constant even when GFR falls to very low levels. Plasma phosphate concentration is also maintained near normal until GFR falls to below 20 to 30 per cent of normal.
TMP11 409, 410

36. (D) Excessive ingestion of aspirin (salicylic acid) causes metabolic acidosis characterized by reductions in plasma HCO_3^- concentration and increased plasma anion gap. The acidosis stimulates respiration, causing a compensatory decrease in plasma PCO_2. The acidosis also increases renal reabsorption of HCO_3^-, leading to decreased urine HCO_3^- excretion. Finally, the acidosis also stimulates a compensatory increase in renal tubular NH_4^+ production.
TMP11 398, 400

Step 1. Initial Conditions

	Volume (L)	Concentration (mOsm/L)	Total (mOsm)
Extracellular fluid	12	260	3120
Intracellular fluid	24	260	6240
Total body water	36	260	9360

Step 2. Effect of Adding 2 Liters of 3 Per Cent Sodium Chloride after Osmotic Equilibrium

	Volume (L)	Concentration (mOsm/L)	Total (mOsm)
Extracellular fluid	17.2	300	3120 + 2052 = 5172
Intracellular fluid	20.8	300	6240
Total body water	36 + 2 = 38	300	9360 + 2052 = 11,412

37. (C) Calculation of fluid shifts and osmolarities after infusion of hypertonic saline is discussed in Chapter 25 of TMP11. The tables shown above represent the initial conditions and the final conditions after infusion of 2 liters of 3 per cent NaCl and osmotic equilibrium. Three per cent NaCl is equal to 30 g NaCl/L, or 0.513 mol/L (513 mmol/L). Because NaCl has two osmotically active particles per mole, the net effect is to add a total of 2052 millimoles in 2 liters of solution. As an approximation, one can assume that cell membranes are impermeable to the NaCl and that the NaCl infused remains in the extracellular fluid compartment.
TMP11 299-301

38. (B) Extracellular fluid volume is calculated by dividing the total milliosmoles in the extracellular compartment (5172 mOsm) by the concentration after osmotic equilibrium (300 mOsm/L) to give 17.2 liters.
TMP11 299-301

39. (C) Urine flow rate is equal to GFR minus tubular fluid reabsorption rate. Therefore, if GFR is reduced to 50 ml/min and tubular reabsorption rate is also 50 ml/min, urine flow rate will be zero.
TMP11 314, 327

40. (C) A large increase in aldosterone secretion combined with a high sodium intake would cause severe hypokalemia. Aldosterone stimulates potassium secretion and causes a shift of potassium from the extracellular fluid into the cells, and a high sodium intake increases the collecting tubular flow rate, which also enhances potassium secretion. In normal persons, potassium intake can be reduced to as low as one-fourth of normal with only a mild decrease in plasma potassium concentration (for further information, see TMP11 Figure 29-7). A low sodium intake would tend to oppose aldosterone's hypokalemic effect, because a low sodium intake would reduce the collecting tubular flow rate and thus tend to reduce potassium secretion. Patients with Addison's disease have a deficiency of aldosterone secretion and therefore tend to have hyperkalemia.
    TMP11 366, 369-371

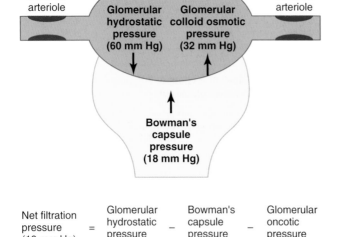

$$\begin{array}{l} \text{Net filtration} \\ \text{pressure} \\ \text{(10 mm Hg)} \end{array} = \begin{array}{l} \text{Glomerular} \\ \text{hydrostatic} \\ \text{pressure} \\ \text{(60 mm Hg)} \end{array} - \begin{array}{l} \text{Bowman's} \\ \text{capsule} \\ \text{pressure} \\ \text{(18 mm Hg)} \end{array} - \begin{array}{l} \text{Glomerular} \\ \text{oncotic} \\ \text{pressure} \\ \text{(32 mm Hg)} \end{array}$$

41. (A) The net filtration pressure at the glomerular capillaries is equal to the sum of the forces favoring filtration (glomerular capillary hydrostatic pressure) minus the forces that oppose filtration (hydrostatic pressure in Bowman's space and glomerular colloid osmotic pressure). Therefore, the net pressure driving glomerular filtration is 50 – 12 – 30 = 8 mm Hg.
    TMP11 317, 318

42. (D) Uncontrolled diabetes mellitus results in increased blood acetoacetic acid levels, which in turn cause metabolic acidosis and decreased plasma HCO_3^- and pH. The acidosis causes several compensatory responses, including increased respiratory rate, which reduces plasma PCO_2; increased renal NH^+ production, which leads to increased NH^+ excretion; and increased phosphate buffering of hydrogen ions secreted by the renal tubules, which increases titratable acid excretion.
    TMP11 396, 398

43. (B) Infusion of a hypotonic solution of NaCl would initially increase extracellular fluid volume and

decrease extracellular fluid osmolarity. The reduction in extracellular fluid osmolarity would cause osmotic flow of fluid into the cells, thereby increasing intracellular fluid volume and decreasing intracellular fluid osmolarity after osmotic equilibrium.
    TMP11 299-301

44. (D) The tubular fluid–plasma ratio of inulin concentration is 4 in the early distal tubule, as shown in the question's figure. Because inulin is not reabsorbed from the tubule, this means that water reabsorption must have concentrated the inulin to four times the level in the plasma that was filtered. Therefore, the amount of water remaining in the tubule is only one fourth of what was filtered, indicating that 75 per cent of the water has been reabsorbed prior to the distal convoluted tubule.
    TPM11 339

45. (B) Potassium secretion by the cortical collecting ducts is stimulated by (1) aldosterone, (2) increased plasma potassium concentration, (3) increased flow rate in the cortical collecting tubules, and (4) alkalosis. Therefore, a diuretic that inhibits aldosterone, decreased plasma potassium concentration, acute acidosis, and low sodium intake would all tend to decrease potassium secretion by the cortical collecting tubules. A diuretic that decreases loop of Henle sodium reabsorption, however, would tend to increase the flow rate in the cortical collecting tubule and therefore stimulate potassium secretion.
    TMP11 369-371

46. (B) Excessive secretion of aldosterone stimulates sodium reabsorption and potassium secretion in the principal cells of the collecting tubules, causing a transient reduction in urinary sodium excretion and expansion of extracellular fluid volume, as well as a transient increase in potassium excretion rate. Sodium retention raises blood pressure and decreases renin secretion. However, under steady-state conditions, sodium and potassium excretion would return to normal, so that intake and output of these electrolytes are balanced. Excess aldosterone excretion would cause a marked reduction in plasma potassium concentration because of the transient increase in potassium excretion, as well as aldosterone's effect of shifting potassium from the extracellular fluid into the cells.
    TMP11 342, 378, 379

47. (B) This patient with diabetes mellitus and chronic renal disease has a reduction in creatinine clearance to 40 per cent of normal, implying a marked reduction in glomerular filtration rate. He also has acidosis, as evidenced by a plasma pH of 7.14. The decrease in creatinine clearance would cause only a transient reduction in sodium excretion and creatinine excretion rate. As the plasma creatinine concentration increased, the urinary creatinine excretion rate would return to normal, despite the sustained decrease in creatinine clearance (creatinine excretion

rate/plasma concentration of creatinine). Diabetes is associated with increased production of acetoacetic acid, which would cause metabolic acidosis and decreased plasma HCO_3^- concentration, as well as a compensatory increase in renal NH_4^+ production and increased NH_4^+ excretion rate.
TMP11 396-398, 410

48. (C) A reduction in plasma protein concentration to 3.6 g/dl would increase the capillary filtration rate, thereby raising interstitial fluid volume and interstitial fluid hydrostatic pressure. The increased interstitial fluid pressure would, in turn, increase the lymph flow rate and reduce the interstitial fluid protein concentration ("washout" of interstitial fluid protein).
TMP11 303, 305

49. (B) The most likely diagnosis for this patient is diabetes insipidus, which can account for the polyuria and the fact that her urine osmolarity is very low (80 mOsm/L) despite overnight water restriction. In many patients with diabetes insipidus, the plasma sodium concentration can be maintained relatively close to normal by increasing fluid intake (polydipsia). When water intake is restricted, however, the high urine flow rate leads to rapid depletion of extracellular fluid volume and severe hypernatremia, as occurred in this patient. The fact that she has no glucose in her urine rules out diabetes mellitus. Neither primary aldosteronism nor a renin-secreting tumor would lead to an inability to concentrate the urine after overnight water restriction. Syndrome of inappropriate antidiuretic hormone would cause excessive fluid retention and increased urine osmolarity.
TMP11 357, 362, 363

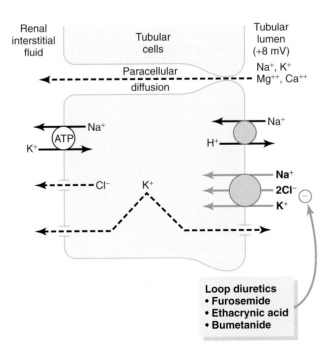

50. (D) Furosemide (Lasix) inhibits the Na^+-2 Cl^--K^+ co-transporter in the ascending limb of the loop of Henle. This not only causes marked natriuresis and diuresis but also reduces the urine concentrating ability. Furosemide does not cause edema; in fact, it is often used to treat severe edema and heart failure. Furosemide also increases the renal excretion of potassium and calcium and therefore tends to cause hypokalemia and hypocalcemia rather than increasing the plasma concentrations of potassium and calcium.
TMP11 335, 350, 351, 370, 371

51. (A) Excessive secretion of renin leads to the formation of large amounts of angiotensin II, which in turn causes marked constriction of efferent arterioles. This reduces renal blood flow, increases glomerular hydrostatic pressure, and decreases peritubular capillary hydrostatic pressure. Because constriction of efferent arterioles reduces renal blood flow more than GFR, the filtration fraction (ratio of GFR to renal plasma flow) increases.
TMP11 320, 322

52. (D) Most of the daily variation in potassium excretion is caused by changes in potassium secretion in the late distal tubules and collecting tubules. Therefore, when the dietary intake of potassium increases, the total body balance of potassium is maintained primarily by an increase in potassium secretion in these tubular segments. Increased potassium intake has little effect on glomerular filtration rate or on reabsorption of potassium in the proximal tubule and loop of Henle. Although high potassium intake may cause a slight shift of potassium into the intracellular compartment, a balance between intake and output must be achieved by increasing the excretion of potassium during high potassium intake.
TMP11 367

53. (B) Hypernatremia can be caused by excessive sodium retention or water loss. The fact that the patient has large volumes of dilute urine suggests excessive urinary water excretion. Of the three possible disturbances listed that could cause excessive urinary water excretion (dehydration, nephrogenic diabetes insipidus, and central diabetes insipidus), nephrogenic diabetes insipidus is the most likely cause. Central diabetes insipidus (decreased ADH secretion) is not the correct answer because plasma ADH levels are markedly elevated. Simple dehydration due to decreased water intake is unlikely because the patient is excreting large volumes of dilute urine.
TMP11 302, 357-359

54. (C) High urine flow occurs in type I diabetes because the filtered load of glucose exceeds the renal threshold, resulting in an increase in glucose concentration in the tubule, which decreases the osmotic driving force for water reabsorption. Increased urine flow reduces extracellular fluid volume and stimulates the release of antidiuretic hormone.
TMP11 331, 360

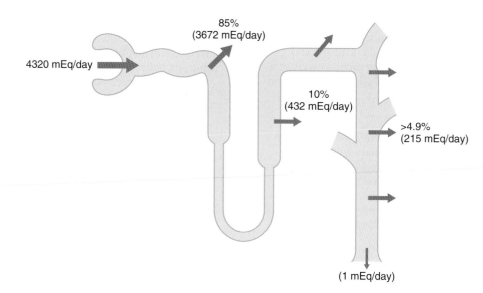

55. (C) Diuretics that inhibit loop of Henle sodium reabsorption are used to treat conditions associated with excessive fluid volume (e.g., hypertension and heart failure). Diuretics initially cause an increase in sodium excretion that reduces extracellular fluid volume and blood pressure, but under steady-state conditions, the urinary sodium excretion returns to normal, due in part to the fall in blood pressure. One of the important side effects of loop diuretics is hypokalemia that is caused by the inhibition of Na^+-2 Cl^--K^+ co-transport in the loop of Henle and by the increased tubular flow rate in the cortical collecting tubules, which stimulates potassium secretion.
    TMP11 370, 403

56. (C) Approximately 80 to 90 per cent of bicarbonate reabsorption occurs in the proximal tubule under normal conditions as well as in acidosis (see above). For each bicarbonate ion reabsorbed, there must also be a hydrogen ion secreted. Therefore, about 80 to 90 per cent of the hydrogen ions secreted are normally used for bicarbonate reabsorption in the proximal tubules.
    TMP11

57. (A) Thiazide diuretics inhibit NaCl co-transport in the luminal membrane of the early distal tubules. (For further information, see TMP11 Table 31-1.)
    TMP11 403-404

58. (C) Reducing the renal perfusion pressure to 80 mm Hg (within the range of autoregulation) would cause only a transient decrease in GFR, renal blood flow, and sodium excretion and a transient increase in renin secretion. The decreased sodium excretion and increased renin secretion would raise arterial pressure, thereby restoring renal perfusion pressure toward normal and returning renal function toward normal. As long as renal perfusion pressure is not reduced below the range of autoregulation, GFR and renal blood flow are returned to normal within minutes after renal artery constriction.
    TMP11 323

59. (C) Phosphate excretion by the kidneys is controlled by an overflow mechanism. When the transport maximum for reabsorbing phosphate is exceeded, the remaining phosphate in the renal tubules is excreted in the urine and can be used to buffer hydrogen ions and form titratable acid. Phosphate normally begins to spill into the urine when the concentration of extracellular fluid rises above a threshold of 0.8 mmol/L, which is usually exceeded.
    TMP11 372, 373

60. (A) A reduction in the number of functional nephrons to 25 per cent of normal would cause a compensatory increase in GFR and urine flow rate of the surviving nephrons and decreased urine concentrating ability. Under steady-state conditions, the urinary creatinine excretion rate and sodium excretion rate would be maintained at normal levels. (For further information, see TMP11 Table 31-6.)
    TMP11 409-411

61. (C) With excessive secretion of ADH, there is a marked increase in water permeability in the late distal tubules and collecting tubules, resulting in water retention, volume expansion, and decreased sodium and protein concentrations in the extracellular fluid. Plasma renin activity and aldosterone concentrations are also decreased because of the volume expansion. Although excessive ADH secretion initially causes a marked reduction in urine flow rate, as volume expansion occurs and as blood pressure increases, there is an "escape" from volume retention, so that urine flow rate returns to normal to match fluid intake.
    TMP11 348-363

62. (A) Excessive secretion of antidiuretic hormone increases water reabsorption by the renal collecting tubules, which reduces extracellular fluid sodium concentration (hyponatremia). Restriction of fluid intake, excessive aldosterone secretion, or administration of hypertonic 3 per cent NaCl solution would all cause increased plasma sodium concentration

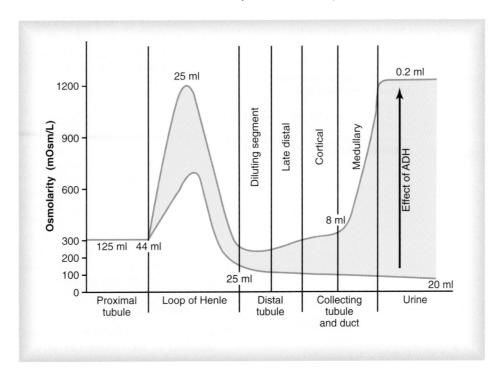

(hypernatremia), whereas administration of 0.9 per cent NaCl (an isotonic solution) would cause no major changes in plasma osmolarity.
TMP11 299, 301, 302, 358

63. (E) In the absence of ADH, the late distal tubule and collecting tubules are not permeable to water (see above). Therefore, the tubular fluid, which is already dilute when it leaves the loop of Henle (about 100 mOsm/L), becomes further diluted as it flows through the late distal tubule and collecting tubules as electrolytes are reabsorbed. Therefore, the final urine osmolarity in the complete absence of ADH is less than 100 mOsm/L.
TMP 11 356

64. (A) About 65 per cent of the filtered potassium is reabsorbed in the proximal tubule, and another 20 to 30 per cent is reabsorbed in the loop of Henle. Although most of the daily variation in potassium excretion is caused by changes in potassium secretion in the distal and collecting tubules, only a small percentage of the filtered potassium load can be reabsorbed in these nephron segments. (For further information, see TMP11 Figure 29-2.)
TMP11 367

65. (A) The proximal tubule normally absorbs approximately 65 per cent of the filtered water, with much smaller percentages being reabsorbed in the descending loop of Henle and in the distal and collecting tubules. The ascending limb of the loop of Henle is relatively impermeable to water and therefore reabsorbs very little water.
TMP11 333, 355

66. (C) The thick ascending limb of the loop of Henle is relatively impermeable to water even under conditions of maximal antidiuresis. The proximal tubule

and descending limb of the loop of Henle are highly permeable to water under normal conditions as well as during antidiuresis. Water permeability of the late distal and collecting tubules increases markedly during antidiuresis owing to the effects of increased levels of antidiuretic hormone.
TMP11 355, 356

67. (D) Interstitial fluid volume is equal to extracellular fluid volume minus plasma volume. Extracellular fluid volume can be estimated from the distribution of inulin or ^{22}Na, whereas plasma volume can be estimated from ^{125}I-albumin distribution. Therefore, interstitial fluid volume is calculated from the difference between the inulin distribution space and the ^{125}I-albumin distribution space.
TMP11 295-296

68. (D) Dehydration due to water deprivation decreases extracellular fluid volume, which in turn increases renin secretion and decreases plasma atrial natriuretic peptide. Dehydration also increases the plasma sodium concentration, which stimulates the secretion of ADH. The increased ADH increases water permeability in the collecting ducts. The ascending limb of the loop of Henle is relatively impermeable to water, and this low permeability is not altered by water deprivation or increased levels of ADH.
TMP11 350, 351, 358-360

69. (E) A 50 per cent reduction in renal efferent arteriolar resistance would reduce glomerular capillary hydrostatic pressure (upstream from the efferent arterioles) and therefore reduce glomerular filtration rate, while increasing hydrostatic pressure in peritubular capillaries (downstream from the efferent arterioles) and increasing renal blood flow.
TMP11 319, 320, 340

Factors That Can Alter Potassium Distribution Between the Intra- and Extracellular Fluid

Factors That Shift K⁺ into Cells (Decrease Extracellular [K⁺])	Factors That Shift K⁺ Out of Cells (Increase Extracellular [K⁺])
• Insulin	• Insulin deficiency (diabetes mellitus)
• Aldosterone	• Aldosterone deficiency (Addison's disease)
• β-adrenergic stimulation	• β-adrenergic blockade
• Alkalosis	• Acidosis
	• Cell lysis
	• Strenuous exercise
	• Increased extracellular fluid osmolarity

70. (E) Metabolic alkalosis is associated with hypokalemia due to a shift of potassium from the extracellular fluid into the cells. ß-adrenergic blockade, insulin deficiency, strenuous exercise, and aldosterone deficiency all cause hyperkalemia due to a shift of potassium out of the cells into the extracellular fluid.
TMP11 366

71. (B) Fluid entering the early distal tubule is almost always hypotonic because sodium and other ions are actively transported out of the thick ascending loop of Henle, whereas this portion of the nephron is virtually impermeable to water. For this reason, the thick ascending limb of the loop of Henle and the early part of the distal tubule are often called the diluting segment.
TMP11 334-336

72. (D) In this example, the filtered load of glucose is equal to GFR (100 ml/min) × plasma glucose (150 mg/dl), or 150 mg/min. If there is no detectable glucose in the urine, the reabsorption rate is equal to the filtered load of glucose, or 150 mg/min.
TMP11 344

73. (D) The patient has classic symptoms of diabetes mellitus: increased thirst, breath smelling of acetone (due to increased acetoacetic acids in the blood), high fasting blood glucose concentration, and glucose in the urine. The acetoacetic acids in the blood cause metabolic acidosis that leads to a compensatory decrease in renal HCO_3^- excretion, decreased urine pH, and increased renal production of ammonium and HCO_3^-. The high level of blood

glucose increases the filtered load of glucose, which exceeds the transport maximum for glucose, causing an osmotic diuresis (increased urine volume) due to the unreabsorbed glucose in the renal tubules acting as an osmotic diuretic.
TMP11 331, 396, 398

74. (D) Approximately 40 to 50 per cent of the filtered urea is reabsorbed in the proximal tubule. The distal convoluted tubule and the cortical collecting tubules are relatively impermeable to urea, even under conditions of antidiuresis; therefore, little urea reabsorption takes place in these segments. Likewise, very little urea reabsorption takes place in the thick ascending limb of the loop of Henle. Under conditions of antidiuresis, the concentration of urea in the renal medullary interstitial fluid is markedly increased because of reabsorption of urea from the collecting ducts, which contributes to the hyperosmotic renal medulla.
TMP11 353, 354

75. (A) Under normal conditions as well as during antidiuresis, most of the filtered water is reabsorbed in the proximal tubule (approximately 60 to 65 per cent). Although dehydration markedly increases water permeability in the cortical and medullary collecting ducts, these segments reabsorb a relatively small (albeit important) fraction of the filtered water.
TMP11 355, 356

76. (C) Intracellular fluid volume is calculated as the difference between total body fluid (0.57 × 60 kilograms = 34.2 kilograms, or approximately 34.2 liters) and extracellular fluid volume (12.8 liters), which equals 21.4 liters.
TMP11 295, 296

77. (C) Plasma volume is calculated as blood volume (4.3 liters) × (1.0 – hematocrit), which is 4.3 × 0.6 = 2.58 liters (rounded up to 2.6).
TMP11 295, 296

78. (C) Interstitial fluid volume is calculated as the difference between extracellular fluid volume (12.8 liters) and plasma volume (2.6 liters), which is equal to 10.2 liters.
TMP11 295, 296

79. (C) The primary site of reabsorption of magnesium is in the loop of Henle, where about 65 per cent of the filtered load of magnesium is reabsorbed. The proximal tubule normally reabsorbs only about 25 per cent of filtered magnesium, and the distal and collecting tubules reabsorb less than 5 per cent.
TMP11 373

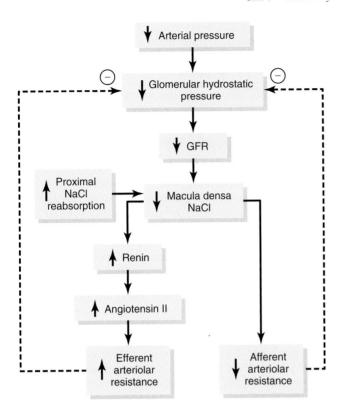

80. (D) The tubuloglomerular feedback mechanism for renal autoregulation involves signaling from the macula densa to the juxtaglomerular cells. Increased arterial pressure raises sodium chloride delivery to the macula densa, which initiates vasoconstriction of renal afferent arterioles and decreased release of renin.
TMP11 323, 324

81. (C) A plasma glucose concentration of 300 mg/dl would increase the filtered load of glucose above the renal tubular transport maximum and therefore increase urinary glucose excretion. The unreabsorbed glucose in the renal tubules would also cause an osmotic diuresis, increased urine volume, and decreased extracellular fluid volume, which would stimulate thirst. Increased glucose delivery to the tubules also causes vasodilatation of afferent arterioles, which increases glomerular filtration rate.
TMP11 325, 331, 361

82. (B) GFR is approximately equal to the clearance of creatinine. Creatinine clearance = urine creatinine concentration (32 mg/dl) × urine flow rate (3600 ml/24 hr, or 2.5 ml/min) ÷ plasma creatinine concentration (4 mg/dl) = 20 ml/min.
TMP11 343-347

83. (D) The net renal tubular reabsorption rate is the difference between the filtered load of potassium (glomerular filtration rate × plasma potassium concentration) and the urinary excretion of potassium (urine potassium concentration × urine flow rate). Therefore, the net tubular reabsorption of potassium is 0.075 mmol/min.
TMP11 343-347

84. (D) Severe diarrhea would result in loss of HCO_3^- in the stool, thereby causing metabolic acidosis that is characterized by low plasma HCO_3^- and low pH. Respiratory compensation would reduce PCO_2. The plasma anion gap would be normal, and the plasma chloride concentration would be elevated (hyperchloremic metabolic acidosis) in metabolic acidosis caused by HCO_3^- loss in the stool.
TMP11 397, 400

85. (E) Primary excessive secretion of aldosterone causes metabolic alkalosis due to increased secretion of hydrogen ions by the intercalated cells of the collecting tubules. Therefore, the metabolic alkalosis would be associated with increases in plasma pH and HCO_3^-, with a compensatory reduction in respiration rate and increased PCO_2. The plasma anion gap would be normal, with a slight reduction in plasma chloride concentration.
TMP11 398, 400

86. (D) Proximal tubular acidosis results from a defect of renal secretion of hydrogen ions, reabsorption of bicarbonate, or both. This leads to increased renal excretion of HCO_3^- and metabolic acidosis characterized by low plasma HCO_3^- concentration, low plasma pH, a compensatory increase in respiration rate and low PCO_2, and a normal anion gap with an increased plasma chloride concentration.
TMP11 397, 400

87. (F) A patient with diabetic ketoacidosis and emphysema would be expected to have metabolic acidosis (due to excess ketoacids in the blood caused by diabetes) as well as increased plasma PCO_2 due to impaired pulmonary function. Therefore, the patient would be expected to have decreased plasma pH, decreased HCO_3^-, increased PCO_2, and an increased anion gap ($Na^+ - Cl^- - HCO_3^-$ >10-12 mEq/L) due to the addition of ketoacids to the blood.
TMP11 399, 400

88. (D) Secretion of hydrogen ions and reabsorption of HCO_3^- depend critically on the presence of carbonic anhydrase in the renal tubules. After inhibition of carbonic anhydrase, renal tubular secretion of hydrogen ions and reabsorption of HCO_3^- would decrease, leading to increased renal excretion of HCO_3^-, reduced plasma HCO_3^- concentration, and metabolic acidosis. The metabolic acidosis, in turn, would stimulate the respiration rate, leading to decreased PCO_2. The plasma anion gap would be within the normal range.
TMP11 391, 392, 397, 400

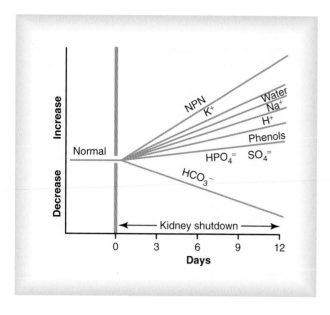

and increased plasma anion gap. The acidosis stimulates respiration, resulting in a compensatory decrease in plasma P_{CO_2}.
TMP11 396, 400

92. (E) Intracellular and extracellular body fluids have the same total osmolarity under steady-state conditions because the cell membrane is highly permeable to water. Therefore, water flows rapidly across the cell membrane until osmotic equilibrium is achieved. The colloid osmotic pressure is determined by the protein concentration, which is considerably higher inside the cell. The cell membrane is also relatively impermeable to potassium, sodium, and chloride, and active transport mechanisms maintain low intracellular concentrations of sodium and chloride and a high intracellular concentration of potassium.
TMP11 296-298

93. (E) Although aldosterone is one of the body's most potent sodium-retaining hormones, it stimulates sodium reabsorption only in the late distal tubule and collecting tubules, which together reabsorb much less than 10 per cent of the filtered load of sodium. Therefore, the maximum percentage of the filtered load of sodium that could be reabsorbed in the distal convoluted tubule and collecting duct, even in the presence of high levels of aldosterone, would be less than 10 per cent.
TMP11 336-338, 342

94. (D) In a dehydrated person, osmolarity in the early distal tubule is less than 300 mOsm/L because the ascending limb of the loop of Henle and the early distal tubule are relatively impermeable to water, even in the presence of ADH. Therefore, the tubular fluid becomes progressively more dilute in these segments, compared with plasma. ADH does not influence water reabsorption in the ascending limb of the loop of Henle. The ascending limb, however, reabsorbs sodium to a much greater extent than does the descending limb. Another important action of ADH is to increase the urea permeability in the medullary collecting ducts, which contributes to the hyperosmotic renal medullary interstitium in antidiuresis.
TMP11 354-356

95. (A) In the proximal tubule, calcium reabsorption usually parallels sodium and water reabsorption. With extracellular volume expansion or increased blood pressure, proximal sodium and water reabsorption is reduced, and there is also a reduction in calcium reabsorption, causing increased urinary excretion of calcium. Increased parathyroid hormone, increased plasma phosphate concentration, and metabolic acidosis all tend to decrease the renal excretion of calcium.
TMP11 371, 372

96. (B) A moderate degree of renal artery stenosis that reduces renal artery pressure distal to the stenosis to 85 mm Hg would result in an autoregulatory response that decreases afferent arteriolar resistance. The decreased renal perfusion pressure would stimulate

89. (B) Acute renal failure caused by tubular nephrosis would cause the rapid development of metabolic acidosis due to the kidneys' failure to rid the body of the acid waste products of metabolism. The metabolic acidosis would lead to a decreased plasma HCO_3^- concentration. Acute renal failure would also lead to a rapid increase in blood urea nitrogen concentration and a significant increase in plasma potassium concentration due to the kidneys' failure to excrete electrolytes or nitrogenous waste products. Necrosis of the renal epithelial cells causes them to slough away from the basement membrane and plug up the renal tubules, thereby increasing hydrostatic pressure in Bowman's capsule and decreasing glomerular filtration rate.
TMP11 406, 411, 412

90. (A) In this example, the plasma sodium concentration is markedly increased, but the urine sodium concentration is relatively normal, and urine osmolarity is almost maximally increased to 1200 mOsm/L. In addition, there are increases in plasma renin, ADH, and aldosterone, which is consistent with dehydration caused by decreased fluid intake. The syndrome of inappropriate ADH would result in a decrease in plasma sodium concentration, as well as suppression of renin and aldosterone secretion. Nephrogenic diabetes insipidus, caused by the kidneys' failure to respond to ADH, would also be associated with dehydration, but urine osmolarity would be reduced rather than increased. Primary aldosteronism would tend to cause sodium and water retention with only a modest change in plasma sodium concentration and a marked reduction in the secretion of renin. Likewise, a renin-secreting tumor would be associated with increases in plasma aldosterone concentration and plasma renin activity, but only a modest change in plasma sodium concentration.
TMP11 348-363

91. (B) This diabetic patient has metabolic acidosis characterized by a low HCO_3^-, decreased plasma pH,

renin secretion, which in turn would increase angiotensin II formation and cause constriction of efferent arterioles. Increased angiotensin II formation would also tend to increase aldosterone secretion.
TMP11 324

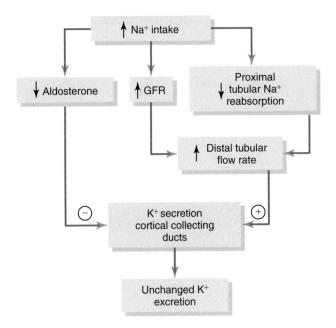

97. (C) Increasing sodium intake would decrease renin secretion and plasma renin activity, as well as reduce plasma aldosterone concentration and increase plasma atrial natriuretic peptide owing to a modest expansion of extracellular fluid volume. Although a high sodium intake would initially increase distal sodium chloride delivery, which would tend to increase potassium excretion, the decrease in aldosterone concentration would offset this effect, resulting in no change in potassium excretion under steady-state conditions. Even very large increases in sodium intake cause only minimal changes in plasma sodium concentration as long as the antidiuretic hormone–thirst mechanisms are fully operative.
TMP11 370, 371

98. (D) This patient is severely dehydrated as a result of sweating and lack of adequate fluid intake. This has also resulted in hyperthermia. The dehydration markedly stimulates the release of ADH and renin secretion, which in turn stimulates the formation of angiotensin II and aldosterone secretion.
TMP11 342, 343, 358, 359

Blood Cells, Immunity, and Blood Clotting

You may refer to the following table of normal test values throughout Unit VI.

Test	Normal Values
Erythrocyte count	Male: 4.3-5.9 million/mm^3
	Female: 3.5-5.5 million/mm^3
Hematocrit	Male: 41-53%
	Female: 36-46%
Hemoglobin, blood	Male: 13.5-17.5 g/dl
	Female: 12.0-16.0 g/dl
Mean corpuscular hemoglobin	25.4-34.6 pg/cell
Mean corpuscular hemoglobin (Hb) concentration	31-36% Hb/cell
Mean corpuscular volume	80-100 fL
Reticulocyte count	0.5-1.5% of red cells
Platelet count	150,000-400,000/mm^3
Leukocyte count and differential	
Leukocyte count	4500-11,000/mm^3
Neutrophils	54-62%
Eosinophils	1-3%
Basophils	0-0.75%
Lymphocytes	25-33%
Monocytes	3-7%
Partial thromboplastin time (activated)	25-40 sec
Prothrombin time	11-15 sec
Bleeding time	2-7 min

1. A 24-year-old man comes to the emergency room with a broken leg. A blood test is ordered, and his white blood cell (WBC) count is 22×10^3/mm^3. Five hours later, a second blood test results in a WBC count of 7×10^3/mm^3. What was the cause of the high WBC count with the first test?
   (A) Increased production of WBCs by the bone marrow
   (B) Shift of WBCs from the marginated pool to the circulating pool
   (C) Decreased destruction of WBCs
   (D) Increased production of selectins

2. What is the proper pathway for the extrinsic clotting pathway?
   (A) Contact of blood with collagen, formation of prothrombin activator, conversion of prothrombin into thrombin, conversion of fibrinogen into fibrin threads
   (B) Tissue trauma, formation of prothrombin activator, conversion of prothrombin into thrombin, conversion of fibrinogen into fibrin threads
   (C) Activation of platelets, formation of prothrombin activator, conversion of prothrombin into thrombin, conversion of fibrinogen into fibrin threads.
   (D) Trauma to the blood, formation of prothrombin activator, conversion of prothrombin into thrombin, conversion of fibrinogen into fibrin threads

3. Which of the following transfusions would result in an immediate transfusion reaction?
   (A) Type O, Rh-negative whole blood to an O, Rh-positive patient
   (B) Type A, Rh-negative whole blood to a B, Rh-negative patient
   (C) Type AB, Rh-negative whole blood to an AB, Rh-positive patient
   (D) Type B, Rh-negative whole blood to a B, Rh-negative patient

4. During the second trimester of pregnancy, where is the predominant site of red blood cell production?
   (A) Yolk sac
   (B) Bone marrow
   (C) Lymph nodes
   (D) Liver

5. Which of the following applies to AIDS patients?
   (A) They are able to generate a normal antibody response
   (B) They have increased helper T cells
   (C) They have increased secretion of interleukins
   (D) They have decreased helper T cells

6. How long do monocytes-macrophages remain in the tissue?
   (A) Several minutes
   (B) Several hours
   (C) Several days
   (D) Several months to years

7. What condition leads to a deficiency in factor IX that can be corrected by an intravenous injection of vitamin K?
   (A) Classic hemophilia
   (B) Hepatitis B
   (C) Bile duct obstruction
   (D) Genetic deficiency in antithrombin III

8. What occurs following presentation of antigen by an infected cell?
   (A) Generation of antibodies
   (B) Activation of cytotoxic T cells
   (C) Increase in phagocytosis
   (D) Release of histamine by mast cells

9. Which of the following is a true statement?
   (A) In a transfusion reaction, there is agglutination of the recipient blood
   (B) Shutdown of the kidneys following a transfusion reaction occurs slowly
   (C) Transfusion of Rh-positive blood into any Rh-negative recipient will result in an immediate transfusion reaction
   (D) A person with type AB blood is considered to be a universal recipient

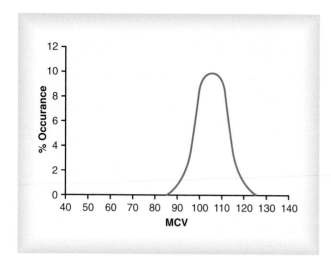

10. A blood sample is taken and the red cells are analyzed for mean corpuscular volume (MCV). Which condition is shown on the graph above?
    (A) Normal red cells
    (B) Acute blood loss
    (C) High vitamin B_{12} diet
    (D) Folic acid deficiency
    (E) Hereditary spherocytosis

11. A patient suffers from a congenital deficiency of factor XIII (fibrin-stabilizing factor). What would analysis of his blood reveal?
    (A) Prolonged prothrombin time
    (B) Prolonged whole blood clotting time
    (C) Prolonged partial thromboplastin time
    (D) Easily breakable clot

12. During an inflammatory response, which is the correct order for cellular events?
    (A) Filtration of monocytes from blood, increased production of neutrophils, activation of tissue macrophages, infiltration of neutrophils from blood
    (B) Activation of tissue macrophages, infiltration of neutrophils from blood, infiltration of monocytes from blood, increased production of neutrophils
    (C) Increased production of neutrophils, activation of tissue macrophages, infiltration of neutrophils from blood, infiltration of monocytes from blood
    (D) Infiltration of neutrophils from blood, activation of tissue macrophages, infiltration of monocytes from blood, increased production of neutrophils

13. Which of the following statements about erythroblastosis fetalis (hemolytic disease of the newborn) is true?
    (A) There is increased folic acid in the fetus
    (B) There are increased numbers of macrophages in the mother
    (C) The erythropoietin level of the fetus is increased
    (D) The free hemoglobin level of the fetus is decreased

14. In a normal, healthy person, which of the following blood components has the shortest life span?
    (A) Macrophages
    (B) Memory T cells
    (C) Erythrocytes
    (D) Memory B lymphocytes

15. A 2-year-old boy bruises easily and has previously had bleeding gums. The maternal grandfather has a bleeding disorder. The boy's physical examination shows several small bruises on the legs. You suspect that this patient has a deficiency of which coagulation factor?
    (A) Prothrombin activator
    (B) Factor II
    (C) Factor VIII
    (D) Factor X

16. A previously healthy 45-year-old woman is admitted to the hospital because of lower gastrointestinal bleeding for 3 days. She has a hematocrit of 25 per cent. Her blood type is O, Rh-positive. Three units of blood are administered over a 3-day period. During administration of a fourth unit, she develops shortness of breath and severe back pain. Her temperature is elevated, she is hypotensive, and she has reddish brown urine. Which of the following is the most likely cause of these findings?
    (A) ABO transfusion incompatibility
    (B) Bacterial contamination of the fourth unit of blood
    (C) Rh factor incompatibility
    (D) Elevated IgE

17. A 65-year-old man complains of dizziness and visual disturbances. His laboratory values are as follows:
    Red blood cell count = $8.5 \times 10^6/mm^3$
    Hemoglobin = 21 g/dl
    Hematocrit = 60 per cent
    Plasma osmolality = 295 mOsm/L
    What is the most likely explanation for this presentation?
    (A) End-stage renal disease
    (B) Polycythemia
    (C) Vitamin B_{12} deficiency
    (D) Dehydration

18. A 45-year-old man presents to the emergency room with a 2-week history of diarrhea that has gotten progressively worse over the last several days. He has minimal urine output and is admitted to the hospital for dehydration. His stool specimen is positive for parasitic eggs. Which type of white blood cells would be elevated in number?
    (A) Eosinophils
    (B) Neutrophils
    (C) T lymphocytes
    (D) B lymphocytes
    (E) Monocytes

19. A 40-year-old woman visits a clinic complaining of fatigue. She has recently been treated for an infection. Her laboratory values are as follows:
    Red blood cell count = $1.8 \times 10^6/mm^3$
    Hemoglobin = 5.2 g/dl
    Hematocrit = 15 per cent
    White blood cell count = $7.6 \times 10^3/mm^3$
    Platelet count = 320,000/mm^3
    Mean corpuscular volume = 92 fL
    Reticulocyte count = 24 per cent
    What is the most likely explanation for this presentation?
    (A) Aplastic anemia
    (B) Hemolytic anemia
    (C) Hereditary spherocytosis
    (D) Vitamin B_{12} deficiency

20. A healthy 3-year-old girl is brought to the emergency department because of a severe, uncontrolled nosebleed. Six months ago, she had an ear infection that improved after treatment. Her temperature is 39°C. Her color is pale, and she has numerous small bruises on her arms and legs. Her laboratory values are as follows:
    Hemoglobin = 4.6 g/dl
    Leukocyte count = 4000/mm^3
    Reticulocyte count = 0.1 per cent
    Platelet count = 14,000/mm^3
    Which of the following is the most likely explanation for these findings?
    (A) Anemia due to blood loss
    (B) Aplastic anemia
    (C) Sickle cell disease
    (D) Mononucleosis

21. What is the term for adhesion of an invading microbe with IgG and complement to facilitate recognition?
    (A) Chemokinesis
    (B) Opsonization
    (C) Phagolysosome fusion
    (D) Signal transduction

22. Which of the following substances cannot prevent coagulation when added to a blood sample (i.e., in a test tube)?
    (A) Heparin
    (B) Citrate
    (C) Coumarins
    (D) Calcium chelators

23. A 34-year-old man with schizophrenia has had chronic fatigue for 6 months. He has a good appetite but has refused to eat vegetables for 1 year because he hears voices that tell him the vegetables are poisoned. His physical and neurological examinations are normal. His hemoglobin level is 9.1 g/dl, leukocyte count is 10,000/mm^3, and mean corpuscular volume is 122. Which of the following is the most likely diagnosis?
    (A) Acute blood loss
    (B) Sickle cell
    (C) Aplastic anemia
    (D) Hemolytic anemia
    (E) Folic acid deficiency

24. Interleukin-2 (IL-2) is an important molecule in the immune response. What is its function?
    (A) It binds to and presents antigen
    (B) It stimulates proliferation of cytotoxic T cells
    (C) It kills virus-infected cells
    (D) It is required for proliferation of helper T cells.

25. A patient presents with a platelet count of $275 \times 10^3/mm^3$ and a bleeding time of 5 minutes. What is the diagnosis?
    (A) Decreased platelet production
    (B) Defective platelet function
    (C) Increased platelet production
    (D) Normal platelet function

26. What is the cause of the initial increase in fluid filtration in the acute inflammatory reaction?
    (A) Increased vascular permeability
    (B) Decreased vascular oncotic pressure
    (C) Increased interstitial oncotic pressure
    (D) Decreased interstitial hydrostatic pressure
    (E) Increased lymphatic pumping

27. A 24-year-old African American man comes to the emergency room 3 hours after the onset of severe back and chest pain, which started while he was skiing. He lives in Los Angeles and had an episode of the same symptoms 5 years ago while visiting Wyoming. He is in obvious pain. Laboratory studies show the following:
    Hemoglobin = 11 g/dl
    Leukocyte count = 22,000/mm^3
    Reticulocyte count = 25 per cent
    What is the diagnosis of this patient?
    (A) Acute blood loss
    (B) Sickle cell anemia
    (C) Anemia of chronic disease
    (D) End-stage renal disease

28. Which cells secrete circulating antibodies?
    (A) T helper lymphocytes
    (B) T suppressor lymphocytes
    (C) Dormant B lymphocytes
    (D) Plasma cells
    (E) T killer lymphocytes

29. Which of the following treatments would prevent a transfusion reaction?
    (A) Administration of plasma-free blood
    (B) Administration of washed erythrocytes
    (C) Treatment with immunoglobulins
    (D) Treatment with mannitol
    (E) Strict adherence to labeling and identification

30. A 63-year-old woman returned to work following a vacation in New Zealand. Several days afterward, she awoke with swelling and pain in her right leg, which was blue. She immediately went to the emergency room, where an examination showed an extensive deep vein thrombosis involving the femoral and iliac veins on the right side. Following resolution of the clot, this patient will require which treatment?
    (A) Continual heparin infusion
    (B) Warfarin
    (C) Aspirin
    (D) Vitamin K

31. A 62-year-old man complains of headaches, visual difficulties, and chest pain. His examination shows a red complexion and a large spleen. A complete blood count shows the following:
    Hematocrit = 58 per cent
    White blood cell count = 13,300/mm^3
    Platelets = 600,000/mm^3
    His arterial oxygen saturation is 97 per cent on room air. Which of the following would you recommend as treatment?
    (A) Chemotherapy
    (B) Phlebotomy
    (C) Iron supplement
    (D) Inhaled oxygen therapy

32. Which of the following would most likely be used for prophylaxis of transient ischemic heart attack?
    (A) Heparin
    (B) Warfarin
    (C) Aspirin
    (D) Streptokinase

33. A 45-year-old woman developed fatigue in July but reportedly had normal blood counts. She is hospitalized with a severe headache in December and has a blood pressure of 175/90 mm Hg. Her laboratory values are as follows:
    Hemoglobin = 8.3 g/dl
    Red blood cell count = 2.2 × 10^6/mm^3
    Hematocrit = 23 per cent
    Mean corpuscular volume = 89 fL
    White blood cell count = 5100/mm^3
    Platelets = 262 × 10^3/mm^3
    Reticulocyte count = 0.8 per cent
    What is the diagnosis for this patient?
    (A) Folic acid deficiency
    (B) Iron deficiency
    (C) Hemolytic anemia
    (D) End-stage renal disease

34. Which of the following is appropriate therapy for massive pulmonary embolism?
    (A) Heparin
    (B) Warfarin
    (C) Aspirin
    (D) Tissue plasminogen activator

Questions 35-38

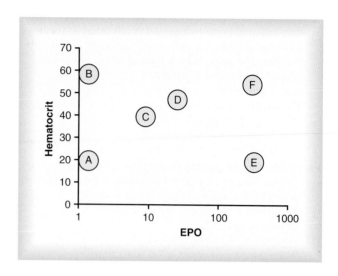

Which point on the graph above most closely defines the following conditions? Normal erythropoietin (EPO) levels are approximately 10.

35. Olympic marathoner ( )

36. Aplastic anemia ( )

37. End-stage renal disease ( )

38. Polycythemia vera ( )

39. Where does the transmigration of white blood cells occur in response to infectious agents?
    (A) Arterioles
    (B) Lymphatic ducts
    (C) Venules
    (D) Inflamed arteries

40. What happens following presentation of antigen by a macrophage?
    (A) Direct generation of antibodies
    (B) Activation of cytotoxic T cells
    (C) Increase in phagocytosis
    (D) Activation of helper T cells

41. Which of the following statements concerning erythroblastosis fetalis (hemolytic disease of the newborn) is true?
    (A) It occurs when an Rh-positive mother has an Rh-negative child
    (B) It is prevented by giving the mother a blood transfusion
    (C) A complete blood transfusion of the first child after birth will prevent the disease
    (D) The father of the child has to be Rh-positive

42. A 65-year-old alcoholic develops chest pain and a cough with the expectoration of sputum. A blood sample reveals that his white blood cell count is 42,000/mm^3. What is the origin of these white blood cells?
    (A) Pulmonary alveoli
    (B) Bronchioles
    (C) Bronchi
    (D) Trachea
    (E) Bone marrow

43. An 85-year-old African American woman complains of feeling tired during the day and sleeping more than she did in the past. She quit smoking 20 years ago, and she has been treated for hypertension and chronic obstructive pulmonary disease for the past several years. In the past year, her mean corpuscular volume has increased from 91 to 100. She is not overweight. Her blood work is as follows:
Hemoglobin = 13 g/dl
Hematocrit = 39 per cent
Mean corpuscular volume = 100 fL
White blood cell count and differential = normal
Platelet count = within normal limits
What would you do for the patient at this time?
    (A) Treat with erythropoietin
    (B) Treat with vitamin B_{12}
    (C) Treat with iron supplements
    (D) Do nothing
    (E) Give a blood transfusion

44. Which of the following best explains a prolonged bleeding time test?
    (A) Hemophilia A
    (B) Hemophilia B
    (C) Thrombocytopenia
    (D) Coumarin use

45. Which of the following would result in a transfusion reaction? Assume that the patient has never had a transfusion.
    (A) Type O, Rh-negative packed cells to an AB, Rh-positive patient
    (B) Type A, Rh-positive packed cells to an A, Rh-negative patient
    (C) Type AB, Rh-positive packed cells to an AB, Rh-positive patient
    (D) Type A, Rh-positive packed cells to an O, Rh-positive patient

46. Activation of the complement system results in which of the following actions?
    (A) Binding of the invading microbe with IgG
    (B) Inactivation of eosinophils
    (C) Decreased tissue levels of complement
    (D) Generation of chemotaxic substances

47. A healthy mother with type A-positive blood has just delivered her second child. The father's blood type is O-negative. Knowing that the child has type O, Rh-negative blood, what would you expect to find?
    (A) The child will have erythroblastosis fetalis due to Rh incompatibility
    (B) The child will have erythroblastosis fetalis due to ABO blood group incompatibility
    (C) The child will have both (A) and (B)
    (D) The child has no chance of developing erythroblastosis fetalis

48. A patient presents complaining of extreme fatigue and shortness of breath on exertion that has gradually worsened over the past 2 weeks. On physical examination, you observe a well-nourished woman who appears to be comfortable but somewhat short of breath. Her vital signs include a pulse of 120, respiratory rate of 20, and blood pressure of 120/70. When she stands up, her pulse increases to 150 and her blood pressure falls to 80/50. Her hematological values are as follows:
Hemoglobin = 7 g/dl
Hematocrit = 20 per cent
Red blood cell count = $2 \times 10^6/mm^3$
Platelet count = $400,000/mm^3$
On a peripheral smear, her red blood cells are microcytic and hypochromic. What is your diagnosis?
    (A) Aplastic anemia
    (B) Renal failure
    (C) Iron deficiency anemia
    (D) Sickle cell anemia
    (E) Megaloblastic anemia

49. A 26-year-old man received a paper cut. What substance is the major cause of pain in this acute inflammatory response?
    (A) Platelet-activating factor
    (B) Bradykinin
    (C) Interleukin-1
    (D) Tumor necrosis factor

50. Why do some malnourished patients bleed excessively when injured?
    (A) Vitamin K deficiency
    (B) Platelet sequestration by fatty liver
    (C) Increased serum bilirubin, neutralizing thrombin
    (D) Low serum protein levels, causing factor XIII problems

51. What causes the release of histamine in an allergic reaction?
    (A) Binding of IgM to basophils
    (B) Binding of IgE to mast cells
    (C) Release of histamine by helper T cells
    (D) Free radical stimulation of endothelial cells

52. After a person is placed in an atmosphere with low oxygen, how long does it take for the number of reticulocytes to increase?
    (A) 6 hours
    (B) 12 hours
    (C) 3 days
    (D) 5 days
    (E) 2 weeks

53. Which of the following blood units carries the least risk of inducing an immediate transfusion reaction in a type B, Rh-positive recipient?
    (A) Type A-positive whole blood
    (B) Type O-positive whole blood
    (C) Type AB-positive whole blood
    (D) Type O-positive packed red cells
    (E) Type AB-negative packed red cells

54. A dentist notices a sore on his patient's lip. The sore is unusual, in that there is no pain or drainage. The patient is subsequently admitted to the hospital with a violent shaking chill. His laboratory values are as follows:
Hematocrit = 30 per cent
Platelets = 400,000/mm^3
White blood cell count = 3100/mm^3
Lymphocytes = 68 per cent
Neutrophils = 20 per cent
What is the diagnosis?
(A) Mild, nontreatable infection
(B) Leukopenia
(C) Aplastic anemia
(D) Acute leukemia

55. Which of the following applies to cytotoxic T cells?
(A) They require the presence of a competent B-lymphocyte system
(B) They require the presence of a competent suppressor T-lymphocyte system
(C) They are activated by the presentation of antigen by an infected cell
(D) They destroy bacteria by initiating macrophage phagocytosis

56. What occurs following activation of basophils?
(A) Decreased diapedesis of neutrophils
(B) Decreased ameboid motion
(C) Contraction of blood vessels
(D) Increased capillary permeability

57. Over the past 12 weeks, a 75-year-old man with moderate aortic stenosis has developed shortness of breath and chest pain during exertion. He appears pale. His stool tests positive for blood. Laboratory studies show the following:
Hemoglobin = 7.2 g/dl
Mean corpuscular volume = 75 fL
A blood smear shows microcytic, hypochromic erythrocytes. Which of the following is the most likely diagnosis?
(A) Vitamin B$_{12}$ deficiency
(B) Autoimmune hemolytic anemia
(C) Folate deficiency anemia
(D) Iron deficiency anemia

58. A pregnant woman is blood type AB, Rh-negative; her husband is type A, Rh-positive.
This is her first child. What should be done?
(A) Nothing
(B) Administer anti-D immunoglobulin to the mother now
(C) Administer anti-D immunoglobulin to the mother after delivery if the child is Rh-positive
(D) Administer anti-D immunoglobulin to the child after delivery
(E) Administer anti-D immunoglobulin to the child if the child is Rh-positive

59. How long do neutrophils remain in the tissue of a healthy human?
(A) Several minutes
(B) Several hours
(C) Several days
(D) Several months to years

60. A 10-year-old boy with a prolonged prothrombin time (25 seconds; control, 11 to 15 seconds) is referred to a hematologist before undergoing surgery. The patient's bleeding time is normal. Which coagulation system is abnormal in this case?
(A) Platelet production
(B) Platelet function
(C) Extrinsic pathway
(D) Generation of clotting factors by the liver

Answers

1. (B) The majority of WBCs are stored in the bone marrow, waiting for an increased level of cytokines to stimulate their release. However, trauma to bone can result in a release of WBCs into the circulation. This increase in WBC count is due to mechanical trauma, not an inflammatory response.
TMP11 431

2. (B) The extrinsic pathway involves damage to the tissue, then the subsequent formation of prothrombin activator. Tissue trauma results in the release of tissue factor or tissue thromboplastin, which functions as a proteolytic enzyme. The binding of tissue factor with factor VII results in an activation of factor X. There is a subsequent activation of prothrombin activator, conversion of prothrombin to thrombin, and conversion of fibrinogen into fibrin threads. Activation of the extrinsic pathway is very fast because of the small number of enzymatic reactions.
TMP11 459-462

3. (B) Transfusion of Rh-negative blood into an Rh-positive person with the same ABO type will not result in any reaction. Type A blood has A antigen on the surface and type B antibodies. Type B blood has B antigens and A antibodies. Therefore, transfusing type A blood into a person with type B blood will cause the A antibodies in the type B person to react with the donor blood.
TMP11 453-455

4. (D) Red blood cell production begins in the yolk sac during the first trimester. Production in the yolk sac decreases at the beginning of the second trimester, and the liver becomes the predominant source of red cell production. During the third trimester, red cell production increases from the bone marrow and continues throughout life.
TMP11 420

5. (D) Helper T cells are destroyed by the AIDS virus, leaving the patient unprotected against infectious diseases.
TMP11 447

6. (D) Monocytes circulate and then move into the interstitium, where they expand to become macrophages. Macrophages, if not activated, can remain in the tissue for the life of a person.
TMP11 431-433

7. (C) Hemophilia is due to a genetic loss of clotting factor VIII. Most clotting factors are formed in the liver. If a vitamin K injection can correct the problem, this implies that the liver is working and that the patient does not have hepatitis. Vitamin K is a fat-soluble vitamin and is absorbed from the intestine, along with fats. Bile secreted by the gallbladder is required for the absorption of fats. If the patient is deficient in vitamin K, the clotting deficiency can be corrected by an injection of vitamin K. Antithrombin III has no relationship to factor IX.
   TMP11 464-465

8. (B) Presentation of an antigen on an infected cell results in activation of the cytotoxic T cells to kill the infected cell. Presentation of an antigen by macrophages activates helper T cells, leading to antibody formation.
   TMP11 446-448

9. (D) The recipient blood has the greater amount of plasma and thus antibodies. These antibodies act on the donor red blood cells. The donor's plasma is diluted and has a minimal effect on the recipient's red blood cells. With any antigen-antibody transfusion reaction, there is a rapid breakdown of red blood cells, releasing hemoglobin into the plasma, which can cause rapid and acute renal shutdown. Transfusion of Rh-positive blood will result in a transfusion reaction only if the Rh-negative person was previously transfused or exposed to Rh-positive antibodies. A type AB person has no AB antibodies in the plasma, so he or she can receive any blood type.
   TMP11 454, 455

10. (D) Normal red cells have an MCV of 90 fL. The red cells shown in the graph have an increased MCV and are considered to be macrocytic. There are several conditions that could cause macrocytic red cells, including vitamin B_{12} and folic acid deficiency. With acute blood loss, red cell production is increased, and the cells are normal or slightly smaller. Hereditary spherocytosis is a condition in which the red blood cells are rounded and smaller.
    TMP11 427

11. (D) Fibrin monomers polymerize to form a clot. A strong clot requires the presence of fibrin-stabilizing factor, which is released from platelets within the clot. The other clotting tests determine the activation of extrinsic and intrinsic pathways or the number of platelets.
    TMP11 457, 458, 460, 467-468

12. (B) The first cellular event during an inflammatory state is activation of the tissue macrophages. This is followed by invasion of neutrophils and monocytes, in that order, and finally there is an increase in the production of white blood cells by the bone marrow.
    TMP11 434, 435

13. (C) In erythroblastosis fetalis, an antigen-antibody reaction in the fetus results in the destruction of red

blood cells and an increase in free hemoglobin. There is no increase in folic acid. There is no immune response in the mother because the fetal red blood cells do not cross the placenta. Because the fetus is anemic, the erythropoietin level will be elevated.
   TMP11 454

14. (C) Macrophages last for many years. T and B memory cells last the life of an individual. Erythrocytes last about 120 days and are then destroyed during passage through the spleen.
    TMP11 431

15. (C) A young boy with a bleeding disorder and a family history of bleeding disorders in male relatives would lead one to suspect hemophilia A, a deficiency of factor VIII.
    TMP11 465

16. (A) The patient exhibits the classic signs of an ABO transfusion reaction. She had an immediate and massive immune response resulting in the destruction of red blood cells, release of hemoglobin into the plasma, and excretion of hemoglobin in the urine. Bacterial complications take place over time. Antigen–antibody reactions to minor blood groups result in minor immune reactions.
    TMP11 454, 455

17. (B) The patient presents with an elevated hematocrit and increased hemoglobin concentration. The laboratory values show increased production of red blood cells by the bone marrow. Patients with end-stage renal disease or vitamin B_{12} deficiency are anemic. Dehydration could result in an increased hematocrit, but this patient's osmolality is normal, so he is not dehydrated. Polycythemia results in an increase in red blood cells, which is the condition of this patient.
    TMP11 427, 428

18. (A) Eosinophils constitute about 2 per cent of the total white blood cell count, but they are produced in large numbers in people with parasitic infections.
    TMP11 436

19. (B) This patient has a decreased number of red blood cells, as confirmed by the anemia (low hemoglobin and hematocrit), yet the red blood cells being produced have a normal size (mean corpuscular volume = 92). Therefore, the patient does not have spherocytosis (small red cells) or vitamin B_{12} deficiency (large red cells). The normal white blood cell count and the increased reticulocyte count suggest that the bone marrow is functioning. The increased reticulocyte count means that a large number of red cells are being produced. These laboratory values support an anemia due to some type of blood loss—in this case, an anemia due to hemolysis.
    TMP11 427

20. (B) This patient has a severely decreased number of blood cells, including red cells, white cells, and

platelets. The low reticulocyte count shows that she is not producing any red blood cells. Her bone marrow is not producing any cells; therefore, she has aplastic anemia.

TMP11 426, 427

21. (B) One of the products of the complement cascade activates phagocytosis of the bacteria to which the antigen–antibody complex is attached. This is called opsonization.

TMP11 445

22. (C) The clotting process involves the formation of thrombin. Additionally, calcium is involved in the clotting cascade. Any compound that decreases thrombin or calcium will prevent clotting. Heparin is used to prevent clot formation by binding to antithrombin III and the subsequent inactivation of thrombin. Citrate and calcium chelators bind calcium and prevent the clotting cascade. Coumarins prevent the clotting process in vivo by inhibiting the formation of vitamin K–dependent clotting factors in the liver. Coumarins have no effect on already formed clotting factors that would be present in blood in a test tube.

TMP11 466, 467

23. (E) This patient is anemic (hemoglobin <14 g/dl). The white count is normal, suggesting a normal bone marrow. His red cells are considerably larger than normal (normal mean corpuscular volume = 90). The lack of vegetables in his diet suggests either a vitamin B_{12} or a folic acid deficiency. However, the body has sufficient stores of vitamin B_{12} to last 4 to 5 years. The body stores folic acid for only 3 to 6 months, so 1 year of not eating vegetables would result in folic acid deficiency.

TMP11 423, 427

24. (B) IL-2 is secreted by helper T cells when the T cells are activated by specific antigens. IL-2 plays a specific role in the growth and proliferation of both cytotoxic and suppressor T cells, and activation of helper T cells.

TMP11 447

25. (D) The normal platelet count is between 150,000 and 400,000. The bleeding time is used to test platelet function, and a normal value is between 2 and 7 minutes. This patient is within the normal range for both values.

TMP11 457, 467

26. (A) All the options increase fluid filtration under normal circumstances. However, in the acute inflammatory phase, there is a release of several tissue products, including histamine and bradykinin, which increases vascular permeability.

TMP11 434

27. (B) This African American man has anemia, as determined by his decreased hemoglobin concentration and elevated reticulocyte count. He also has some type of infectious or inflammatory response, as

evidenced by the elevated white cell count. The high altitude was the stimulus for a hypoxic episode that caused sickling of his red cells. This patient has sickle cell anemia.

TMP11 427

28. (D) Upon exposure to a specific antigen, B lymphocytes enlarge and differentiate into lymphoblasts. Some lymphoblasts differentiate into plasmablasts, which are the precursors of plasma cells. The mature plasma cells then produce gamma globulins at an extremely rapid rate.

TMP11 443

29. (E) Transfusion reactions are caused by an immune response. The health care provider should make sure that an immune response is unlikely. The only way to do this is to make sure that the patient receives a compatible blood type.

TMP11 455

30. (B) This clot is due to stasis of blood flow in the venous circulation (likely caused by the long plane ride from New Zealand). Heparin is used for the prevention of clot formation; this anticoagulation occurs when heparin binds to antithrombin III, leading to the subsequent inactivation of thrombin. A continuous heparin infusion would be impractical, however. Warfarin is used to inhibit the formation of vitamin K clotting factors and would prevent the formation of any clot. Aspirin is used to prevent the activation of platelets, but the current clot is not due to platelet activation. Vitamin K would be used to restore clotting factors that may be decreased after warfarin treatment, but this patient has sufficient clotting factors, as evidenced by her venous clot.

TMP11 465-466

31. (B) This patient has polycythemia vera: increased red blood cells, white blood cells, and platelets. His increased hematocrit also increases the viscosity of the blood, resulting in an increased afterload for the heart. This is probably the reason for his chest pain. Thus, a phlebotomy (bleeding) is needed to decrease the elevated blood count.

TMP11 428

32. (C) Heparin is used for the prevention of clot formation (binding to antithrombin III and the subsequent inactivation of thrombin), but it has to be infused, making it impractical. Warfarin is used to inhibit the formation of vitamin K clotting factors, and takes time (days) to take effect. Aspirin is used to prevent the activation of platelets; platelet activation following exposure to atherosclerotic plaque and the formation of a platelet plug impede blood flow and result in an ischemic heart attack. Streptokinase is used to break down an already formed clot, which is appropriate therapy for a pulmonary embolus.

TMP11 457, 458, 463, 464, 466, 467

33. (D) This patient is anemic, but the red blood cells being produced are normal (normal mean corpuscu-

lar volume). The overall production of red blood cells is decreased (low reticulocyte count). White blood cells and platelets are normal, suggesting a normal bone marrow. Folic acid and iron deficiency anemia would result in a lower mean corpuscular volume. Hemolytic anemia would result in an increased reticulocyte count. The elevated blood pressure provides evidence of renal disease. This patient has end-stage renal disease and decreased erythropoietin production.
TMP11 423

34. (D) Heparin is used for the prevention of a clot; this occurs by binding to antithrombin III and the subsequent inactivation of thrombin. Warfarin is used to inhibit the formation of vitamin K clotting factors. Aspirin is used to prevent the activation of platelets. Tissue plasminogen activator is used to break down an already formed clot, which is appropriate therapy for a pulmonary embolus.
TMP11 457, 458, 465, 466

35. (D) A well-trained athlete will have a slightly elevated EPO level, and the hematocrit will be elevated up to a value of 50 per cent. A hematocrit higher than 50 per cent suggests EPO treatment.
TMP11 427

36. (E) In aplastic anemia, bone marrow production is decreased, but it does not respond to EPO. Therefore, a person with aplastic anemia would have a low hematocrit and an elevated EPO level.
TMP11 426

37. (A) With end-stage renal disease, the EPO level is decreased owing to impaired release from the diseased kidneys. As a result of the decreased EPO level, the hematocrit will be decreased.
TMP11 422, 423

38. (B) With polycythemia vera, the bone marrow produces red blood cells without a stimulus from EPO. The hematocrit is very high, even up to 60 per cent. With the elevated hematocrit, there is a feedback suppression of EPO, so the EPO level is very low.
TMP11 427, 428

39. (C) Transmigration of white blood cells occurs through parts of the vasculature that have very thin walls and minimal vascular smooth muscle layers. This includes capillaries and venules.
TMP11 431, 434, 435

40. (D) Presentation of an antigen on the surface of macrophages or dendritic cells results in the activation of helper T cells. Activation of helper T cells then initiates the release of lymphokines, which stimulates cytotoxic T-cell activation along with the activation of B cells and the generation of antibodies.
TMP11 446, 447

41. (D) Hemolytic disease of the newborn occurs when an Rh-negative mother gives birth to a second Rh-positive child. Therefore, the father has to be Rh-positive. The mother becomes sensitized to the Rh antigens following the birth of the first Rh-positive child. Hemolytic disease of the newborn is prevented by treating the mother with antibodies against Rh antigen after the birth of each Rh-positive child. This destroys all fetal red blood cells in the mother and prevents her from being sensitized to the Rh antigen. A complete blood transfusion of the mother would be required to prevent the formation of Rh antibodies, but that is impractical. A transfusion of the first child after birth would not accomplish anything, because the mother was exposed to the Rh-positive antigen during the birth process.
TMP11 454

42. (E) All white blood cells originate from the bone marrow, from myelocytes or lymphocytes.
TMP11 430, 431

43. (D) This is an elderly patient who, except for a slightly elevated MCV, has normal hematological values. Her slightly high MCV may suggest a vitamin B_{12} or folic acid deficiency; however, if there is a deficiency, it has not led to any type of anemia. Appropriate treatment would be to follow the patient to see whether she develops anemia. Her fatigue may be a consequence of her age and pulmonary disease.
TMP11 423-428

44. (C) There are three major tests used to determine coagulation defects. Prothrombin time is used to test the extrinsic pathway and is based on the time required for the formation of a clot following the addition of tissue thromboplastin. Bleeding time following a small cut is used to test for several clotting factors, but it is especially prolonged by a lack of platelets. Partial thromboplastin time is used to test the intrinsic pathway and is based on the addition of plasma thromboplastin to blood.
TMP11 467, 468

45. (D) Type O red blood cells are considered to be universal donor blood. Reactions occur between the recipient antibody and the donor antigen as shown in the following table:

Donor	Donor Antigen	Recipient	Recipient Antibody	Reaction
O–	None	AB+	None	None
A+	A, Rh	A–	B	None
AB+	A, B, Rh	AB+	None	None
A+	A, Rh	O+	A, B	A (antigen) and A (antibody)

TMP11 452, 453

46. (D) Activation of the complement system results in a series of actions. These include opsonization and phagocytosis by neutrophils, lysis of bacteria, agglutination of organisms, activation of basophils and mast cells, and chemotaxis. Fragment C5a of the complement system causes chemotaxis of neutrophils and macrophages.
TMP11 444, 445

47. (D) Erythroblastosis fetalis occurs when the mother is Rh-negative and the father is Rh-positive, resulting in an Rh-negative child. Because the child is O-negative and the father is Rh-negative, there is no chance of the disease.
    TMP11 454

48. (C) The blood count values show that the patient is anemic. Her bone marrow is functioning and she has a normal platelet count, but she is generating a decreased number of abnormal red blood cells (RBCs). The finding of microcytic (small), hypochromic (decreased intracellular hemoglobin) RBCs is classic for iron deficiency anemia. With renal failure, the patient would be anemic with normal RBCs. Sickle cell anemia results in mis-shapen RBCs. Megaloblastic anemia is characterized by macrocytic (large) RBCs.
    TMP11 423-427

49. (B) There are several factors that can cause and initiate pain. These include histamine, bradykinin, and prostaglandins. Platelet-activating factor activates platelets during the clotting process. Interleukin and tumor necrosis factor are involved in the inflammatory response and control of macrophages.
    TMP11 434, 435

50. (A) The clotting factors are formed in the liver and require vitamin K. Vitamin K is a fat-soluble vitamin, and its absorption is dependent on adequate fat digestion and absorption. Therefore, any state of malnutrition would result in decreased fat absorption, leading to decreased vitamin K absorption and decreased synthesis of clotting factors.
    TMP11 464, 465

51. (B) The allergic tendency is passed from parent to child and is characterized by large quantities of IgE antibodies in the plasma. One characteristic of IgE antibodies is the attachment to mast cells and basophils. When an allergen (antigen) binds to IgE, there is a release of granules containing histamine and other factors from the mast cells.
    TMP11 444, 449

52. (C) Erythropoietin levels increase following a decreased arterial oxygen level, with maximal erythropoietin production occurring within 24 hours. It takes 5 days for the production of new erythrocytes, and it takes 1 to 2 days for a reticulocyte to become an erythrocyte. Therefore, the correct answer is 3 days until there are increased numbers of reticulocytes.
    TMP11 422

53. (D) In any patient, transfusion of type O packed cells would minimize the chance of a transfusion reaction because the antibodies are removed along with the plasma. If the Rh factor is matched, this would also minimize the possibility of a transfusion reaction. Therefore, in a B-positive patient, an O-positive transfusion (as well as a B-positive transfusion) would elicit no transfusion reaction.
    TMP11 452-454

54. (B) The patient has a slightly decreased red cell count and a normal platelet count. This suggests that the bone marrow is working properly. His white count is low, and the percentage of cells is not normal. He should have 60 per cent neutrophils. The 68 per cent lymphocytes (normal = 30 per cent) suggests that the patient has leukopenia.
    TMP11 436-437

55. (C) Cytotoxic cells act on infected cells when the cells have the appropriate antigen located on the surface. Cytotoxic T cells are stimulated by lymphokines generated by the activation of helper T cells. Cytotoxic T cells destroy infected cells by releasing proteins that punch large holes in the membrane of the infected cells. There is no interaction between cytotoxic T cells and B cells.
    TMP11 447-448

56. (D) Basophils release heparin, histamine, and a series of activating factors. The histamine acts to increase capillary permeability, and the heparin prevents clotting. Substances released from basophils also attract neutrophils.
    TMP11 436

57. (D) This patient is anemic; he has low hemoglobin and small red blood cells (RBCs). Vitamin B_{12} and folic acid deficiency would result in macrocytic RBCs. His white blood cell and platelet counts are normal, suggesting normal bone marrow. The positive stool shows a gastrointestinal blood loss. A person can be anemic from blood loss and have normal-size RBCs as long as there is enough iron in the body. The microcytic and hypochromic RBCs are classic signs of iron deficiency anemia.
    TMP11 425-427

58. (C) An Rh-negative mother will generate antibodies to Rh-positive red blood cells (RBCs) after the birth of her first child that is Rh-positive. In the scenario presented, the mother has not been exposed to Rh-positive RBCs, so she has not developed antibodies. However, after the birth of this child, if the child is found to be Rh-positive, anti-D immunoglobulin should be administered to the mother to destroy any fetal RBCs and to prevent her from forming antibodies to the Rh-positive D antigen.
    TMP11 454

59. (C) Neutrophils circulate 4 to 8 hours in the blood and then enter the tissue, where they remain for another 4 to 5 days. Monocytes-macrophages remain in the tissue for months.
    TMP11 431

60. (C) The prothrombin time is the time required for clot formation following the addition of tissue thromboplastin. Because the extrinsic pathway is short, only two factors—X and prothrombin activator—are activated before the activation of prothrombin. Thus, in the extrinsic pathway, the time for prothrombin activation is short; and the prothrombin time is the same as the activation time of the extrinsic pathway. Because the boy's prothrombin time is longer than normal, there is a defect in the extrinsic pathway.

TMP11 467, 468

Respiration

1. A 67-year-old man is admitted to University Hospital because of severe chest pain. A Swan-Ganz catheter is floated into the pulmonary artery, the balloon is inflated, and the pulmonary wedge pressure is measured. The pulmonary wedge pressure is used clinically to monitor which of the following pressures?
   (A) Left atrial pressure
   (B) Left ventricular pressure
   (C) Pulmonary artery diastolic pressure
   (D) Pulmonary artery systolic pressure
   (E) Pulmonary capillary pressure

2. Which of the following sets of differences best describes the hemodynamics of the pulmonary circulation when compared with the systemic circulation?

	Flow	Resistance	Arterial Pressure
(A)	Higher	Higher	Higher
(B)	Higher	Lower	Lower
(C)	Lower	Higher	Lower
(D)	Lower	Lower	Lower
(E)	Same	Higher	Lower
(F)	Same	Lower	Lower

3. A 43-year-old woman is biking in the mountains, where the atmospheric pressure is 700 mm Hg and the relative humidity is close to zero. What is the partial pressure of oxygen and nitrogen in the mountain air?

	Oxygen (mm Hg)	Nitrogen (mm Hg)
(A)	100	500
(B)	110	590
(C)	133	576
(D)	147	553
(E)	92	608

4. A healthy, 45-year-old man is reading the newspaper. Which of the following muscles are used for quiet breathing?
   (A) Diaphragm and external intercostals
   (B) Diaphragm and internal intercostals
   (C) Diaphragm only
   (D) Internal intercostals and rectus abdominis
   (E) Scalene muscles
   (F) Sternocleidomastoid muscles

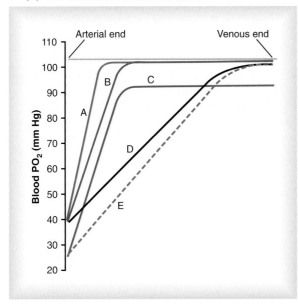

5. A 32-year-old medical student has a fourfold increase in cardiac output during strenuous exercise. Which of the curves on the previous diagram best represents the changes in oxygen tension that occur as blood flows from the arterial end to the venous end of the pulmonary capillaries in this student? ( )

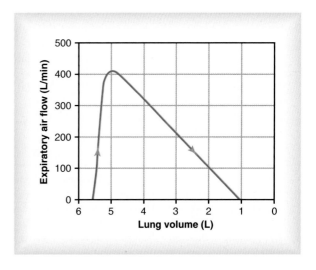

6. A 45-year-old man inhales as much air as possible and then expires with a maximum effort until no more air can be expired. This produces the maximum expiratory flow-volume curve shown in the diagram above. What is the forced vital capacity of this man?
   (A) 1.5 liters
   (B) 2.5 liters
   (C) 3.5 liters
   (D) 4.5 liters
   (E) 5.5 liters
   (F) 6.5 liters

7. The basic rhythm of respiration is generated by neurons located in the medulla. Which of the following limits the duration of inspiration and increases respiratory rate?
   (A) Apneustic center
   (B) Dorsal respiratory group
   (C) Nucleus of the tractus solitarius
   (D) Pneumotaxic center
   (E) Ventral respiratory group

8. When respiratory drive for increased pulmonary ventilation becomes greater than normal, a special set of respiratory neurons that are inactive during normal, quiet breathing becomes active, contributing to respiratory drive. These neurons are located in which of the following structures?
   (A) Apneustic center
   (B) Dorsal respiratory group
   (C) Nucleus of the tractus solitarius
   (D) Pneumotaxic center
   (E) Ventral respiratory group

9. A healthy, 25-year-old medical student participates in a 10-kilometer run to benefit the American Heart Association. Which of the following muscles are used during expiration?
(A) Diaphragm and external intercostals
(B) Diaphragm and internal intercostals
(C) Diaphragm only
(D) Internal intercostals and rectus abdominis
(E) Scalene muscles
(F) Sternocleidomastoid muscles

10. The forces governing the diffusion of a gas through a biological membrane include the pressure difference across the membrane (ΔP), the cross-sectional area of the membrane (A), the solubility of the gas (S), the distance of diffusion (d), and the molecular weight of the gas (MW). Which of the following changes decreases the diffusion of a gas through a biological membrane?

	ΔP	A	S	d	MW
(A)	Decrease	Decrease	Decrease	Decrease	Decrease
(B)	Decrease	Decrease	Decrease	Increase	Increase
(C)	Decrease	Decrease	Increase	Decrease	Decrease
(D)	Decrease	Increase	Increase	Decrease	Decrease
(E)	Increase	Increase	Increase	Increase	Increase

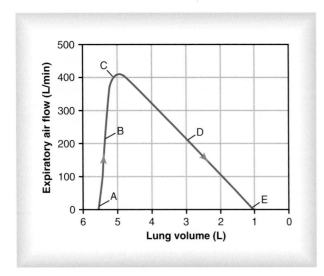

11. The maximum expiratory flow-volume curve is used as a diagnostic tool to identify obstructive and restrictive lung diseases. In the diagram above, at which point on the curve does airway collapse limit the maximum expiratory air flow? ( )

12. The pleural pressure of a normal 56-year-old woman is approximately -5 cm H_2O during resting conditions immediately before inspiration (i.e., at functional residual capacity). What is the pleural pressure during inspiration?
(A) $+1$ cm H_2O
(B) $+4$ cm H_2O
(C) 0 cm H_2O
(D) -3 cm H_2O
(E) -7 cm H_2O

13. The Hering-Breuer inflation reflex is mainly a protective mechanism that controls ventilation under certain conditions. Which of the following best describe the effect of this reflex on inspiration and expiration and the location of the stretch receptors that initiate the reflex?

	Location of Stretch Receptors	Inspiration	Expiration
(A)	Alveolar wall	No effect	Switches off
(B)	Alveolar wall	Switches off	No effect
(C)	Alveolar wall	Switches on	Switches on
(D)	Bronchi/bronchioles	No effect	Switches off
(E)	Bronchi/bronchioles	Switches off	No effect
(F)	Bronchi/bronchioles	Switches on	Switches on
(G)	Chest wall	No effect	Switches off
(H)	Chest wall	Switches off	No effect
(I)	Chest wall	Switches on	Switches on

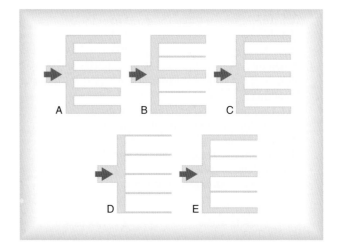

14. Which of the diagrams above best illustrates the pulmonary vasculature when the cardiac output has increased to the maximum extent? ( )

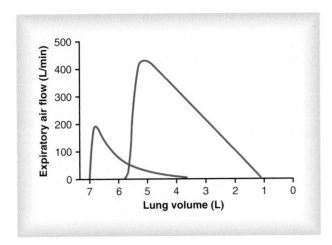

15. The maximum expiratory flow-volume curves in the diagram above were obtained from a healthy individual (red curve) and a 57-year-old man who complains of shortness of breath (green curve). Which of the following disorders does the man most likely have?
    (A) Asbestosis
    (B) Emphysema
    (C) Kyphosis
    (D) Scoliosis
    (E) Silicosis
    (F) Tuberculosis

16. A 10-year-old boy is at the top of Pikes Peak, where the barometric pressure is 462 mm Hg and the ambient oxygen concentration is 97 mm Hg. The partial pressures of the various gases in his alveolar air are as follows:
    Nitrogen   328 mm Hg
    Carbon dioxide   20 mm Hg
    Water vapor pressure   47 mm Hg
    What is the oxygen partial pressure (P_{O_2}) in his alveoli?
    (A) 52 mm Hg
    (B) 67 mm Hg
    (C) 75 mm Hg
    (D) 96 mm Hg
    (E) 104 mm Hg

17. The alveolar pressure of a normal 77-year-old woman is approximately 1 cm H_2O during expiration. What is the alveolar pressure during inspiration?
    (A) +0.5 cm H_2O
    (B) +1 cm H_2O
    (C) +2 cm H_2O
    (D) 0 cm H_2O
    (E) −1 cm H_2O
    (F) −5 cm H_2O

18. A chemosensitive area located in the medulla modulates respiration when the blood level of certain substances is not optimal. The chemosensitive area responds to changes in the blood levels of which of the following substances?

	Oxygen	Carbon Dioxide	Hydrogen Ion
(A)	No	No	No
(B)	No	No	Yes
(C)	No	Yes	No
(D)	No	Yes	Yes
(E)	Yes	No	No
(F)	Yes	No	Yes
(G)	Yes	Yes	No
(H)	Yes	Yes	Yes

19. A 76-year-man who has smoked 40 cigarettes a day for the past 50 years has developed severe emphysema. Which of the following sets of changes is present in him, compared with a healthy nonsmoker?

	Alveolar Surface Area	Arterial Oxygen Tension
(A)	Decreased	Decreased
(B)	Decreased	Increased
(C)	Increased	Decreased
(D)	Increased	Increased
(E)	No change	Decreased

20. A 30-year-old woman performs a Valsalva maneuver about 30 minutes after eating lunch. Which of the following best describes the changes in pulmonary and systemic blood volumes that occur in this woman?

	Pulmonary Volume	Systemic Volume
(A)	Decreased	Decreased
(B)	Decreased	Increased
(C)	Decreased	No change
(D)	Increased	Decreased
(E)	Increased	Increased
(F)	Increased	No change
(G)	No change	Decreased
(H)	No change	Increased
(I)	No change	No change

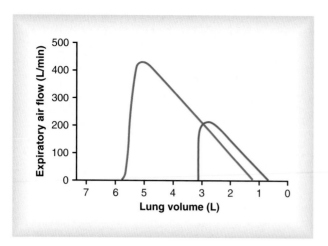

21. A 62-year-old man complains to his physician that he has difficulty breathing. The diagram above shows a maximum expiratory flow-volume (MEFV) curve from the patient (green curve) and from a typical healthy individual (red curve). Which of the following best explains the MEFV curve of the patient?
    (A) Asbestosis
    (B) Asthma
    (C) Bronchospasm
    (D) Emphysema
    (E) Old age

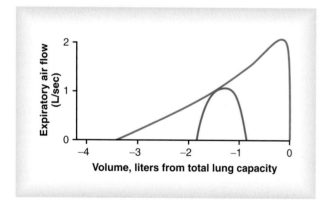

22. The maximum expiratory flow-volume curves in the diagram above were obtained from a 75-year-old man who has smoked 40 cigarettes a day for the past 60 years (red curve) and from the same man during resting conditions (green curve). Which of the following sets of changes most likely applies to this man?

	Exercise Tolerance	Total Lung Capacity	Residual Volume
(A)	Decreased	Decreased	Decreased
(B)	Decreased	Increased	Increased
(C)	Decreased	Normal	Normal
(D)	Increased	Increased	Increased
(E)	Normal	Decreased	Decreased

23. A 37-year-old man has a static pulmonary compliance of 0.25 L/cm H_2O. His pleural pressure changes from –4 cm H_2O to –8 cm H_2O when he inhales. How much air did he inhale?
    (A) 0.5 liter
    (B) 0.75 liter
    (C) 1.0 liter
    (D) 1.5 liters
    (E) 2.0 liters

24. Blood oxygenation is increased during exercise, not only by increased alveolar ventilation but also by a greater diffusing capacity of the respiratory membrane for transporting oxygen into the blood. Which of the following sets of changes occurs during exercise?

	Surface Area of Respiratory Membrane	Ventilation-Perfusion Ratio
(A)	Decreased	Improved
(B)	Increased	Improved
(C)	Increased	No change
(D)	No change	Improved
(E)	No change	No change

25. Excess carbon dioxide (CO_2) or excess hydrogen ions (H^+) in the blood or in the vicinity of the chemosensitive area of the respiratory center can lead to an increase in ventilation. Which of the following best describes the relative effectiveness of CO_2 and H^+ in increasing ventilation by their presence in blood and by their direct effect on chemosensitive neurons?

	Presence in Blood	Direct Effect on Chemosensitive Neurons
(A)	$CO_2 < H^+$	$CO_2 < H^+$
(B)	$CO_2 < H^+$	$CO_2 = H^+$
(C)	$CO_2 < H^+$	$CO_2 > H^+$
(D)	$CO_2 = H^+$	$CO_2 < H^+$
(E)	$CO_2 = H^+$	$CO_2 = H^+$
(F)	$CO_2 = H^+$	$CO_2 > H^+$
(G)	$CO_2 > H^+$	$CO_2 < H^+$
(H)	$CO_2 > H^+$	$CO_2 = H^+$
(I)	$CO_2 > H^+$	$CO_2 > H^+$

26. A 22-year-old woman has a pulmonary compliance of 0.2 L/cm H_2O and a pleural pressure of –4 cm H_2O. What is the pleural pressure when the woman inhales 1.0 liter of air?
    (A) –6 cm H_2O
    (B) –7 cm H_2O
    (C) –8 cm H_2O
    (D) –9 cm H_2O
    (E) –10 cm H_2O

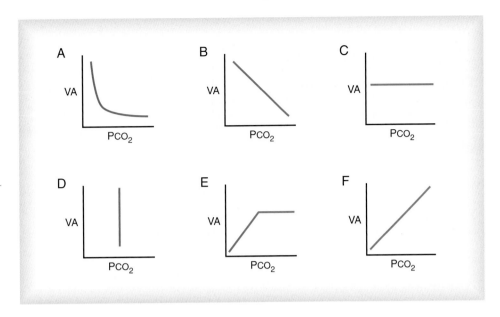

27. Which diagram above best describes the relationship between alveolar ventilation (VA) and arterial carbon dioxide tension (PCO_2) when the PCO_2 is changed acutely over a range of 35 to 75 mm Hg? ( )

28. A 32-year-old man drives to the top of Pikes Peak, where the oxygen tension is 85 mm Hg. Which of the following best describes the effects of a hypoxic environment on the pulmonary and systemic vascular resistances?

	Pulmonary Vascular Resistance	Systemic Vascular Resistance
(A)	Decreased	Decreased
(B)	Decreased	Increased
(C)	Decreased	No change
(D)	Increased	Decreased
(E)	Increased	Increased
(F)	Increased	No change
(G)	No change	Decreased
(H)	No change	Increased
(I)	No change	No change

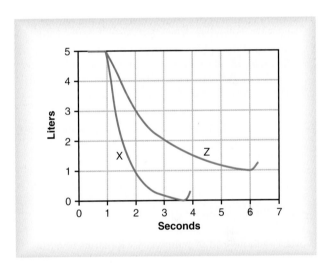

29. The diagram above shows a forced expiration for a healthy person (curve X) and a person with a pulmonary disease (curve Z). What is the ratio of forced expiratory volume in 1 second to forced vital capacity (FEV_1/FVC), as a percentage, in these individuals?

	Person X (%)	Person Z (%)
(A)	80	50
(B)	80	40
(C)	100	80
(D)	100	60
(E)	90	50
(F)	90	60

30. The diffusing capacity of a gas is the volume of gas that will diffuse through a membrane each minute for a pressure difference of 1 mm Hg. Which of the following gases is often used to estimate the oxygen diffusing capacity of the lungs?
    (A) Carbon dioxide
    (B) Carbon monoxide
    (C) Cyanide gas
    (D) Nitrogen
    (E) Oxygen

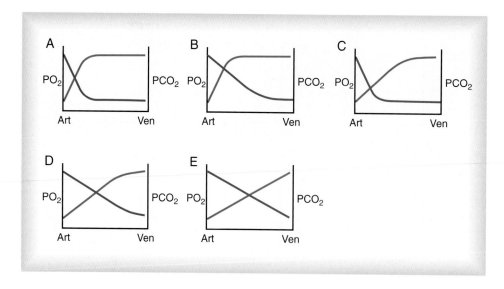

31. The diagrams above show changes in the partial pressures of oxygen (PO₂; red curves) and carbon dioxide (PCO₂; green curves) as blood flows from the arterial end to the venous end of the pulmonary capillaries. Which diagram best depicts the normal relationship between P_{O_2} and P_{CO_2} during resting conditions? ( )

32. The largest change in the P_{O_2} of blood occurs during its transit through which of the following vascular segments under resting conditions?
    (A) Aorta to pulmonary artery
    (B) Pulmonary artery to venous end of pulmonary capillary
    (C) Systemic arterioles to systemic venules
    (D) Vena cava to aorta
    (E) Venous end of pulmonary capillaries to aorta

33. A 23-year-old medical student has mixed venous oxygen and carbon dioxide tensions of 40 mm Hg and 45 mm Hg, respectively. A group of alveoli is not ventilated in this student because mucus blocks a local airway. What are the alveolar oxygen and carbon dioxide tensions distal to the mucous block?

	Oxygen (mm Hg)	Carbon Dioxide (mm Hg)
(A)	100	40
(B)	40	40
(C)	40	45
(D)	50	50
(E)	40	90

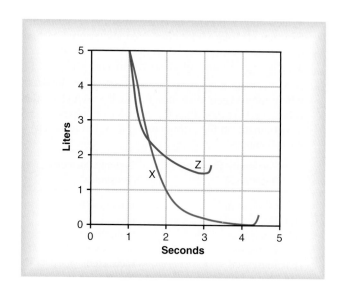

34. The diagram above shows forced expirations from a person with healthy lungs (curve X) and from a patient with a pulmonary disorder (curve Z). Which of the following is most likely present in the patient?
    (A) Asthma
    (B) Bronchospasm
    (C) Emphysema
    (D) Old age
    (E) Silicosis

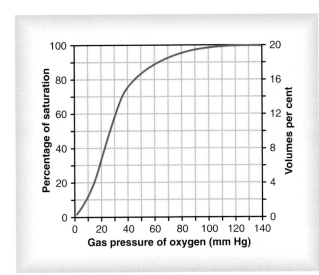

35. The diagram above shows a normal oxygen-hemoglobin dissociation curve. Which of the following are the approximate values of hemoglobin saturation (% Hb-O$_2$), oxygen partial pressure (PO$_2$), and oxygen (O$_2$) content for oxygenated blood leaving the lungs and reduced blood returning to the lungs from the tissues?

| | Oxygenated Blood | | | Reduced Blood | | |
	% Hb-O$_2$	PO$_2$	O$_2$ Content	% Hb-O$_2$	PO$_2$	O$_2$ Content
(A)	100	104	15	80	42	16
(B)	100	104	20	30	20	6
(C)	100	104	20	75	40	15
(D)	90	100	16	60	30	12
(E)	98	140	20	75	40	15

36. A 45-year-old man at sea level has an inspired oxygen tension of 149 mm Hg, nitrogen tension of 563 mm Hg, and water vapor pressure of 47 mm Hg. A small tumor pushes against a pulmonary blood vessel, completely blocking the blood flow to a small group of alveoli. What are the carbon dioxide and oxygen tensions of the alveoli that are not perfused?

	Carbon Dioxide (mm Hg)	Oxygen (mm Hg)
(A)	0	0
(B)	0	149
(C)	40	104
(D)	47	149
(E)	45	149

37. A preterm infant has a surfactant deficiency. Without surfactant, many of the alveoli collapse at the end of each expiration, which leads to pulmonary failure. Which of the following sets of changes is present in a preterm infant, compared with a normal infant?

	Alveolar Surface Tension	Pulmonary Compliance
(A)	Decreased	Decreased
(B)	Decreased	Increased
(C)	Decreased	No change
(D)	Increased	Decreased
(E)	Increased	Increased
(F)	Increased	No change
(G)	No change	No change

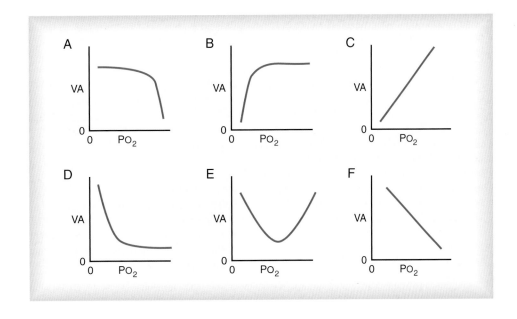

38. Which of the diagrams (A to F, page 119) best describes the relationship between alveolar ventilation (VA) and arterial oxygen tension (PO_2) when the PO_2 is changed acutely over a range of 0 to 160 mm Hg and the arterial PCO_2 and hydrogen ion concentration remain normal? ( )

39. Mountain climbers have found that acclimatization to a hypoxic environment occurs within 2 to 3 days. Which of the following best describes the alveolar ventilation and sensitivity of the respiratory center to changes in arterial PCO_2 after acclimatization has occurred?

	Alveolar Ventilation	Sensitivity to PCO_2
(A)	Higher	Higher
(B)	Higher	Lower
(C)	Higher	Same
(D)	Lower	Higher
(E)	Lower	Lower

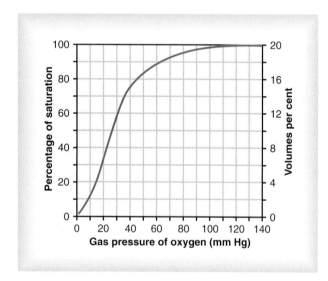

40. The diagram above shows a normal oxygen-hemoglobin dissociation curve during resting conditions. What is the P_{50} of the curve during resting conditions and during exercise?

	Rest	Exercise
(A)	25	15
(B)	25	35
(C)	40	20
(D)	40	60
(E)	50	25
(F)	50	50

Glucose:	100 mg/dl
Urea nitrogen:	20 mg/dl
Potassium:	4.8 mmol/L
Chloride:	104 mmol/L
Sodium:	143 mmol/L
Total protein:	6.7 g/dl
Hemoglobin:	7.2 g/dl
Albumin:	4.2 g/dl

41. A 65-year-old man visits his physician for an annual checkup. Selected laboratory results from a venous blood sample are shown in the table above. Which of the following sets of changes is most likely to have occurred in this man, compared with normal values?

	Arterial O_2 Content	Arterial O_2 Saturation of Hemoglobin	Arterial O_2 Tension
(A)	Decreased	Decreased	Decreased
(B)	Decreased	Decreased	Normal
(C)	Decreased	Normal	Normal
(D)	Increased	Increased	Normal
(E)	Increased	Normal	Normal
(F)	Normal	Decreased	Decreased
(G)	Normal	Normal	Decreased
(H)	Normal	Normal	Normal

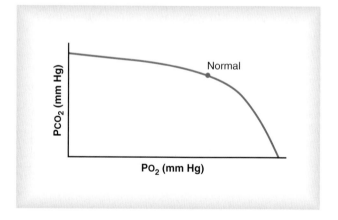

42. The O_2-CO_2 diagram above shows a ventilation-perfusion ratio line for the normal lung. Which of the following best describes the effect of decreasing the ventilation-perfusion ratio on the alveolar PCO_2 and PO_2?

	CO_2 Tension	O_2 Tension
(A)	Decreased	Decreased
(B)	Decreased	Increased
(C)	Decreased	No change
(D)	Increased	Decreased
(E)	Increased	Increased

43. The distribution of pulmonary blood flow in the upright lung is dictated by differences between the pulmonary arterial and venous blood pressures, as well as the alveolar air pressure. Which of the following best describes the relative differences in blood flow among the upper, middle, and lower portions of the lung during resting conditions in a standing person and during exercise in a running person?

	Standing Still	Running
(A)	Upper < middle < lower	Upper < middle < lower
(B)	Upper < middle < lower	Upper = middle = lower
(C)	Upper = middle = lower	Upper < middle < lower
(D)	Upper > middle > lower	Upper = middle = lower
(E)	Upper > middle > lower	Upper > middle > lower

44. A normal 22-year-old man breathes in as much air as he can and then exhales as much air as possible. The lung volume at maximum inspiration is 6.0 liters, and the lung volume after maximum expiration is 1.0 liter. His tidal volume at rest is 0.5 liter, and his functional residual capacity is 3.5 liters. What is his vital capacity?
(A) 3.0 liters
(B) 3.5 liters
(C) 4.0 liters
(D) 5.0 liters
(E) 5.5 liters
(F) 6.0 liters

45. A 50-year-old woman who has smoked 60 cigarettes a day for the past 30 years complains of shortness of breath. Which of the following sets of changes best describes the effects of emphysema on physiologic shunt and physiologic dead space?

	Physiologic Shunt	Physiologic Dead Space
(A)	Decreased	Decreased
(B)	Decreased	Increased
(C)	Decreased	No change
(D)	Increased	Decreased
(E)	Increased	Increased

46. During strenuous exercise, oxygen consumption and carbon dioxide formation can increase up to 20-fold. Alveolar ventilation increases almost exactly in step with this increase in oxygen consumption. Which of the following best describes what happens to the mean arterial oxygen tension (PO_2), carbon dioxide tension (PCO_2), and pH in a healthy athlete during strenuous exercise?

	Arterial PO_2	Arterial PCO_2	Arterial pH
(A)	Decreased	Decreased	Decreased
(B)	Decreased	Increased	Decreased
(C)	Increased	Decreased	Increased
(D)	Increased	Increased	Increased
(E)	No change	No change	No change

47. Alveolar ventilation increases severalfold during strenuous exercise. Which of the following factors is most likely to stimulate ventilation during strenuous exercise?
(A) Collateral impulses from higher brain centers
(B) Decreased mean arterial pH
(C) Decreased mean arterial PO_2
(D) Decreased mean venous PO_2
(E) Increased mean arterial PCO_2

Questions 48 and 49

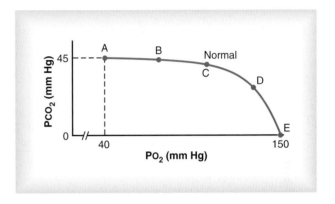

48. A 67-year-old man has a solid tumor that pushes against an airway, partially obstructing air flow to the distal alveoli. Which point on the ventilation-perfusion line of the O_2-CO_2 diagram above corresponds to the alveolar gas of these distal alveoli? ( )

49. A 55-year-old man has a pulmonary embolism that partially blocks the blood flow to his right lung. Which point on the ventilation-perfusion line of the O_2-CO_2 diagram above corresponds to the alveolar gas of his right lung? ( )

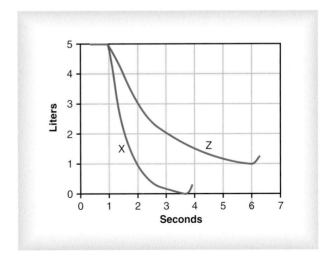

50. The previous diagram (page 121) shows forced expirations from a person with healthy lungs (curve X) and from a patient with a pulmonary disorder (curve Z). Which of the following best explains the results from the patient?
    (A) Asbestosis
    (B) Emphysema
    (C) Fibrotic pleurisy
    (D) Pleural effusion
    (E) Pneumothorax
    (F) Silicosis
    (G) Tuberculosis

51. A 34-year-old woman is anemic, with a blood hemoglobin concentration of 7.1 g/dl. Which of the following sets of changes has occurred in this woman, compared with normal values?

	Arterial P_{O_2}	Mixed Venous P_{O_2}	2,3-Diphosphoglycerate
(A)	Decreased	Decreased	Increased
(B)	Decreased	Decreased	Normal
(C)	Decreased	Normal	Decreased
(D)	Increased	Decreased	Normal
(E)	Increased	Increased	Increased
(F)	Increased	Normal	Decreased
(G)	Normal	Decreased	Decreased
(H)	Normal	Decreased	Increased
(I)	Normal	Normal	Normal

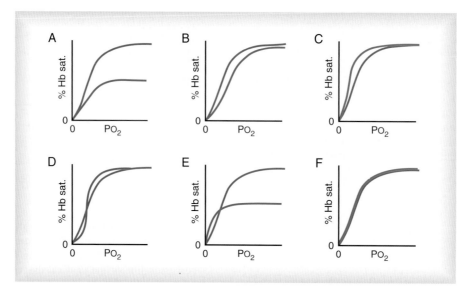

52. Which of the oxygen-hemoglobin dissociation curves above corresponds to normal blood (red line) and blood containing carbon monoxide (green line)?
    ( )

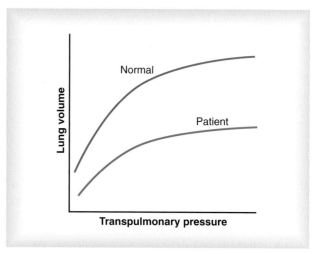

53. The volume-pressure curves in the diagram above were obtained from a young, healthy subject and a patient with a pulmonary disorder. Which of the following best describes the condition of the patient?
    (A) Asthma
    (B) Bronchospasm
    (C) Emphysema
    (D) Old age
    (E) Silicosis

Questions 54 and 55

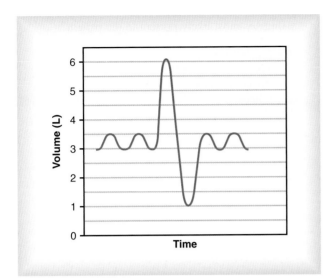

54. A 27-year-old man is breathing quietly. He then inhales as much air as possible and exhales as much air as he can, producing the spirogram shown (left). What is his expiratory reserve volume?
    (A) 2.0 liters
    (B) 2.5 liters
    (C) 3.0 liters
    (D) 3.5 liters
    (E) 4.0 liters
    (F) 5.0 liters

55. A 22-year-old woman inhales as much air as possible and exhales as much air as she can, producing the spirogram shown (left). A residual volume of 1.5 liters was determined using the helium dilution technique. What is her functional residual capacity?
    (A) 2.0 liters
    (B) 2.5 liters
    (C) 3.0 liters
    (D) 3.5 liters
    (E) 4.0 liters
    (F) 5.0 liters

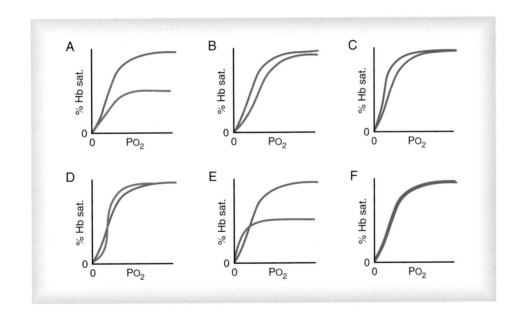

56. Which of the oxygen-hemoglobin dissociation curves (A to F, above) above corresponds to blood during resting conditions (red line) and blood during exercise (green line)? ( )

124   Unit VII   *Respiration*

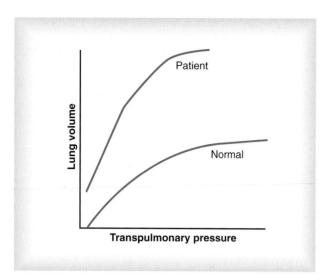

57. The volume-pressure curves (left) were obtained from a normal subject and a patient suffering from a pulmonary disease. Which of the following abnormalities is most likely present in the patient?
(A) Asbestosis
(B) Emphysema
(C) Mitral obstruction
(D) Rheumatic heart disease
(E) Silicosis
(F) Tuberculosis

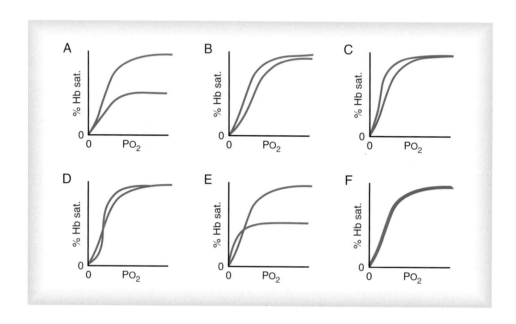

58. Which of the oxygen-hemoglobin dissociation curves (A to F, above) above corresponds to blood from an adult (red line) and blood from a fetus (green line)? ( )

59. A normal 22-year-old medical student in the upright position is breathing against a positive pressure, which causes the intra-alveolar pressure to increase. Other values are as follows:

Cardiac output	6 L/min
Pulmonary systolic pressure	25 mm Hg
Pulmonary diastolic pressure	8 mm Hg
Mean pulmonary artery pressure	15 mm Hg
Intra-alveolar pressure	12 mm Hg

What is the pulmonary blood flow in the upper one third of the lungs of this student?
(A) <1.0 L/min
(B) 2.0 L/min
(C) 2.5 L/min
(D) 3.0 L/min
(E) 3.5 L/min
(F) 4.0 L/min

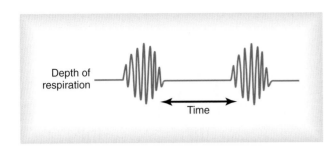

60. The diagram above shows the depth of respiration of a 45-year-old man who suffered a head injury in an automobile accident. This "crescendo-decrescendo" pattern of breathing is called which of the following?
    (A) Apnea
    (B) Biot's breathing
    (C) Cheyne-Stokes breathing
    (D) Hyperpnea
    (E) Tachypnea

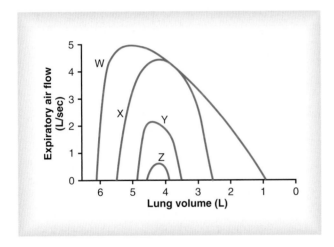

61. A 34-year-old medical student generates the flow-volume curves in the diagram above. Curve W is a normal maximum expiratory flow-volume curve generated when the student is healthy. Which of the following can best explain curve X?
    (A) Asthma attack
    (B) Aspiration of meat into the trachea
    (C) Heavy exercise
    (D) Light exercise
    (E) Normal breathing at rest
    (F) Pneumonia
    (G) Tuberculosis

62. A 55-year-old man has a hematocrit of 28 and a blood hemoglobin concentration of 10 g/dl. His arterial oxygen tension is 100 mm Hg, and the arterial blood is fully saturated with oxygen. Which of the following best describes his arterial oxygen content, mixed venous oxygen content, and oxygen usage by the tissues during resting conditions (in ml O_2/dl)?

	Arterial Oxygen Content	Venous Oxygen Content	Oxygen Usage by Tissues
(A)	10.0	5.0	5.0
(B)	10.0	6.0	3.0
(C)	13.4	7.4	7.0
(D)	13.4	10.4	3.0
(E)	20.0	10.0	8.0
(F)	20.0	15.0	5.0

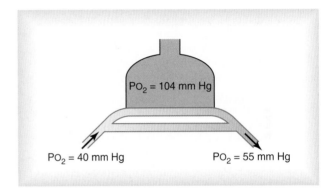

63. The diagram above shows a lung with a large shunt in which mixed venous blood bypasses the oxygen exchange areas of the lung. Breathing room air produces the oxygen partial pressures shown on the diagram. What is the oxygen tension of the arterial blood when the person breathes 100 per cent oxygen and the inspired oxygen tension is over 600 mm Hg?
    (A) 40 mm Hg
    (B) 55 mm Hg
    (C) 60 mm Hg
    (D) 175 mm Hg
    (E) 200 mm Hg
    (F) 400 mm Hg
    (G) 600 mm Hg

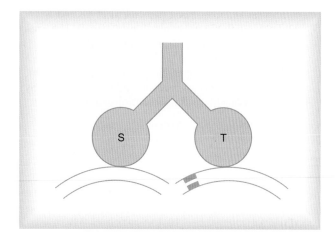

64. The diagram above shows two lung units (S and T) with their blood supplies. Lung unit S has an ideal relationship between blood flow and ventilation. Lung unit T has a compromised blood flow. What is the relationship between alveolar dead space (D_{ALV}), physiologic dead space (D_{PHY}), and anatomic dead space (D_{ANAT}) for these lung units?

	Lung Unit S	Lung Unit T
(A)	$D_{PHY} < D_{ANAT}$	$D_{PHY} = D_{ANAT}$
(B)	$D_{PHY} = D_{ALV}$	$D_{PHY} > D_{ALV}$
(C)	$D_{PHY} = D_{ANAT}$	$D_{PHY} < D_{ANAT}$
(D)	$D_{PHY} = D_{ANAT}$	$D_{PHY} > D_{ANAT}$
(E)	$D_{PHY} > D_{ANAT}$	$D_{PHY} < D_{ANAT}$

65. The various lung volumes and capacities include total lung volume (TLC), vital capacity (VC), inspiratory capacity (IC), tidal volume (VT), expiratory capacity (EC), expiratory reserve volume (ERV), inspiratory reserve volume (IRV), functional residual capacity (FRC), and residual volume (RV). Which of the following lung volumes and capacities can be measured using direct spirometry without additional methods?

	TLC	VC	IC	VT	EC	ERV	IRV	FRC	RV
(A)	No	No	Yes	No	Yes	No	Yes	No	No
(B)	No	Yes	Yes	Yes	Yes	Yes	Yes	No	No
(C)	No	Yes	Yes	Yes	Yes	Yes	Yes	Yes	No
(D)	Yes	Yes	Yes	Yes	Yes	Yes	Yes	No	Yes
(E)	Yes	Yes	Yes	Yes	Yes	Yes	Yes	Yes	Yes

66. A 25-year-old medical student participates in a treadmill exercise study. The student has a dead space volume of 150 milliliters, a tidal volume of 1150 milliliters, and a respiratory rate of 20 breaths/min. What is the student's rate of alveolar ventilation?
   (A) 5 liters
   (B) 10 liters
   (C) 15 liters
   (D) 20 liters
   (E) 25 liters
   (F) 30 liters

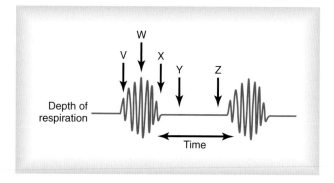

67. Cheyne-Stokes breathing is an abnormal breathing pattern characterized by a gradual increase in the depth of breathing, followed by a progressive decrease in the depth of breathing, that repeats about every minute. Which of the time points (V through Z) on the diagram above are associated with the highest P_{CO_2} of lung blood and the highest P_{CO_2} of neurons in the respiratory center?

	Lung Blood	Respiratory Center
(A)	V	V
(B)	V	W
(C)	W	W
(D)	X	Z
(E)	Y	Z

68. A 78-year-old man who has smoked 60 cigarettes a day for 55 years complains of shortness of breath. The patient is diagnosed with chronic pulmonary emphysema. Which of the following sets of changes is present in this man, compared with a healthy nonsmoker?

	Pulmonary Compliance	Lung Elastic Recoil	Total Lung Capacity
(A)	Decreased	Decreased	Decreased
(B)	Decreased	Decreased	Increased
(C)	Decreased	Increased	Increased
(D)	Increased	Decreased	Decreased
(E)	Increased	Decreased	Increased
(F)	Increased	Increased	Increased

69. Carbon dioxide is transported in the blood in the dissolved state, in the form of bicarbonate ion, and in combination with hemoglobin (carbaminohemoglobin). Which of the following best describes the quantitative relationship of these three mechanisms for transporting carbon dioxide in the venous blood under normal conditions?

	Dissolved State (%)	Bicarbonate Ion (%)	Carbamino-hemoglobin (%)
(A)	7	70	23
(B)	70	23	7
(C)	23	70	7
(D)	7	23	70
(E)	70	7	23
(F)	23	7	70

70. A 30-year-old man participates in a pulmonary function laboratory exercise. He has a dead space volume of 200 milliliters, a tidal volume of 200 milliliters, and a respiratory rate of 40 breaths/min. What is his rate of alveolar ventilation?
    (A) 0 liters
    (B) 1 liter
    (C) 2 liters
    (D) 3 liters
    (E) 4 liters
    (F) 5 liters

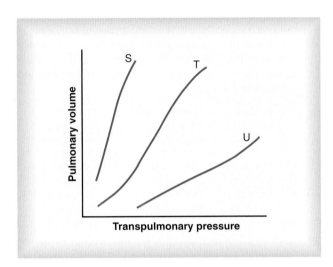

71. The diagram shows three different compliance curves (S, T, and U) for isolated lungs subjected to various transpulmonary pressures. Which of the following best describe the relative compliance for the three curves?
    (A) S < T < U
    (B) S < T > U
    (C) S = T = U
    (D) S > T < U
    (E) S > T > U

72. The patient is a 75-year-old man. When he was in his 40s, he worked for 5 years in a factory where asbestos was used as an insulator. He is diagnosed with asbestosis. Which of the following sets of changes is present in this man, compared with a person with healthy lungs?

	Pulmonary Compliance	Lung Elastic Recoil	Total Lung Capacity
(A)	Decreased	Decreased	Decreased
(B)	Decreased	Increased	Increased
(C)	Decreased	Increased	Decreased
(D)	Increased	Decreased	Decreased
(E)	Increased	Decreased	Increased
(F)	Increased	Increased	Increased

73. A 66-year-old woman suffers a myocardial infarction that immediately reduces cardiac output to about one third of normal. Which of the following sets of changes best describes the pulmonary capillary hydrostatic pressure (PCP), left atrial pressure (LAP), pulmonary interstitial hydrostatic pressure (PIP), and pulmonary lymph flow (PLF) during acute left ventricular failure?

	PCP	LAP	PIP	PLF
(A)	Decreased	Decreased	Decreased	Decreased
(B)	Increased	Increased	Decreased	Decreased
(C)	Increased	Increased	Decreased	Increased
(D)	Increased	Increased	Increased	Decreased
(E)	Increased	Increased	Increased	Increased

74. A 50-year-old woman is diagnosed with pneumonia that is localized to one lung. Which of the following sets of changes is most likely to be present in this woman, compared with a healthy person?

	Surface Area of Pulmonary Membrane	Ventilation-Perfusion Ratio	Arterial P_{CO_2}	Arterial P_{O_2}
(A)	Decreased	Decreased	Decreased	Decreased
(B)	Decreased	Decreased	Increased	Decreased
(C)	Decreased	Increased	Decreased	Increased
(D)	Decreased	Increased	Increased	Decreased
(E)	Increased	Decreased	Increased	Decreased
(F)	Increased	Increased	Increased	Decreased

75. An experiment is conducted in two individuals (subjects T and V) with identical tidal volumes (1000 milliliters), dead space volumes (200 milliliters), and ventilation frequencies (20 breaths/min). Subject T doubles his tidal volume and reduces his ventilation frequency by 50 per cent. Subject V doubles his ventilation frequency and reduces his tidal volume by 50 per cent. Which of the following best describes the total ventilation (also called minute ventilation) and alveolar ventilation of subjects T and V?

	Total Ventilation	Alveolar Ventilation
(A)	T < V	T = V
(B)	T < V	T > V
(C)	T = V	T < V
(D)	T = V	T = V
(E)	T = V	T > V
(F)	T > V	T < V
(G)	T > V	T = V

76. A 26-year-old medical student on a normal diet has a respiratory exchange ratio of 0.8. How much oxygen and carbon dioxide are transported between the lungs and tissues of this student (in ml gas/100 ml blood)?

	Oxygen	Carbon Dioxide
(A)	4 in ml gas	4 ml
(B)	5 in ml gas	3 ml
(C)	5 in ml gas	4 ml
(D)	5 in ml gas	5 ml
(E)	6 in ml gas	3 ml
(F)	6 in ml gas	4 ml

77. Carbon dioxide is transported from the tissues to the lungs predominantly in the form of bicarbonate ion. Compared with arterial red blood cells, which of the following best describes venous red blood cells?

	Intracellular Chloride Concentration	Cell Volume
(A)	Decreased	Decreased
(B)	Decreased	Increased
(C)	Decreased	No change
(D)	Increased	Decreased
(E)	Increased	No change
(F)	Increased	Increased
(G)	No change	Decreased
(H)	No change	Increased
(I)	No change	No change

78. The entire right lung of a 44-year-old man is collapsed because of a tumor that totally obstructs the airway. Blood flow is reduced to zero in the collapsed lung. Which of the following sets of changes is most likely to be present in this man during resting conditions, compared with a healthy person?

	Surface Area of Pulmonary Membrane	Arterial P_{CO_2}	Arterial P_{O_2}
(A)	Decreased	Decreased	Increased
(B)	Decreased	Increased	Decreased
(C)	Decreased	Increased	Increased
(D)	Decreased	No change	No change
(E)	Increased	Increased	Decreased
(F)	Increased	No change	No change

79. A healthy 10-year-old boy breathes quietly under resting conditions. His tidal volume is 400 milliliters, and his ventilation frequency is 12 breaths/min. Which of the following best describes the ventilation of the upper, middle, and lower lung zones in this boy?

	Upper Zone	Middle Zone	Lower Zone
(A)	Highest	Lowest	Intermediate
(B)	Highest	Intermediate	Lowest
(C)	Intermediate	Lowest	Highest
(D)	Lowest	Intermediate	Highest
(E)	Same	Same	Same

80. The effectiveness of oxygen therapy is dependent on the cause of the hypoxia. In which of the following conditions would oxygen therapy be of greatest value in alleviating hypoxia in the peripheral tissues?
    (A) Anemia
    (B) Cyanide poisoning
    (C) Localized circulatory deficiencies
    (D) Pulmonary emphysema
    (E) Right-to-left cardiac shunts

81. A 19-year-old man suffers full-thickness burns over 60 per cent of his body surface area. A systemic *Pseudomonas aeruginosa* infection occurs, and severe pulmonary edema follows 7 days later. The following data are collected from the patient:
    Plasma colloid osmotic pressure   19 mm Hg
    Pulmonary capillary hydrostatic pressure   7 mm Hg
    Interstitial fluid hydrostatic pressure   1 mm Hg
    Which of the following sets of changes has occurred in the lungs of this patient as a result of the burn and subsequent infection?

	Lymph Flow	Plasma Colloid Osmotic Pressure	Pulmonary Capillary Permeability
(A)	Decreased	Decreased	Decreased
(B)	Increased	Decreased	Decreased
(C)	Increased	Decreased	Increased
(D)	Increased	Increased	Decreased
(E)	Increased	Increased	Increased

82. A 34-year-old man sustains a bullet wound to the chest that causes a pneumothorax. Which of the following best describes the changes in lung volume and thoracic volume in this man, compared with normal values?

	Lung Volume	Thoracic Volume
(A)	Decreased	Decreased
(B)	Decreased	Increased
(C)	Decreased	No change
(D)	Increased	Decreased
(E)	Increased	Increased
(F)	No change	Decreased

83. The resistance of the pulmonary tree is so low that a 1 cm H_2O pressure gradient is sufficient to cause normal air flow during resting conditions. Which of the following often has substantial resistance during pulmonary disease states that can limit alveolar ventilation?
    (A) Alveoli
    (B) Bronchioles
    (C) Large bronchi
    (D) Small bronchi
    (E) Trachea

84. A healthy native of the Andes Mountains has a hematocrit of 60 and blood hemoglobin of 22.5 g/dl. While visiting his cousin in Florida, he develops a blue tint to his skin and lips (cyanosis). Which of the following sets of differences is present in the Andes native at sea level, compared with a healthy sea-level native?

	Arterial Oxygen Content	Arterial Oxygen Tension	Arterial Oxygen Saturation
(A)	Decreased	Decreased	Decreased
(B)	Decreased	No difference	No difference
(C)	Increased	Increased	Increased
(D)	Increased	No difference	No difference
(E)	No difference	No difference	No difference

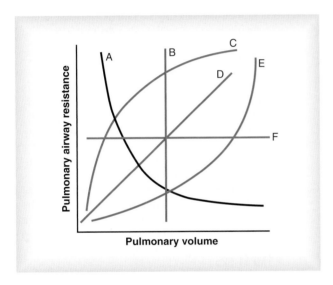

85. The diagram above shows pulmonary airway resistance expressed as a function of pulmonary volume. Which relationship best describes the normal lung? ( )

86. The respiratory passageways have smooth muscle in their walls. Which of the following best describes the effect of acetylcholine and epinephrine on the respiratory passageways?

	Acetylcholine	Epinephrine
(A)	Constricts	Constricts
(B)	Constricts	Dilates
(C)	Constricts	No effect
(D)	Dilates	Constricts
(E)	Dilates	Dilates
(F)	Dilates	No effect
(G)	No effect	Constricts
(H)	No effect	Dilates

Answers

1. (A) It is usually not feasible to measure the left atrial pressure directly in normal human beings because it is difficult to pass a catheter through the heart chambers into the left atrium. The balloon-tipped, flow-directed Swan-Ganz catheter was developed nearly 30 years ago to estimate left atrial pressure for the management of acute myocardial infarction. When the balloon is inflated on a Swan-Ganz catheter, the pressure measured through the catheter, called the wedge pressure, approximates the left atrial pressure for the following reason: blood flow distal to the catheter tip has been stopped all the way to the left atrium, which allows left atrial pressure to be estimated. The wedge pressure is actually a few mm Hg higher than the left atrial pressure, depending on where the catheter is wedged, but this still allows changes in left atrial pressure to be monitored in patients with left ventricular failure.
   TMP11 484

2. (F) The pulmonary and systemic circulations both receive about the same amount of blood flow because the lungs receive the entire cardiac output. (However, the output of the left ventricle is actually 1 to 2 per cent higher than that of the right ventricle because the bronchial arterial blood originates from the left ventricle and the bronchial venous blood empties into the pulmonary veins.) The pulmonary blood vessels have a relatively low resistance, allowing the entire cardiac output to pass through them without increasing the pressure to a great extent. The pulmonary artery pressure averages about 15 mm Hg, which is much lower than the systemic arterial pressure of about 100 mm Hg.
   TMP11 483, 484

3. (D) The partial pressure of a gas is calculated by multiplying its fractional concentration by the atmospheric pressure. Dry air has an oxygen concentration of about 21 per cent and a nitrogen concentration of about 79 per cent. Because the atmospheric pressure on the mountain is 700 mm Hg, the partial pressure of oxygen is 147 mm Hg (0.21×700) and the partial pressure of nitrogen is 553 mm Hg (0.79×700).
   TMP11 492

4. (C) The lungs can be expanded and contracted by increasing and decreasing the volume of the chest cavity. The volume of the chest cavity can be changed in two ways: (a) downward and upward movement of the diaphragm increases and decreases the length of the chest cavity, and (b) elevating and depressing the rib cage increases and decreases the anteroposterior diameter of the chest cavity. Normal breathing during resting conditions is accomplished entirely by the diaphragm. The diaphragm contracts, causing inspiration, and relaxes, causing expiration. The other muscles listed in the question elevate or depress the rib cage and are used during heavy breathing associated with exercise, as well as in those with respiratory abnormalities characterized by excessive respiratory effort.
   TMP11 471

5. (E) The P_{O_2} of mixed venous blood entering the pulmonary capillaries is normally about 40 mm Hg, and the P_{O_2} at the venous end of the capillaries is normally equal to that of the alveolar gas (104 mm Hg). The P_{O_2} of the pulmonary blood normally rises to equal that of the alveolar air by the time the blood has moved a third of the distance through the capillaries, becoming almost 104 mm Hg. Thus, curve B represents the normal resting state. During exercise, the cardiac output can increase severalfold, but the pulmonary capillary blood still becomes almost saturated with oxygen during its transit through the lungs. However, because of the faster flow of blood through the lungs during exercise, the oxygen has less time to diffuse into the pulmonary capillary blood; therefore, the P_{O_2} of the capillary blood does not reach its maximum value until it reaches the venous end of the pulmonary capillaries. Although curves D and E both show that oxygen saturation of blood occurs near the venous end, only curve E shows a low P_{O_2} of 25 mm Hg at the arterial end of the pulmonary capillaries, which is typical of mixed venous blood during strenuous exercise.
TMP11 503

6. (D) The forced vital capacity (FVC) is equal to the difference between the total lung capacity (TLC) and the residual volume (RV). The TLC and RV are the points of intersection between the abscissa and flow-volume curve; that is, TLC = 5.5 liters, and RV = 1.0 liter. Therefore, FVC = 5.5 – 1.0 = 4.5 liters.
TMP11 525

7. (D) The pneumotaxic center transmits signals to the dorsal respiratory group that "switch off" inspiratory signals, thus controlling the duration of the filling phase of the lung cycle. This has a secondary effect of increasing the rate of breathing, because limiting inspiration also shortens expiration and the entire period of respiration.
TMP11 515

8. (E) The basic rhythm of respiration is generated in the dorsal respiratory group of neurons, located almost entirely within the nucleus of the tractus solitarius. When the respiratory drive for increased pulmonary ventilation becomes greater than normal, respiratory signals spill over into the ventral respiratory neurons, causing the ventral respiratory area to contribute to respiratory drive. However, neurons of the ventral respiratory group remain almost totally inactive during normal, quiet breathing.
TMP11 515

9. (D) Contraction of the internal intercostals and the rectus abdominis muscles pull the rib cage downward during expiration. The rectus abdominis and other abdominal muscles compress the abdominal contents upward toward the diaphragm, which also helps eliminate air from the lungs. The diaphragm relaxes during expiration. The external intercostals, sternocleidomastoid muscles, and scalene muscles increase the diameter of the chest cavity during exer-

cise and thus assist with inspiration, but only the diaphragm is necessary for inspiration during quiet breathing.
TMP11 471

10. (B) Fick's law of diffusion states that the rate of diffusion (D) of a gas through a biological membrane is proportional to ΔP, A, and S, and inversely proportional to d and the square root of the MW of the gas (i.e., D α [ΔP × A × S] / [d × MW^{-2}]). The lower the solubility of the gas, the fewer the number of gas molecules available to diffuse for a given difference in pressure. The lower the cross-sectional area of the membrane, the fewer the total number of molecules that can diffuse through the membrane. When the distance of the diffusion pathway is longer, it takes more time for the molecules to diffuse the entire distance. When the molecular weight of the gas molecule is higher, the velocity of kinetic movement of the molecule is lower, which also decreases the rate of diffusion.
TMP11 493

11. (D) The maximum expiratory flow-volume curve is created when a person inhales as much air as possible (point A; total lung capacity = 5.5 liters) and then expires the air with a maximum effort until no more air can be expired (point E; residual volume = 1.0 liter). The descending portion of the curve indicated by the downward-pointing arrow represents the maximum expiratory flow at each lung volume. This descending part is sometimes referred to as the "effort-independent" portion of the curve, because a person cannot increase the expiratory flow rate even by making a greater expiratory effort.
TMP11 525

12. (E) The pleural pressure (sometimes called the intrapleural pressure) is the pressure of the fluid in the narrow space between the visceral pleura of the lungs and the parietal pleura of the chest wall. The pleural pressure is normally about –5 cm H_2O immediately before inspiration—that is, at functional residual capacity (FRC)—when all the respiratory muscles are relaxed. During inspiration, the volume of the chest cavity increases, and the pleural pressure becomes more negative. The pleural pressure averages about –7.5 cm H_2O immediately before expiration, when the lungs are fully expanded. The pleural pressure then returns to its resting value of –5 cm H_2O as the diaphragm relaxes and lung volume returns to FRC. Therefore, the intrapleural pressure is always subatmospheric under normal conditions, varying between –5 and –7.5 cm H_2O during quiet breathing.
TMP11 572

13. (E) The muscular walls of the bronchi and bronchioles contain stretch receptors that transmit signals through the vagi into the dorsal respiratory group of neurons when the lungs are overstretched. These signals "switch off" inspiration, thus preventing excess lung inflation in much the same way as

signals from the pneumotaxic center do. The reflex does not have a direct effect on expiration.
TMP11 515

14. (A) The pulmonary blood flow can increase several-fold without causing an excessive increase in pulmonary artery pressure for two reasons: previously closed vessels open up (recruitment), and the vessels enlarge (distention). Both recruitment and distention of the pulmonary blood vessels serve to lower the pulmonary vascular resistance (and thus maintain low pulmonary blood pressures) when the cardiac output has increased.
TMP11 485

15. (B) In obstructive diseases such as emphysema and asthma, the maximum expiratory flow-volume curve begins and ends at abnormally high lung volumes, and the flow rates are lower than normal at any given lung volume. The curve may also have a scooped-out appearance, as shown on the diagram. The other possible answers are constricted (also called restrictive) lung diseases. Lung volumes are lower than normal in constricted lung diseases.
TMP11 526

16. (B) The total pressure of the air in the alveoli is equal to the atmospheric pressure, which is 462 mm Hg, as stated in the problem. Therefore, the oxygen tension of the alveolar air can be determined by simply subtracting the partial pressures of nitrogen, carbon dioxide, and water vapor from the atmospheric pressure: oxygen partial pressure = 462 − (328 + 20 + 47) = 67 mm Hg. The low alveolar carbon dioxide tension caused by hyperventilation is one of the most useful responses to high altitude. For example, with an alveolar carbon dioxide tension of 40 mm Hg (i.e., a normal sea-level value), the alveolar oxygen tension would be only 47 mm Hg.
TMP11 493

17. (E) Alveolar pressure is the pressure of the air inside the lung alveoli. When the glottis is open and no air is flowing into or out of the lungs, the pressures in all parts of the respiratory tree are equal to zero. Expansion of the chest cavity during inspiration causes the alveolar pressure to become subatmospheric, averaging about −1 cm H_2O during quiet breathing; this creates a +1 cm H_2O pressure gradient for air to move into the lungs. Contraction of the chest cavity during expiration causes the alveolar pressure to achieve a positive value of about +1 cm H_2O, which again creates a +1 cm H_2O pressure gradient for air to move out of the lungs. The alveolar pressures become more negative during inspiration and more positive during expiration during heavy breathing associated with exercise, as well as in various disease states.
TMP11 472

18. (D) Excess carbon dioxide or excess hydrogen ions in the blood act on the chemosensitive area of the respiratory center in the medulla to increase the strength of both inspiratory and expiratory motor signals to the respiratory muscles. Oxygen does not have a significant direct effect on the respiratory center in the brain. Instead, it acts almost entirely on peripheral chemoreceptors located in the carotid and aortic bodies.
TMP11 516

19. (A) In emphysema, many of the alveoli coalesce, with dissolution of many alveolar walls. Therefore, the new chambers (air sacs) are larger than the original alveoli, and the total surface area of the respiratory membrane often decreases as much as fivefold because of loss of the alveolar walls. This decrease in the surface area of the respiratory membrane limits oxygen diffusion into the blood, causing a chronic decrease in the arterial oxygen tension.
TMP11 526

20. (B) When a person performs the Valsalva maneuver (forcing air against a closed glottis), high pressure builds up in the lungs that can force as much as 250 milliliters of blood from the pulmonary circulation into the systemic circulation. The lungs have an important blood reservoir function, automatically shifting blood to the systemic circulation as a compensatory response to hemorrhage and other conditions in which the systemic blood volume is too low.
TMP11 484

21. (A) Asbestosis is a constricted lung disease characterized by diffuse interstitial fibrosis. In constricted (also called restrictive) lung diseases, the maximum expiratory flow-volume curve begins and ends at abnormally low lung volumes, and the flow rates are often higher than normal at any given lung volume, as shown on the diagram. Lung volumes are expected to be higher than normal in asthma, bronchospasm, emphysema, old age, and other conditions in which the airways are narrowed or radial traction of the airways is reduced, allowing them to close more easily.
TMP11 526

22. (B) The diagram shows that a maximum respiratory effort is needed during resting conditions because the maximum expiratory flow rate is achieved. It should be clear that this patient's ability to exercise is greatly diminished. The man has smoked for 60 years and is likely to have emphysema. Therefore, the student can surmise that the total lung capacity, functional residual capacity, and residual volume are greater than normal. The vital capacity is only about 3.4 liters, as shown on the diagram.
TMP11 526

23. (C) Compliance (C) is equal to the change in lung volume (ΔV) that occurs for a given change in transpulmonary pressure (ΔP); that is, C = ΔV / ΔP. The transpulmonary pressure is the numerical difference between alveolar pressure and pleural pressure. Because static compliance is measured when air flow

is equal to zero, and therefore alveolar pressure is equal to zero, it should be clear that transpulmonary pressure is equal to pleural pressure under the conditions stated in the problem. The problem provides the compliance (0.25 L/cm H_2O) and the change in pleural pressure (4 cm H_2O) that occurs when the man inhales. Therefore, the man inhales 1.0 liter ($\Delta V = \Delta P \times C = 4$ cm $H_2O \times 0.25$ L/cm $H_2O = 1.0$ liter).
   TMP11 473

24. (B) The diffusing capacity of a gas is the volume of the gas that will diffuse through a membrane each minute for a pressure difference of 1 mm Hg. The diffusing capacity of oxygen is increased during exercise by the opening of previously closed capillaries (recruitment) and the dilation of previously open capillaries (distention), both of which increase the surface area of the blood into which oxygen can diffuse. Improving the ventilation-perfusion ratio, which means improving the match between the ventilation of the alveoli and the perfusion of the alveolar capillaries with blood, can also improve oxygenation during exercise.
   TMP11 486

25. (G) The sensor neurons in the chemosensitive area are especially sensitive to hydrogen ions. In fact, hydrogen ions may be the only important direct stimulus for these neurons. However, hydrogen ions do not easily cross the blood-brain barrier. For this reason, changes in hydrogen ion concentration in the blood have considerably less effect in stimulating the chemosensitive neurons compared with carbon dioxide (which passes easily through the blood-brain barrier). Although carbon dioxide has little direct effect in stimulating the chemosensitive neurons, it does have a potent indirect effect. It does this by reacting with water to form carbonic acid, which in turn dissociates into bicarbonate and hydrogen ions. Therefore, carbon dioxide is the most potent blood factor and hydrogen ion is the most potent direct stimulus of the chemosensitive neurons.
   TMP11 516

26. (D) Because the compliance is 0.2 L/cm H_2O, it should be clear that a 1.0-liter increase in volume will cause a 5 cm H_2O decrease in pleural pressure (1.0 L / 0.2 L/cm H_2O = 5.0 cm H_2O); and, because the initial pleural pressure was –4 cm H_2O before inhalation, the pressure is reduced by 5 cm H_2O (to –9 cm H_2O) when 1.0 liter of air is inhaled.
   TMP11 473

27. (F) Alveolar ventilation can increase by more than eightfold when the arterial carbon dioxide tension is increased over a physiological range from about 35 to 75 mm Hg. This demonstrates the tremendous effect that changes in carbon dioxide have in controlling respiration. By contrast, the change in respiration caused by changing the blood pH over a normal range from 7.3 to 7.5 is more than 10 times less effective.
   TMP11 517

28. (D) It is important for the blood to be distributed to those segments of the lungs where the alveoli are best oxygenated. When the oxygen tension of the alveoli decreases below normal, the adjacent blood vessels constrict, causing their resistance to increase as much fivefold at extremely low oxygen levels. This is opposite to the effect observed in systemic vessels, which dilate in response to low oxygen (i.e., resistance decreases).
   TMP11 485

29. (A) The forced vital capacity (FVC) is the vital capacity measured with a forced expiration. The forced expiratory volume in 1 second (FEV_1) is the amount of air that can be expelled from the lungs during the first second of a forced expiration. The FEV_1/FVC for the normal individual (curve X) is 4 L/5 L = 80 per cent, and it is 2 L/4 L = 50 per cent for the patient (curve Z). The FEV_1/FVC ratio has diagnostic value for differentiating normal, obstructive, and constricted patterns of forced expiration.
   TMP11 526

30. (B) It is not practical to measure the oxygen diffusing capacity directly, because it is not possible to accurately measure the oxygen tension of the pulmonary capillary blood. However, the diffusing capacity for carbon monoxide (CO) can be measured accurately because the CO tension in pulmonary capillary blood is zero under normal conditions. The CO diffusing capacity is then used to calculate the oxygen diffusing capacity by taking into account the differences in diffusion coefficient between oxygen and CO. Knowing the rate of transfer of CO across the respiratory membrane is often helpful for evaluating the presence of parenchymal lung disease when spirometry or lung volume determinations suggest a reduced vital capacity, residual volume, or total lung capacity.
   TMP11 499

31. (A) The PO_2 of mixed venous blood entering the pulmonary capillaries increases during its transit through the pulmonary capillaries (from 40 to 104 mm Hg), and the PCO_2 decreases simultaneously from 45 to 40 mm Hg. During resting conditions, oxygen has a 64 mm Hg pressure gradient (104 – 40 = 64 mm Hg) and carbon dioxide has a 5 mm Hg pressure gradient (45 – 40 = 5 mm Hg) between the blood at the arterial end of the capillaries and the alveolar air. Despite this large difference in pressure gradients between oxygen and carbon dioxide, both gases equilibrate with the alveolar air by the time the blood has moved a third of the distance through the capillaries in the normal resting state (choice A). This is possible because carbon dioxide can diffuse about 20 times as rapidly as oxygen.
   TMP11 502

32. (B) Blood at the venous ends of the pulmonary capillaries has a PO_2 of about 104 mm Hg, which is virtually identical to that of alveolar air. The PO_2 of blood decreases by about 9 mm Hg during its transit

from the venous ends of the pulmonary capillaries (104 mm Hg) to the aorta (95 mm Hg), mostly because venous blood from the bronchial circulation enters the pulmonary veins. The PO_2 of aortic blood remains unchanged during its transit through the arterial system but begins to decrease slightly in the arterioles and then more so in the systemic capillaries, reaching, on average, a mixed venous PO_2 of 40 mm Hg. Therefore, the PO_2 of blood increases by 64 mm Hg as it flows from the pulmonary artery to the venous ends of the pulmonary capillaries (104 − 40 = 64 mm Hg) and decreases by 55 mm Hg as it flows from the aorta to the pulmonary artery (95 − 40 = 55 mm Hg).
TMP11 503

33. (C) Because the blood that perfuses the pulmonary capillaries is venous blood returning to the lungs (i.e., mixed venous blood) from the systemic circulation, the alveolar gases equilibrate with the gases in this blood. Therefore, when an airway is blocked, the alveolar air equilibrates with the mixed venous blood, and the partial pressures of the gases in both the blood and the alveolar air become identical.
TMP11 500

34. (E) The forced vital capacity (FVC) is the vital capacity measured with a forced expiration. The forced expiratory volume in 1 second (FEV_1) is the amount of air that can be expelled from the lungs during the first second of a forced expiration. The FEV_1/FVC ratio for the healthy individual X is 4 L/5 L = 80 percent; the FEV_1/FVC for patient Z is 3.0 L/3.5 L = 86 per cent. FEV_1/FVC is often increased in silicosis and other diseases characterized by interstitial fibrosis because of the increased radial traction of the airways; that is, the airways are held open to a greater extent at any given lung volume, reducing their resistance to air flow. Airway resistance is increased (and therefore FEV_1/FVC is decreased) in asthma, bronchospasm, emphysema, and old age.
TMP11 526

35. (C) Pulmonary venous blood is nearly 100 per cent saturated with oxygen, has a PO_2 of about 104 mm Hg, and each 100 milliliters of blood carries about 20 grams of oxygen (i.e., oxygen content is about 20 volumes per cent). Approximately 25 per cent of the oxygen carried in the arterial blood is used by the tissues under resting conditions. Thus, reduced blood returning to the lungs is about 75 per cent saturated with oxygen, has a PO_2 of about 40 mm Hg, and has an oxygen content of about 15 volumes per cent. Note that it is necessary to know only one value for oxygenated and reduced blood; the other two values requested in the question can be read from the oxygen-hemoglobin dissociation curve.
TMP11 506

36. (B) Alveolar air normally equilibrates with the mixed venous blood that perfuses the alveoli, so the gas composition of alveolar air and pulmonary capillary blood is identical. When a group of alveoli is not perfused, the composition of the alveolar air becomes equal to the inspired gas composition, which has an oxygen tension of 149 mm Hg and a carbon dioxide tension of about 0 mm Hg.
TMP11 500

37. (D) Surfactant is formed relatively late in fetal life. Premature babies born without adequate amounts of surfactant can develop pulmonary failure and die. Surfactant is a surface-active agent that greatly reduces the surface tension of the water lining the alveoli. Water is normally attracted to itself, which is why raindrops are round. By reducing the surface tension of the water lining the alveoli (and thus reducing the tendency of water molecules to coalesce), surfactant reduces the work of breathing; that is, less transpulmonary pressure is required to inhale a given volume of air. Because compliance is equal to the change in lung volume for a given change in transpulmonary pressure, it should be clear that pulmonary compliance is decreased in the absence of surfactant.
TMP11 529

38. (D) The arterial oxygen tension has essentially no effect on alveolar ventilation when it is higher than about 100 mm Hg, but ventilation approximately doubles when the arterial oxygen tension falls to 60 mm Hg, and it can increase as much as fivefold at very low oxygen tensions. This quantitative relationship between arterial oxygen tension and alveolar ventilation was established in an experimental setting in which the arterial carbon dioxide tension and pH were held constant. The student can imagine that the ventilatory response to hypoxia would be blunted if the carbon dioxide tension were permitted to decrease.
TMP11 518

39. (B) The excess ventilatory blow-off of carbon dioxide that normally inhibits an increase in respiration fails to do so after acclimatization has occurred. This allows the low oxygen to drive the respiratory system to a much higher level of alveolar ventilation than under acute low-oxygen conditions.
TMP11 519

40. (B) The P_{50} of the oxygen-hemoglobin dissociation curve is the oxygen partial pressure required to achieve 50 per cent saturation of hemoglobin. The P_{50} is about 25 mm Hg during resting conditions, as shown on the diagram. Exercise causes the oxygen-hemoglobin curve to shift to the right, which increases the P_{50} to a higher value. Factors that cause a rightward shift of the curve include increases in temperature, hydrogen ion concentration, carbon dioxide tension, and 2,3-diphosphoglycerate.
TMP11 506

41. (C) The laboratory results are normal except for hemoglobin, which is reduced to 7.2 g/dl (normal for a male is 13.5 to 17.5 g/dl). A decrease in blood

hemoglobin causes a proportionate decrease in the oxygen carrying capacity of the blood. Each gram of hemoglobin normally carries 1.34 ml of oxygen when the hemoglobin is fully saturated with oxygen. Thus, the arterial blood normally carries about 20 ml of oxygen for each 100 milliliters of blood, assuming a hemoglobin concentration of 15 g/dl ($1.34 \times 15 = 20$). With a blood hemoglobin of 7.2 g/dl, the oxygen content would be 9.6 ml oxygen/100 dl. The oxygen saturation of hemoglobin in the arterial blood and the arterial oxygen partial pressure are not affected by the hemoglobin concentration of the blood.
TMP11 506

42. (D) A decrease in the ventilation-perfusion ratio ($\dot{V}_A/\dot{Q}$) is depicted by moving to the left along the normal ventilation-perfusion line shown in the diagram. Whenever the $\dot{V}_A/\dot{Q}$ is below normal, there is inadequate ventilation to provide the oxygen needed to fully oxygenate the blood flowing through the alveolar capillaries (i.e., alveolar P_{O_2} is low). Therefore, a certain fraction of the venous blood passing through the pulmonary capillaries does not become oxygenated. Poorly ventilated areas of the lung also accumulate carbon dioxide that diffuses into the alveoli from the mixed venous blood. The result of decreasing the $\dot{V}_A/\dot{Q}$ (moving to the left along the $\dot{V}_A/\dot{Q}$ line) on alveolar P_{O_2} and P_{CO_2} is shown on the diagram—P_{O_2} decreases and P_{CO_2} increases.
TMP11 500

43. (A) The difference in hydrostatic pressure between the highest and lowest points in the lungs of an upright person is about 30 cm, which represents a 23 mm Hg difference in blood pressure. This means that the pulmonary arterial pressure at the top of the lungs is about 15 mm Hg less than at the level of the heart, and the arterial pressure is about 8 mm Hg higher at the lowest point in the lungs. These differences in pulmonary blood pressure cause the flow to be highest in the lower portions of the lungs, where the vessels are stretched open to the greatest extent, and the flow at the apex is lowest. The relative differences in blood flow in the upright lung are similar when cardiac output increases during exercise. When the alveolar pressure is increased during positive pressure breathing or when the pulmonary arterial pressure is low during hypovolemic states, the alveolar pressure becomes greater than the arterial pressure, which can decrease blood flow to zero at the top of the lungs (which is then called zone 1).
TMP11 486

44. (D) The vital capacity (VC) is the maximum amount of air a person can expel from the lungs after first filling the lungs to their maximum extent and then expiring to the maximum extent. The total lung capacity (TLC; 6 liters) is the maximum volume to which the lungs can be expanded with the greatest possible effort. The residual volume (RV; 1 liter) is the volume of air remaining in the lungs after the

most forceful expiration. Therefore, VC = TLC − RV = 6 liters − 1 liter = 5 liters.
TMP11 475

45. (E) Physiologic shunt is the total amount of blood per minute that passes through the lungs without being oxygenated. The ventilation-perfusion ratio ($\dot{V}_A/\dot{Q}$) is low when physiologic dead space is high because of inadequate ventilation. Physiologic dead space is the sum of alveolar dead space and anatomic dead space. Alveolar dead space consists of alveoli that are ventilated but are not perfused and thus do not participate in gas exchange. $\dot{V}_A/\dot{Q}$ is high when physiologic dead space is high because of inadequate blood flow. Some of the air that a person breathes in fills the respiratory passageways and never reaches the gas exchange areas of the lungs. This air is called the anatomic dead space because it is not useful for gas exchange. In those who smoke, various degrees of bronchial obstruction occur; this causes air to be trapped in the alveoli, resulting in emphysema. The obstructed areas of the lung without adequate ventilation have a low $\dot{V}_A/\dot{Q}$ (increased physiologic shunt). In those areas of the lung where alveolar walls are mainly destroyed, there is still ventilation, but this is mostly wasted because of inadequate blood flow resulting in a high $\dot{V}_A/\dot{Q}$ (increased physiologic dead space).
TMP11 478

46. (E) It is remarkable that the arterial P_{O_2}, P_{CO_2}, and pH remain almost exactly normal in a healthy athlete during strenuous exercise despite the 20-fold increase in oxygen consumption and carbon dioxide formation. This interesting phenomenon begs the question: What is it that causes the intense ventilation during exercise?
TMP11 520

47. (A) Because strenuous exercise does not significantly change the mean arterial P_{O_2}, P_{CO_2}, or pH, it is unlikely that these play an important role in stimulating the immense increase in ventilation. Although the mean venous P_{O_2} decreases during exercise, the venous vasculature does not contain chemoreceptors that can sense P_{O_2}. The brain, as it transmits motor impulses to the contracting muscles, is believed to transmit collateral impulses to the brain stem to excite the respiratory center. Also, the movement of body parts during exercise is believed to excite joint and muscle proprioceptors, which then transmit excitatory impulses to the respiratory center.
TMP11 520

48. (B) A reduction in $\dot{V}_A/\dot{Q}$ (caused by the partially obstructed airway in this problem) causes the alveolar P_{O_2} and P_{CO_2} to approach the values achieved when $\dot{V}_A/\dot{Q} = 0$. When the ventilation is reduced to zero ($\dot{V}_A/\dot{Q} = 0$), alveolar air equilibrates with the mixed venous blood entering the lung, which causes the gas composition of the alveolar air to become identical to that of the blood. This occurs at point A

on the diagram, where the alveolar P_{O_2} is 40 mm Hg and the alveolar P_{CO_2} is 45 mm Hg.
TMP11 500

49. (D) A pulmonary embolism decreases blood flow to the affected lung, causing ventilation to exceed blood flow. An increase in $\dot{V}_A/\dot{Q}$ caused by the partially obstructed blood flow in this problem causes the alveolar P_{O_2} and P_{CO_2} to approach the values achieved when $\dot{V}_A/\dot{Q} = \infty$. When an embolism completely blocks all blood flow to an area of the lung, the gas composition of the inspired air entering the alveoli equilibrates with the blood trapped in the alveolar capillaries, so that within a short time, the gas composition of the alveolar air is identical to that of inspired air. This situation, in which $\dot{V}_A/\dot{Q}$ is equal to infinity, corresponds to point E on the diagram (inspired gas).
TMP11 500

50. (B) The forced vital capacity (FVC) is the vital capacity measured with a forced expiration (FVC = 4.0 liters for patient Z). The forced expiratory volume in 1 second (FEV_1) is the amount of air that can be expelled from the lungs during the first second of a forced expiration (FEV_1 = 2.0 liters for patient Z). FEV_1/FVC is a function of airway resistance. Airway resistance is often increased in emphysematous lungs, which causes FEV_1/FVC to decrease. Note that FEV_1/FVC is 50 per cent in patient Z and 80 per cent in the healthy individual represented by curve X. The FEV_1/FVC ratio is usually not affected in pleural effusion and pneumothorax because airway resistance is normal. FVC is often decreased in asbestosis, fibrotic pleurisy, silicosis, and tuberculosis, and the FEV_1/FVC ratio is either normal or slightly increased.
TMP11 526

51. (H) The oxygen carrying capacity of the blood is reduced in an anemic person, but the arterial P_{O_2} and oxygen saturation of hemoglobin are both normal. The decrease in arterial oxygen content is compensated for by an increase in the extraction of oxygen from hemoglobin, which reduces the P_{O_2} of the venous blood. The unloading of oxygen at the tissue level is enhanced by increased levels of 2,3-diphosphoglycerate (2,3-DPG) in an anemic patient because 2,3-DPG causes a rightward shift of the oxygen-hemoglobin dissociation curve.
TMP11 506

52. (E) Carbon monoxide (CO) combines with hemoglobin at the same point on the hemoglobin molecule as oxygen does; therefore, CO can displace oxygen from the hemoglobin, reducing its oxygen saturation. Because CO binds with hemoglobin (to form carboxyhemoglobin) with about 250 times as much tenacity as oxygen does, even small amounts of CO in the blood can severely limit its oxygen carrying capacity. The presence of carboxyhemoglobin also shifts the oxygen dissociation curve to the left (which means that oxygen binds more tightly to

hemoglobin), which further limits the transfer of oxygen to the tissues.
TMP11 509

53. (E) Prolonged exposure to silica causes interstitial fibrosis, which in turn decreases pulmonary compliance. Compliance is the change in lung volume for a given change in transpulmonary pressure required to inflate the lungs. The volume-pressure curve indicates that the patient has a lower than normal pulmonary compliance, which is consistent with silicosis. The elastic recoil of the lung is increased when fibrous material is deposited in the interstitium and alveolar walls, reducing the distensibility (compliance) of the lung. The pulmonary compliance is increased in emphysema and old age. Asthma and other diseases characterized by bronchospasm also cause the apparent pulmonary compliance to increase.
TMP11 526

54. (A) The expiratory reserve volume (ERV) is the maximum extra volume of air that can be expired by forceful expiration after the end of a normal tidal expiration. ERV is equal to the difference between the functional residual capacity (FRC; 3 liters) and the residual volume (RV; 1 liter). Although neither FRC nor RV can be determined from a spirogram alone, the relative differences between these two volumes can be determined from a spirogram and can be used to calculate ERV.
TMP11 476

55. (D) The functional residual capacity (FRC) equals the expiratory reserve volume (2 liters) plus the residual volume (1.5 liters). This is the amount of air that remains in the lungs at the end of a normal expiration. FRC is considered to be the resting volume of the lungs, because none of the respiratory muscles is contracted at FRC. This problem illustrates an important point: a spirogram can measure changes in lung volume but not absolute lung volumes. Thus, a spirogram alone cannot be used to determine residual volume, functional residual capacity, or total lung capacity.
TMP11 476

56. (B) In exercise, several factors shift the oxygen-hemoglobin curve to the right, which serves to deliver extra amounts of oxygen to the exercising muscle fibers. These factors include increased quantities of carbon dioxide released from the muscle fibers, increased hydrogen ion concentration in the muscle capillary blood, and increased temperature resulting from heat generated by the exercising muscle. The rightward shift of the oxygen-hemoglobin curve allows more oxygen to be released to the muscle at a given oxygen partial pressure in the blood.
TMP11 508

57. (B) The loss of alveolar walls, with destruction of associated capillary beds in the emphysematous lung, reduces the elastic recoil and increases the

compliance. Recall that compliance is equal to the change in lung volume for a given change in transpulmonary pressure; that is, compliance is equal to the slopes of the volume-pressure relationships shown in the diagram. Asbestosis, silicosis, and tuberculosis are associated with deposition of fibrous tissue in the lungs, which decreases the compliance. Mitral obstruction and rheumatic heart disease can cause pulmonary edema, which also decreases the pulmonary compliance.

TMP11 473

58. (C) Structural differences between fetal hemoglobin and adult hemoglobin make fetal hemoglobin unable to react with 2,3-diphosphoglycerate and thus to have a higher affinity for oxygen at a given partial pressure of oxygen. The fetal dissociation curve is therefore shifted to the left relative to the adult curve. Typically, fetal arterial oxygen pressures are low; hence, the leftward shift enhances the placental uptake of oxygen.

TMP11 506

59. (A) The capillaries in the alveolar walls are distended by the blood pressure within them, but they are simultaneously compressed by the alveolar air pressure outside them. The pulmonary systolic pressure is greater than the alveolar air pressure for at least part of the cardiac cycle, so that normally, all portions of the lung are perfused. However, if an upright person is breathing against a positive pressure, so that the intra-alveolar pressure is at least 10 mm Hg greater than normal but the pulmonary systolic pressure is normal, one would expect blood flow to be zero or close to zero. This is referred to as zone 1 conditions.

TMP11 486

60. (C) Cheyne-Stokes breathing is the most common type of periodic breathing. The person breathes deeply for a short interval and then breathes slightly or not at all for an additional interval. This pattern repeats itself about every minute. Apnea is a transient cessation of respiration, so Cheyne-Stokes breathing is associated with periods of apnea. Biot's breathing refers to sequences of uniformly deep gasps, apnea, and then deep gasps. Hyperpnea means increased breathing and usually refers to increased tidal volume with or without increased frequency. Tachypnea means increased frequency of breathing.

TMP11 522

61. (C) Curve X represents heavy exercise with a tidal volume of about 3 liters. Note that the expiratory flow rate has reached a maximum value of nearly 4.5 L/sec during the heavy exercise. This occurred because maximum expiratory air flow is required to move the air through the airways with the high ventilatory frequency associated with heavy exercise. Normal breathing at rest is represented by curve Z; note that the tidal volume is less than 1 liter during resting conditions. Curve Y was recorded during

mild exercise. An asthma attack or aspiration of meat would increase the resistance to air flow from the lungs, making it unlikely that the expiratory air flow rate could approach its maximum value at a given lung volume. The tidal volume should not increase greatly with pneumonia or tuberculosis, and it should not be possible to achieve a maximum expiratory air flow at a given lung volume with these diseases.

TMP11 525

62. (D) Each gram of hemoglobin normally carries 1.34 milliliters of oxygen. This man has a hemoglobin concentration of 10 g/dl, and his arterial blood is fully saturated with oxygen. Therefore, the arterial oxygen content is $1.34 \times 10 = 13.4$ ml O_2/dl of blood. The mixed venous oxygen content (measured from a blood sample taken from the pulmonary artery) is equal to the arterial oxygen content minus the oxygen usage by the tissues. This latter fact eliminates choice C and leaves choice D as the correct answer. Although about 5 milliliters of oxygen are extracted from each 100 milliliters of blood under normal resting conditions, this is decreased in anemia and is dependent on other considerations, such as how much the cardiac output has increased and how much the oxygen-hemoglobin curve has shifted to the right.

TMP11 506

63. (C) Breathing 100 per cent oxygen has a limited effect on the arterial P_{O_2} when the cause of arterial hypoxemia is a vascular shunt. However, breathing 100 per cent oxygen raises the arterial P_{O_2} to over 600 mm Hg in a normal subject. With a vascular shunt, the arterial P_{O_2} is determined by highly oxygenated end-capillary blood ($P_{O_2} > 600$ mm Hg) that has passed through ventilated portions of the lung and by shunted blood that has bypassed the ventilated portions of the lungs and thus has an oxygen partial pressure equal to that of mixed venous blood ($P_{O_2} = 40$ mm Hg). A mixture of the two bloods causes a large fall in P_{O_2} because the oxygen dissociation curve is so flat in its upper range.

TMP11 500

64. (D) The anatomic dead space (D_{ANAT}) is the air that a person breathes in that fills the respiratory passageways but never reaches the alveoli. Alveolar dead space (D_{ALV}) is the air in the alveoli that are ventilated but not perfused. Physiologic dead space (D_{PHY}) is the sum of D_{ANAT} and D_{ALV}. D_{ALV} is zero in lung unit S (the ideal lung unit), so D_{ANAT} and D_{PHY} are equal to each other. The diagram shows a group of alveoli with a poor blood supply (lung unit T), which means that D_{ALV} is substantial. Thus, D_{PHY} is greater than either D_{ANAT} or D_{ALV} in lung unit T.

TMP11 500

65. (B) A spirometer can be used to measure changes in lung volume but cannot determine absolute volume. It consists of a drum filled with air inverted over a chamber of water. When the person breathes in and

out, the drum moves up and down, recording the changes in lung volume. The spirometer cannot be used to measure residual volume (RV) because the RV of air in the lungs cannot be exhaled into the spirometer. The functional residual capacity (FRC) is the amount of air left in the lungs after a normal expiration. FRC cannot be measured using a spirometer because it contains the RV. The total lung capacity (TLC) is the total amount of air that the lungs can hold after a maximum inspiration. Because the TLC includes the RV, it cannot be measured using a spirometer. TLC, FRC, and RV can be determined using the helium dilution method or a body plethysmograph.
TMP11 475

66. (D) Alveolar ventilation (V_A) per minute is the total volume of new air entering the alveoli and adjacent gas exchange areas each minute. It is equal to the respiratory frequency times the amount of new air that enters these areas with each breath. Thus, $V_A = (V_T - V_D) \times$ Freq, where V_T is the tidal volume, V_D is the dead space volume, and Freq is the frequency of respiration per minute.
TMP11 478

67. (B) The basic mechanism of Cheyne-Stokes breathing can be attributed to a buildup of carbon dioxide, which stimulates overventilation, followed by a depression of the respiratory center due to a low PCO_2 of the respiratory neurons. It should be clear that the greatest depth of breathing occurs when the neurons of the respiratory center are exposed to the highest levels of carbon dioxide (point W). This increase in breathing causes carbon dioxide to be blown off; thus, the PCO_2 of lung blood is at its lowest value at about point Y on the diagram. The PCO_2 of pulmonary blood gradually increases from point Y to point Z, reaching its maximum value at point V. Thus, it is the phase lag between the PCO_2 at the respiratory center and the PCO_2 of the pulmonary blood that leads to this type of breathing. This phase lag often occurs with left heart failure due to enlargement of the left ventricle, which increases the time required for blood to reach the respiratory center. Another cause of Cheyne-Stokes breathing is increased negative feedback gain in the respiratory control areas, which can be caused by head trauma, stroke, and other types of brain damage.
TMP11 522

68. (E) Loss of lung tissue in emphysema leads to an increase in the compliance of the lungs and a decrease in the elastic recoil of the lungs. Pulmonary compliance and elastic recoil always change in opposite directions—that is, compliance is proportional to 1/elastic recoil. The total lung capacity, residual volume, and functional residual capacity are increased in emphysema, but the vital capacity is decreased.
TMP11 471

69. (A) Most of the carbon dioxide (70 per cent) is transported in the blood in the form of bicarbonate ion. Dissolved carbon dioxide reacts with water to form carbonic acid (mostly in red blood cells), which dissociates into bicarbonate and hydrogen ions. Carbon dioxide also reacts with amine radicals of the hemoglobin molecule to form the compound carbaminohemoglobin, which accounts for about 23 per cent of the carbon dioxide transported in the blood. The remaining carbon dioxide (7 per cent) is transported in the dissolved state.
TMP11 510

70. (A) Alveolar ventilation (V_A) per minute is the total volume of new air entering the alveoli and adjacent gas exchange areas each minute. V_A is equal to the respiratory frequency times the amount of new air that enters these areas with each breath. Thus, $V_A = (V_T - V_D) \times$ Freq, where V_T is the tidal volume, V_D is the dead space volume, and Freq is the frequency of respiration per minute. V_A is equal to zero in this problem because V_T is equal to V_D. This problem illustrates an important point: hyperventilation is defined as an increase in alveolar ventilation—it is not defined as an increase in the frequency of ventilation. The most effective way to increase V_A is to increase the tidal volume—by taking long, deep breaths.
TMP11 478

71. (E) Compliance (C) is the change in lung volume (ΔV) that occurs for a given change in transpulmonary pressure (ΔP): $C = \Delta V / \Delta P$. (Transpulmonary pressure is the difference between alveolar pressure and pleural pressure.) Because compliance is equal to the slope of the volume-pressure relationship, it should be clear that curve S represents the highest compliance and that curve U represents the lowest compliance.
TMP11 473

72. (C) Asbestosis is associated with deposition of fibrous material in the lungs. This causes the pulmonary compliance (i.e., distensibility) to decrease and the elastic recoil to increase. Pulmonary compliance and elastic recoil change in opposite directions because compliance is proportional to 1/elastic recoil. It is somewhat surprising to learn that the elastic recoil of a rock is greater than that of a rubber band; that is, the more difficult it is to deform an object, the greater the object's elastic recoil. The total lung capacity, functional residual capacity, residual volume, and vital capacity are decreased in all types of fibrotic lung disease.
TMP11 473

73. (E) Failure of the left ventricle causes blood to dam up in the left atrium and lungs, which leads to increases in the left atrial and pulmonary capillary pressures. When the pulmonary capillary pressure rises to a value approximately equal to that of the plasma colloid osmotic pressure, excess amounts of fluid begin to collect in the lungs. The accumulation

of excess interstitial fluid raises the interstitial fluid hydrostatic pressure from its normal negative value (i.e., subatmospheric value) to a positive value. Lymph flow increases greatly when excess fluid accumulates in the lungs.

TMP11 487

74. (B) In pneumonia, the pulmonary membrane becomes inflamed and highly porous, so that fluid, red blood cells, and white blood cells leak from the blood into the alveoli. The accumulation of fluid and cells in the alveoli results in two major pulmonary abnormalities: reduction in the surface area of the pulmonary membrane, and decreased ventilation-perfusion ratio. Both of these effects cause hypoxemia (low blood oxygen) and hypercapnia (high blood carbon dioxide).

TMP11 527

75. (E) Total ventilation is equal to the tidal volume (V_T) times the ventilation frequency (Freq). Alveolar ventilation = $(V_T - V_D) \times$ Freq, where V_D is the dead space volume. Both individuals have the same total ventilation: subject T, $2,000 \times 10 = 20$ L/min; subject V, $500 \times 40 = 20$ L/min. However, subject T has an alveolar ventilation of 18 liters ($[2000 - 200] \times 10$), whereas subject V has an alveolar ventilation of only 12 liters ($[500 - 200] \times 40$). This problem further illustrates that the most effective means of increasing alveolar ventilation is to increase the tidal volume, not the respiratory frequency.

TMP11 478

76. (C) The respiratory exchange ratio (R) is equal to the rate of carbon dioxide output divided by the rate of oxygen uptake. A value of 0.8 means that the amount of carbon dioxide produced by the tissues is 80 per cent of the amount of oxygen used by the tissues, which also means that the amount of carbon dioxide transported from the tissues to the lungs in each 100 milliliters of blood is 80 per cent of the amount of oxygen transported from the lungs to the tissues in each 100 milliliters of blood. Choice C is the only answer in which the ratio of carbon dioxide to oxygen is 0.8 ($4/5 = 0.8$). Although R changes under different metabolic conditions, ranging from 1.00 in those who consume carbohydrates exclusively to 0.7 in those who consume fats exclusively, the average value for R is close to 0.8.

TMP11 512

77. (F) Dissolved carbon dioxide combines with water in red blood cells to form carbonic acid, which dissociates to form bicarbonate and hydrogen ions. Many of the bicarbonate ions diffuse out of the red blood cells while chloride ions diffuse into the red blood cells to maintain electrical neutrality. This phenomenon, called the chloride shift, is made possible by a special bicarbonate-chloride carrier protein in the red cell membrane that shuttles the ions in opposite directions. Water moves into the red blood

cells to maintain osmotic equilibrium, which results in a slight swelling of the red blood cells in the venous blood.

TMP11 511

78. (D) The surface area of the pulmonary membrane is reduced to half of normal because the right lung is totally nonfunctional. Blood flow is routed through the ventilated lung and therefore becomes well aerated during resting conditions; thus, the arterial PCO_2 and PO_2 are both normal.

TMP11 528

79. (D) The lower zones of the lung ventilate better than the upper zones, and the middle zones have intermediate ventilation. These differences in regional ventilation can be explained by regional differences in pleural pressure. The pleural pressure is typically about -10 cm H_2O in the upper regions and about -2.5 cm H_2O in the lower regions. A less negative pleural pressure in the lower regions of the chest cavity causes less expansion of the lower zones of the lung during resting conditions. Therefore, the bottom of the lung is relatively compressed during rest but expands better during inspiration compared with the apex.

80. (D) The loss of lung tissue associated with emphysema leads to a decrease in the diffusion capacity of the lungs, which results in arterial hypoxemia. Oxygen therapy can return the arterial oxygen levels to normal. Oxygen therapy is of limited value in anemia, right-to-left cardiac shunts, and localized circulatory deficiencies because there is already sufficient oxygen available in the alveoli. Cyanide poisoning blocks the action of cytochrome oxidase to such an extent that the tissues cannot use oxygen regardless of how much is available.

TMP11 530

81. (C) A *Pseudomonas* infection can increase the capillary permeability in the lungs and elsewhere in the body, which leads to excess loss of plasma proteins into the interstitial spaces. This leakage of plasma proteins from the vasculature caused the plasma colloid osmotic pressure to decrease from a normal value of about 28 mm Hg to 19 mm Hg in this patient. The capillary hydrostatic pressure remained at a normal value of 7 mm Hg in this case, but it can sometimes increase to higher levels, exacerbating the formation of edema. The interstitial fluid hydrostatic pressure increased from a normal value of about -5 mm Hg to 1 mm Hg, which tends to decrease fluid loss from the capillaries. Excess fluid in the interstitial spaces (edema) causes lymph flow to increase.

TMP11 488

82. (B) Both the lung and the thoracic cage are elastic. Under normal conditions, the elastic tendency of the lungs to collapse is exactly balanced by the elastic tendency of the thoracic cage to expand. When air is introduced into the pleural space, the pleural pres-

sure becomes equal to atmospheric pressure—the chest wall springs outward, and the lungs collapse.

83. (B) The larger bronchi near the trachea have the greatest resistance to air flow in the healthy lung. However, in disease conditions, the smaller bronchioles often have a far greater role in determining resistance because they are easily occluded, owing to their small size, and they have an abundance of smooth muscle in their walls and therefore constrict easily.
TMP11 529

84. (D) Cyanosis appears whenever the arterial blood contains more than 5 grams of deoxygenated hemoglobin in each 100 milliliters of blood. A person with anemia almost never becomes cyanotic because of the low hemoglobin, whereas a person with polycythemia has so much hemoglobin that cyanosis can occur under normal conditions. The arterial oxygen content is increased because of the high hemoglobin, but the arterial oxygen tension and oxygen saturation are normal because the inspired oxygen tension is normal.
TMP11 531

85. (A) An increase in pulmonary volume causes a decrease in airway resistance, which means that airway diameter increases. The airways are tethered to the surrounding tissues, which causes them to be pulled open when the lungs expand. This so-called radial traction phenomenon explains why it is easier for a person with obstructive pulmonary disease to breathe at higher than normal lung volumes.
TMP11 525

86. (B) Smooth muscle tone in the respiratory passageways is under the control of the autonomic nervous system as well as circulating epinephrine. Motor innervation is by the vagus nerve. Stimulation of adrenergic receptors by norepinephrine and epinephrine causes bronchodilation. Parasympathetic activity (as well as acetylcholine) causes bronchoconstriction. Note that these effects of the autonomic nervous system on the respiratory passageways are opposite to those on peripheral blood vessels.
TMP11 479

Aviation, Space, and Deep-Sea Diving Physiology

1. An aviator is flying at 30,000 feet, where the barometric pressure is 226 mm Hg. He is breathing 100 per cent oxygen, his alveolar P_{CO_2} is 40 mm Hg, and his alveolar water vapor pressure is 47 mm Hg. What is the alveolar P_{O_2} of the aviator? (Assume that the respiratory exchange ratio is equal to 1.)
   (A) 43 mm Hg
   (B) 75 mm Hg
   (C) 99 mm Hg
   (D) 139 mm Hg
   (E) 215 mm Hg

2. A diver carries a 1000-liter metal talk-box with an open bottom to a depth of 66 feet. A person on the surface pumps air into the box until it is completely filled with air, which allows two divers to insert their heads into the box and talk beneath the water. How much air from the surface is required to fill the box?
   (A) 1000 liters
   (B) 2000 liters
   (C) 3000 liters
   (D) 4000 liters
   (E) 5000 liters

3. Which of the following sets of changes best describes a Himalayan native living in the Himalayas compared with a sea-level native living at sea level?

	Hematocrit	Arterial P_{O_2}	Arterial O_2 Content
(A)	Decreased	Decreased	Decreased
(B)	Decreased	Decreased	No difference
(C)	Decreased	Increased	Decreased
(D)	Decreased	Increased	No difference
(E)	Increased	Decreased	Decreased
(F)	Increased	Increased	Decreased
(G)	Increased	Increased	No difference
(H)	Increased	Decreased	No difference

4. A 35-year-old man remains at high altitude too long and develops chronic mountain sickness. Which of the following sets of changes best describes the man with chronic mountain sickness compared with someone living at high altitude who does not develop chronic mountain sickness?

	Hematocrit	Pulmonary Artery Pressure	Blood Viscosity
(A)	Decreased	Decreased	Decreased
(B)	Decreased	Increased	Decreased
(C)	Decreased	No difference	Decreased
(D)	Increased	Decreased	Increased
(E)	Increased	Increased	Increased
(F)	Increased	No difference	Increased

5. A diver breathing compressed air goes to a depth of 100 feet and remains there for 1 hour. What are the nitrogen and oxygen partial pressures in the air at this depth?

	Nitrogen (mm Hg)	Oxygen (mm Hg)
(A)	600	160
(B)	1201	319
(C)	1801	479
(D)	2402	638
(E)	3002	798

6. Exposure to 4 atmospheres of oxygen (P_{O_2} = 3040 mm Hg) can cause death within an hour or so. The acute lethal effects of oxygen poisoning can be attributed to the dysfunction of which of the following organs?
   (A) Brain
   (B) Heart
   (C) Kidneys
   (D) Liver
   (E) Lungs

7. A 35-year-old man travels to Mars. His exercise equipment malfunctions, so he is subjected to prolonged weightlessness without appropriate exercise. Which of the following sets of changes best describes the physiological changes that occur in this man?

	Blood Volume	Red Cell Mass	Maximum Cardiac Output
(A)	Decreased	Decreased	Decreased
(B)	Decreased	Increased	Increased
(C)	Decreased	No change	Decreased
(D)	Increased	Decreased	Decreased
(E)	Increased	Increased	Increased
(F)	Increased	No change	Decreased

8. A diver has the following gaseous pressures in his body fluids:
   H_2O 47 mm Hg
   CO_2 40 mm Hg
   O_2 60 mm Hg
   N_2 3918 mm Hg
   Which of the following best describe the gaseous pressures in his body fluids (in mm Hg) immediately after sudden decompression?

	H_2O	CO_2	O_2	N_2
(A)	0	40	100	1428
(B)	0	40	60	660
(C)	47	40	100	573
(D)	47	40	150	523
(E)	47	40	60	3918

Answers

1. (D) The alveolar oxygen tension (PAO_2) can be calculated using the following formula: $PAO_2 = PIO_2 - (PACO_2 / R) + F$, where PIO_2 is the inspired oxygen tension, $PACO_2$ is the alveolar carbon dioxide tension, R is the respiratory quotient (R = 1, as indicated in the question), and F is a small correction factor that can be ignored. PIO_2 is equal to the barometric pressure minus the water vapor pressure multiplied by the fractional concentration of oxygen in the inspired air: $PIO_2 = (226 - 47) \times 1.00 = 179$ mm Hg. Therefore, $PAO_2 = 179 - 40/1 = 139$ mm Hg.
   TMP11 538

2. (C) Boyle's law states that $P_1 \cdot V_1 = P_2 \cdot V_2$, where P_1 and V_1 are the original pressure and volume and P_2 and V_2 are the new pressure and volume. The atmospheric pressure at a depth of 66 feet is three times greater than the atmospheric pressure at the surface of the water; that is, there is 1 atmosphere at the surface plus an additional atmosphere for each 33 feet below the surface. Therefore, it takes three times as much sea-level air to fill the box when the box is submerged to a depth of 66 feet because the air is subjected to 3 atmospheres.
   TMP11 545

3. (H) Acclimatization to hypoxia includes an increase in pulmonary ventilation, an increase in red blood cells, an increase in diffusion capacity of the lungs, an increase in vascularity of the tissues, and an increase in the cells' ability to use the available oxygen. The increased hematocrit of high-altitude natives allows normal amounts (or even greater than normal amounts) of oxygen to be carried in the blood despite a lower than normal arterial oxygen tension. For example, natives of 15,000 feet have an arterial oxygen tension of only 40 mm Hg, but because of greater amounts of hemoglobin in the blood, the quantity of oxygen carried in the blood is often greater than that carried in the blood of sea-level natives.
   TMP11 539

4. (E) Chronic mountain sickness is characterized by an exceptionally high hematocrit; this increases the blood viscosity so much that blood flow to the peripheral tissues is decreased, and oxygen delivery begins to decrease as well. The pulmonary blood vessels are exceptionally vasospastic because of the lung hypoxia, which raises the pulmonary artery pressure to high levels, causing the right heart to fail. Death often follows unless the person is moved to a lower altitude.
   TMP11 541

5. (D) The atmospheric pressure at a depth of 100 feet is 3040 mm Hg, which is four times greater than the atmospheric pressure at the surface of the water; that is, there is 1 atmosphere (760 mm Hg) at the surface plus an additional atmosphere for each 33 feet below the surface ($4 \times 760 = 3040$ mm Hg). Because about 79 per cent of the air is nitrogen and 21 per cent is oxygen, the partial pressure of nitrogen at 4 atmospheres is $0.79 \times 3040 = 2402$ mm Hg, and the partial pressure of oxygen at 4 atmospheres is $0.21 \times 3040 = 638$ mm Hg.
   TMP11 547

6. (A) Molecular oxygen is converted to "active" forms of oxygen called oxygen free radicals. High concentrations of oxygen free radicals cause cell damage in many ways, but especially by oxidizing polyunsaturated fatty acids, which are essential components of many of the membranous structures of the cells. Nervous tissues are especially susceptible to the acute lethal effects of oxygen because of their high lipid content. Therefore, the acute lethal effects of oxygen toxicity are caused by brain dysfunction.
   TMP11 547

7. (A) The effects of a prolonged stay in space are similar to those of prolonged bed rest—decrease in blood volume, decrease in red cell mass, decrease in muscle strength and work capacity, decrease in maximum cardiac output, and loss of calcium and phosphate from the bones. Most of these problems can be greatly reduced by extensive exercise programs.
   TMP11 544

8. (E) The pressures of the various gases in the body fluids are identical before and immediately after sudden decompression. The pressure on the outside of the body becomes 1 atmosphere (760 mm Hg) after sudden decompression, whereas the pressures of water, carbon dioxide, oxygen, and nitrogen inside the body total 4065 mm Hg. Note that most of the gaseous pressure is caused by nitrogen (3918 mm Hg). This difference in gaseous pressure between the inside and outside of the body causes the gases (especially nitrogen) to form bubbles (or cavitate) in the tissues and blood. This leads to a condition called the "bends."
   TMP11 548

The Nervous System: General Principles and Sensory Physiology

1. After a pain stimulus is applied, fast pain is felt within which of the following time frames?
   (A) About 0.01 second
   (B) About 0.1 second
   (C) About 1 second
   (D) About 1 millisecond
   (E) About 1 nanosecond

2. Slow pain is also referred to as burning, aching, or throbbing pain and can be associated with which of the following?
   (A) Tissue damage or destruction
   (B) Inactivation of warmth receptors
   (C) Type Aδ sensory fibers
   (D) Skin temperatures between 35°C and 45°C
   (E) Certain encapsulated receptors such as pacinian corpuscles

3. The release of a neurotransmitter at a chemical synapse in the central nervous system is dependent on which of the following?
   (A) Synthesis of acetylcholinesterase
   (B) Hyperpolarization of the synaptic terminal
   (C) Fusion of synaptic vesicles with the postsynaptic membrane
   (D) Opening of ligand-gated calcium ion channels
   (E) Influx of calcium into the synaptic terminal

4. Which of the following is best described as an elongated, encapsulated receptor found in the dermal pegs of glabrous skin and is especially abundant on the lips and fingertips?
   (A) Pacinian corpuscle
   (B) Merkel's disc
   (C) Free nerve ending
   (D) Meissner's corpuscle
   (E) Ruffini's ending

5. Pain receptors in the skin are typically classified as which of the following?
   (A) Encapsulated nerve endings
   (B) A single class of morphologically specialized receptors
   (C) The same type of receptor that detects position sense
   (D) Free nerve endings
   (E) Pacinian corpuscles

6. Which of the following best describes an expanded tip tactile receptor found in the dermis of hairy skin that is specialized to detect continuously applied touch sensation?
   (A) Free nerve ending
   (B) Merkel's disc
   (C) Pacinian corpuscle
   (D) Ruffini's ending
   (E) Muscle spindle

7. Which of the following is a nonencapsulated receptor found in the epidermis of skin throughout the body as well as in the cornea, where it signals touch, pressure, and pain sensations?
   (A) Merkel's disc
   (B) Pacinian corpuscle
   (C) Free nerve ending
   (D) Golgi tendon organ
   (E) Muscle spindle

8. Which of the following best describes the concept of specificity in sensory nerve fibers that transmit only one modality of sensation?
   (A) Frequency coding principle
   (B) Concept of specific nerve energy
   (C) Unity theory
   (D) Singularity principle
   (E) Labeled line principle

9. Which of the following is an encapsulated receptor found deep in the skin throughout the body as well as in fascial layers, where it detects indentation of the skin (pressure) and movement across the surface (vibration)?
   (A) Pacinian corpuscle
   (B) Meissner's corpuscle
   (C) Free nerve ending
   (D) Ruffini's ending
   (E) Muscle spindle

10. Which of the following substances enhances the sensitivity of pain receptors but does not directly excite them?
    (A) Bradykinin
    (B) Serotonin
    (C) Histamine
    (D) Potassium ions
    (E) Prostaglandins

11. Which of the following is an important functional parameter of pain receptors?
    (A) Exhibit little or no adaptation
    (B) Are not affected by muscle tension
    (C) Signal only flexion at joint capsules
    (D) Can be inhibited voluntarily
    (E) Give rise to signals that rarely, if ever, convey the location of tissue ischemia

12. The excitatory or inhibitory action of a neurotransmitter is determined by which of the following?
    (A) Function of its postsynaptic receptor
    (B) Its molecular composition
    (C) Shape of the synaptic vesicle in which it is contained
    (D) Distance between the pre- and postsynaptic membranes
    (E) Influx of chloride ions into the synaptic terminal

13. Which of the following statements concerning the transmission of pain signals into the central nervous system is correct?
    (A) The "fast" pain fibers that conduct at about 6 to 30 m/sec are classified as type C fibers
    (B) Type Aδ pain fibers are responsible for the localization of a pain stimulus
    (C) Upon entering the spinal cord dorsal horn, the fast and slow pain fibers synapse with the same populations of neurons
    (D) The paleospinothalamic tract is specialized to rapidly conduct pain signals to the thalamus
    (E) The neospinothalamic tract carries pain signals that are responsible for chronic, lingering pain

14. Which of the following is the system that transmits somatosensory information with the highest degree of temporal and spatial fidelity?
    (A) Anterolateral system
    (B) Dorsal column–medial lemniscal system
    (C) Corticospinal system
    (D) Spinocerebellar system
    (E) Vestibulospinal system

15. Which of the following pathways crosses in the ventral white commissure of the spinal cord within a few segments of entry and then courses to the thalamus contralateral to the side of the body from which the signal originated?
    (A) Anterolateral system
    (B) Dorsal column–medial lemniscal system
    (C) Corticospinal system
    (D) Spinocerebellar system
    (E) Vestibulospinal system

16. Which transmitter agent is used by the fast pain fibers at their synapses in the dorsal horn?
    (A) Glutamate
    (B) Acetylcholine
    (C) GABA
    (D) Substance P
    (E) Calcitonin gene-related peptide

17. In chemical synapses that involve a so-called second messenger, typically a G protein linked to the post-synaptic receptor is activated when neurotransmitter binds to that receptor. Which of the following represents an activity performed by the activated second messenger?
    (A) Closure of a membrane channel for sodium or potassium
    (B) Activation of cyclic adenosine monophosphate (cAMP) or cyclic guanosine monophosphate (cGMP)
    (C) Inactivation of enzymes that initiate biochemical reactions in the postsynaptic neuron
    (D) Inactivation of gene transcription in the postsynaptic neuron
    (E) Inactivation of the neurotransmitter agent

18. Which transmitter agent used by the slow pain fibers is released slowly over a period of seconds or minutes at synapses in the dorsal horn?
    (A) Acetylcholine
    (B) Calcitonin gene-related peptide
    (C) GABA
    (D) Substance P
    (E) Glutamate

19. Which of the following systems conveys information concerning highly localized touch sensation and body position (proprioceptive) sensation?
    (A) Anterolateral system
    (B) Dorsal column–medial lemniscal system
    (C) Corticospinal system
    (D) Spinocerebellar system
    (E) Vestibulospinal system

20. Which of the following explains why individuals in severe pain have difficulty sleeping without sedative medication?
    (A) The somatosensory cortical area for pain perception blocks the sleep-generating circuits
    (B) Pain fibers entering the dorsal horn and the ascending pain pathways block the sleep-generating circuits
    (C) Ascending pain pathways provide excitatory input to brain stem reticular formation areas that are involved in maintenance of the alert, waking state
    (D) Neurotransmitters used in the slow pain pathway diffuse into neighboring cell groups and generally raise the excitability of the brain
    (E) Neurotransmitters used in the fast pain pathway diffuse into neighboring cell groups and block the sleep-generating circuits

21. The first-order (primary afferent) cell bodies of the dorsal column–medial lemniscal system are found in which of the following structures?
    (A) Spinal cord dorsal horn
    (B) Spinal cord ventral horn
    (C) Dorsal root ganglia
    (D) Nucleus cuneatus
    (E) Sympathetic chain ganglia

22. Which of the following structures carries axons from the nucleus gracilis to the thalamus?
    (A) Fasciculus gracilis
    (B) Fasciculus lemniscus
    (C) Lateral spinothalamic tract
    (D) Medial lemniscus
    (E) Medial longitudinal fasciculus

23. Which of the following represents the basis for transduction of a sensory stimulus into nerve impulses?
    (A) Change in the ion permeability of the receptor membrane
    (B) Generation of an action potential
    (C) Inactivation of a G protein–mediated response
    (D) Protein synthesis
    (E) Conversion of electrical energy to mechanical energy

24. Which of the following structures carries axons from neurons in the ventral posterolateral nucleus of the thalamus to the primary somatosensory cortex?
    (A) Medial lemniscus
    (B) External capsule
    (C) Internal capsule
    (D) Extreme capsule
    (E) Lateral lemniscus

25. Which of the following is characteristic of the events occurring at an excitatory synapse?
    (A) There is a massive efflux of calcium from the presynaptic terminal
    (B) Synaptic vesicles bind to the postsynaptic membrane
    (C) Voltage-gated potassium channels are closed
    (D) Ligand-gated channels are opened to allow sodium to enter the postsynaptic neuron
    (E) Electrical changes occurring at the postsynaptic membrane have no effect on other parts of the postsynaptic neuron

26. For the past 2 years, a 57-year-old man has suffered from severe pain resulting from a tumor involving the ascending colon. To relieve the pain, a surgeon is contemplating an anterolateral cordotomy. This procedure involves sectioning the anterolateral tract in the spinal cord to interrupt the ascending pain transmission pathway. Which of the following is the most appropriate site for this procedure?
    (A) L-5 region on left side
    (B) L-5 region on right side
    (C) T-6 region on left side
    (D) T-6 region on right side
    (E) Right lateral medulla

27. Which group of neurons in the brain's endogenous pain suppression system has cell bodies located in a portion of the midbrain?
    (A) Periaqueductal gray
    (B) Nucleus raphes magnus
    (C) Dorsal horn of spinal cord

28. Which of the following body parts is represented superiorly and medially within the postcentral gyrus?
    (A) Upper limb
    (B) Lower limb
    (C) Abdomen
    (D) Genitalia
    (E) Face

29. In which of the following regions of the pain suppression pathway do neurons use serotonin as a neurotransmitter?
    (A) Postcentral gyrus
    (B) Nucleus raphes magnus
    (C) Periaqueductal gray

30. As the receptor potential rises higher above a threshold, which of the following best characterizes the new frequency of action potentials?
    (A) Decreased
    (B) Increased
    (C) Unchanged
    (D) Increased only when the receptor potential increases to twice the threshold level
    (E) Unchanged until the receptor potential increases to twice the threshold level

31. An interneuron in which region uses enkephalin to inhibit pain transmission?
    (A) Nucleus raphes magnus
    (B) Postcentral gyrus
    (C) Dorsal horn of spinal cord

32. What is the Brodmann number designation for the primary somatosensory cortex?
    (A) 4
    (B) 6
    (C) 3, 1, 2
    (D) 41, 42
    (E) 17, 18, 19

33. Inhibition of pain signals by tactile stimulation of a skin surface involves which of the following?
    (A) Type Aα fibers in peripheral nerves
    (B) Type Aβ fibers in peripheral nerves
    (C) Type Aδ fibers in peripheral nerves
    (D) Type C fibers in peripheral nerves
    (E) Golgi tendon organs

34. Within the primary somatosensory cortex, the various parts of the contralateral body surface are represented in areas of varying size that reflect which of the following?
    (A) Relative size of the body parts
    (B) Density of the specialized peripheral receptors
    (C) Size of the muscles in that body part
    (D) Conduction velocity of the primary afferent fibers
    (E) Size of the primary afferent fibers

35. The gray matter of the primary somatosensory cortex contains six layers of cells. Which of the following layers receives the bulk of incoming signals from the somatosensory nuclei of the thalamus?
    (A) Layer I
    (B) Layers II and III
    (C) Layer III only
    (D) Layer IV
    (E) Layer VI

36. Which of the following statements concerning the neuronal membrane at rest is correct?
    (A) The extracellular sodium concentration is less than its intracellular concentration
    (B) The concentration of chloride is greatest inside the cell
    (C) If the resting potential is moved to a more negative value, the cell becomes more excitable
    (D) The sodium pump moves sodium in and potassium out of the cell
    (E) The concentration gradient for potassium is such that it tends to move out of the cell

37. Which of the following is the basis for referred pain?
    (A) Visceral pain signals and pain signals from the skin synapse with separate populations of neurons in the dorsal horn
    (B) Visceral pain transmission and pain transmission from the skin are received by a common set of neurons in the thalamus
    (C) Visceral pain signals are rarely of sufficient magnitude to exceed the threshold of activation of dorsal horn neurons
    (D) Some visceral pain signals and pain signals from the skin provide convergent input to a common set of neurons in the dorsal horn
    (E) A population of neurons in the somatosensory cortex is responsible for integrating visceral pain signals and pain signals from the skin

38. The cells in the six layers of the primary somatosensory cortex are functionally organized into which of the following?
    (A) Vertical columns of cells extending through all six layers
    (B) Vertical columns of cells occupying layers IV through VI
    (C) Vertical columns of cells occupying layers I through IV
    (D) Tangential nets of cells in layer IV
    (E) Tangential nets of cells occupying all six layers

39. Which of the following statements best describes the effect on sensory receptors subjected to an increase in the frequency of stimulation?
    (A) Immediate inactivation
    (B) Continuously increasing level of response activity
    (C) Variable rate of adaptation
    (D) No change in their response characteristics
    (E) Gradual increase in permeability to calcium

40. Which of the following statements concerning visceral pain signals is correct?
    (A) They are transmitted along sensory fibers that course mainly with sympathetic nerves in the abdomen and thorax
    (B) They are not stimulated by ischemia in visceral organs
    (C) They are transmitted only by the lightly myelinated type Aδ sensory fibers
    (D) They are typically well localized
    (E) They are not initiated by the leakage of chemical substances from pathological perforations in the wall of the gastrointestinal tract

Questions 41-43

Each of the disorders in the next three questions is characterized by either the production of excessive pain (hyperalgesia) or the loss of pain sensation.

41. Which disorder is characterized by excessive pain in a skin dermatomal distribution resulting from a viral infection of a dorsal root ganglion?
    (A) Tic douloureux
    (B) Thalamic pain syndrome
    (C) Lateral medullary syndrome
    (D) Brown-Séquard syndrome
    (E) Herpes zoster

42. Which disorder involves a loss of pain sensation on one side of the body coupled with the loss of proprioception, precise tactile localization, and vibratory sensations on the contralateral side of the body?
    (A) Herpes zoster
    (B) Thalamic pain syndrome
    (C) Lateral medullary syndrome
    (D) Brown-Séquard syndrome
    (E) Tic douloureux

43. Which disorder is characterized by the loss of pain sensation throughout one entire side of the body and the opposite side of the face?
    (A) Brown-Séquard syndrome
    (B) Thalamic pain syndrome
    (C) Herpes zoster
    (D) Lateral medullary syndrome
    (E) Tic douloureux

44. Which of the following electrical events is characteristic of inhibitory synaptic interactions?
    (A) A neurotransmitter agent that selectively opens ligand-gated chloride channels is the basis for an inhibitory postsynaptic potential
    (B) Because the Nernst potential for chloride is about –70 millivolts, chloride ions tend to move out of the cell along its electrochemical gradient
    (C) A neurotransmitter that selectively opens potassium channels allows potassium to move into the cell
    (D) An increase in the extracellular sodium concentration usually leads directly to an inhibitory postsynaptic potential
    (E) Inhibitory postsynaptic potentials result from the inability of a neurotransmitter agent to bind to a receptor in the postsynaptic membrane

45. Which of the following somatosensory deficits is typically not seen with lesions that involve the postcentral gyrus?
    (A) Inability to discretely localize touch sensation over the contralateral face and upper limb
    (B) Inability to judge the weight of easily recognizable objects
    (C) Inability to recognize the position of the contralateral arm and leg
    (D) Inability to accurately assess the texture of common objects by touching them with the fingers
    (E) Inability to move the contralateral arm and leg

46. The ability to detect two points simultaneously applied to the skin is based on which of the following physiological mechanisms?
    (A) Presynaptic inhibition
    (B) Lateral inhibition
    (C) Medial inhibition
    (D) Feed-forward inhibition
    (E) Feedback inhibition

47. Stimulation by touching or pulling on which of the following structures is least likely to cause a painful sensation?
    (A) Postcentral gyrus
    (B) Dura overlying the postcentral gyrus
    (C) Branches of the middle meningeal artery that lie superficial to the dura over the postcentral gyrus
    (D) Branches of the middle cerebral artery that supply the postcentral gyrus
    (F) Veins draining into the superior sagittal sinus from the region over the postcentral gyrus

48. Vibratory sensation is dependent on the detection of rapidly changing, repetitive sensations. The high-frequency end of the repetitive stimulation scale is detected by which of the following?
   (A) Merkel's discs
   (B) Meissner's corpuscles
   (C) Pacinian corpuscles
   (D) Free nerve endings
   (E) End bulbs of Krause

49. Synapses that involve a G protein as a second messenger are characterized by which of the following events occurring in the postsynaptic cell that is directly attributable to the G protein?
   (A) Rapid closure of an open ion channel
   (B) Inactivation of cAMP or cGMP in the postsynaptic cell
   (C) Massive efflux of calcium from the postsynaptic cell
   (D) Activation of gene transcription
   (E) Production of a "fast" excitatory postsynaptic potential

50. Which of the following correctly pairs a small-molecule rapidly acting transmitter with its most common source or action?
   (A) Glutamate—inhibition
   (B) Glycine—inhibition
   (C) Serotonin—locus ceruleus
   (D) Dopamine—choroid plexus
   (E) Norepinephrine—raphe nuclei

51. Which one of the following statements concerning sensory neurons or their functional properties is true?
   (A) All sensory fibers are unmyelinated
   (B) In spatial summation, increasing signal strength is transmitted by using progressively greater numbers of sensory fibers
   (C) Increased stimulus intensity is signaled by a progressive decrease in the receptor potential
   (D) Continuous subthreshold stimulation of a pool of sensory neurons results in disfacilitation of those neurons
   (E) In temporal summation, increased stimulus strength is signaled by decreasing the frequency of action potentials in the sensory fibers

52. In comparison to the intensities detected by other sensory systems such as vision or audition, which of the following terms best describes the range of stimulus intensities that can be detected by the somatosensory system (using the pacinian corpuscle as an example)?
   (A) Greater than
   (B) Less than
   (C) Equivalent to
   (D) Several orders of magnitude greater than
   (E) Several orders of magnitude less than

53. Migraine headaches typically begin with a prodromal symptom such as nausea, loss of vision, visual aura, or other sensory hallucinations. Which of the following is thought to be the cause of such prodromes?
   (A) Increased blood flow to brain tissue in the visual or other sensory cortex
   (B) Selective loss of GABA neurons in the various sensory areas of cortex
   (C) Constipation
   (D) Vasospasm leading to ischemia and disruption of neuronal activity in the relevant sensory areas of cortex
   (E) Excessive sleep and relative inactivity

54. Which statement concerning the generation of an action potential is correct?
   (A) When the membrane potential in the soma-axon hillock dips below "threshold," an action potential is initiated
   (B) The action potential is initiated in synaptic boutons
   (C) The fewest voltage-gated sodium channels in an axon are found near the node of Ranvier
   (D) Once an action potential is initiated, it always runs its course to completion
   (E) The action potential is propagated along dendrites until it reaches the cell body

55. Position sense or, more commonly, proprioceptive sensation involves muscle spindles and which of the following?
   (A) Skin tactile receptors
   (B) Deep receptors in joint capsules
   (C) Both tactile and joint capsule receptors
   (D) Pacinian corpuscles
   (E) Meissner's corpuscles

56. The sensation of temperature is signaled mainly by warm and cold receptors whose sensory fibers travel in association with the sensory fibers carrying pain signals. Which of the following statements best characterizes the transmission of signals from warm receptors?
   (A) Warm receptors are well characterized histologically
   (B) Signals from warm receptors are transmitted mainly along slow-conducting type C sensory fibers
   (C) Warm receptors are located well below the surface of the skin in the subcutaneous connective tissue
   (D) There are 3 to 10 times more warm receptors than cold receptors in most areas of the body
   (E) The fingertips contain fewer warm receptors than does the upper posterior portion of the shoulders and back

57. Like other sensory systems, the somatosensory system has a descending component that functions to regulate its overall sensitivity. Which of the following best describes the function of the corticofugal signals transmitted from the somatosensory cortex downward to the thalamus and dorsal column nuclei?
    (A) Increase or decrease the perception of signal intensity
    (B) Decrease the ability to sense body position
    (C) Remove the thalamus from the processing of somatosensory signals
    (D) Allow ascending information to bypass the nucleus cuneatus and nucleus gracilis
    (E) Block transmission of somatosensory signals entering the spinal cord

58. Which of the following statements accurately describes a feature of temperature sensation by the nervous system?
    (A) Cold receptors continue to be activated even if skin temperature is well below its freezing point
    (B) Cold and warm receptors have very specific, nonoverlapping ranges of temperature sensitivity
    (C) Warm and cold receptors respond to both steady-state temperatures and changes in temperature
    (D) Temperature receptor function is the result of ion conduction changes and not changes in their metabolic rate
    (E) Warm but not cold receptors exhibit spatial summation

59. Which of the following statements concerning synaptic transmission is correct?
    (A) When a specific population of synaptic terminals is spread over the considerable surface of a neuron, their collective effects cannot spatially summate and lead to initiation of an action potential
    (B) Even if the successive discharges of an excitatory synapse occur sufficiently close in time, they cannot temporally summate and initiate an action potential
    (C) A neuron is "facilitated" when its membrane potential is moved in the hyperpolarizing direction
    (D) Even when rapidly stimulated by excitatory synaptic input for a prolonged period, neurons typically do not exhibit synaptic fatigue
    (E) Dendrites cannot propagate action potentials, but they can transmit electrical potentials by electrotonic conduction

60. Which of the following statements regarding the processing of sensory signals by a pool of neurons is correct?
    (A) Convergence of input signals to individual neurons in the pool, each of which contributes to the same output channel, can lead to amplification of the signal
    (B) Divergence of input signals to multiple neurons in the pool, each of which leads to a different output channel, can lead to diffusion of the signal
    (C) The combination of multiple input signals from multiple sources onto a single neuron in the pool is an example of divergence
    (D) The distribution of multiple input signals from a single source onto many neurons in the pool is an example of convergence
    (E) In some instances, a sensory input to a neuronal pool causes a prolonged pause in the generation of output signals, called an afterdischarge

Answers

1. (B) Fast pain is perceived within 0.1 second of stimulus application.
   TMP11 598

2. (A) Slow or burning-type pain is associated with tissue damage.
   TMP11 598, 599

3. (E) The release of neurotransmitter is dependent on the influx of calcium through voltage-gated channels. When this occurs, synaptic vesicles fuse with the presynaptic membrane and release the transmitter agent into the synaptic cleft.
   TMP11 559, 560

4. (D) Meissner's corpuscles are found in the dermal pegs.
   TMP11 586

5. (D) Pain receptors in the skin are free nerve endings.
   TMP11 598

6. (B) Merkel's discs are found in the dermis of hairy skin and signal continuous touch.
   TMP11 586

7. (C) Free nerve endings are the nonencapsulated (receptor) terminal ends of sensory nerve fibers located in the epidermis.
   TMP11 586

8. (E) The association of one sensory modality with one type of nerve fiber is the basis for the labeled line theory.
   TMP11 572, 573

9. (A) Pacinian corpuscles detect pressure and movement across the skin surface and are encapsulated receptors found deep in the skin throughout the body.
TMP11 586

10. (E) Prostaglandins are believed to enhance the sensitivity of pain receptors but do not actually excite them.
TMP11 598

11. (A) Pain receptors exhibit little or no functional adaptation.
TMP11 598, 599

12. (A) The function of a transmitter agent is solely dependent on the postsynaptic receptor to which it binds.
TMP11 560, 561

13. (B) Type Aδ fibers, not type C fibers, are responsible for pain localization.
TMP11 600, 601

14. (B) Temporal and spatial fidelity is enhanced in the dorsal column–medial lemniscal system compared with the anterolateral system.
TMP11 588, 589

15. (A) Fibers in the anterolateral system cross in the anterior white commissure within a few segments of their entry before ascending on the contralateral side. Signals ascending in the dorsal column–medial lemniscal system do not cross until they reach the dorsal column nuclei in the medulla.
TMP11 588, 589

16. (A) Glutamate is the transmitter agent used by fast pain fibers.
TMP11 600, 601

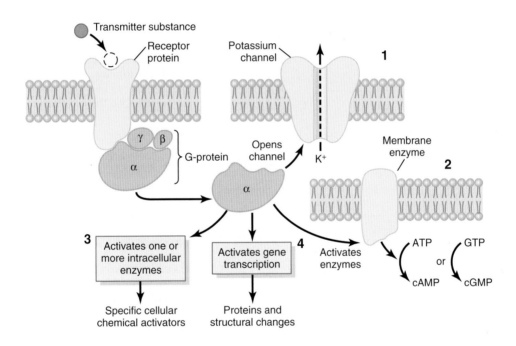

17. (B) The binding of G proteins can lead to the activation of cAMP or cGMP. Such proteins do not close sodium or potassium channels, nor do they inactivate various enzymes, gene transcription, or transmitter agents (see the figure above).
TMP11 561, 562

18. (D) Substance P is the transmitter agent used by slow pain fibers.
TMP11 601

19. (B) The sensations of highly localized touch and body position are carried in the dorsal column–medial lemniscal system.
TMP11 588

20. (C) Individuals experiencing severe, chronic pain have difficulty sleeping because the ascending pain

pathways provide input to reticular formation elements that constitute the reticular activating system. The latter system maintains the alert, waking state.
TMP11 602, 603

21. (C) Primary afferent neuronal cell bodies are found in the dorsal root ganglia.
TMP11 588, 589

22. (D) The medial lemniscus conveys axons from the nucleus gracilis and nucleus cuneatus to the thalamus.
TMP11 589

23. (A) A central factor in the sensory transduction mechanism is the change (increase) in ion permeability that occurs in the receptor membrane.
TMP11 567

24. (C) The internal capsule conveys axons from the ventral posterolateral thalamic nucleus to the primary somatosensory cortex.
   TMP11 589

25. (D) Ligand-gated channels open and allow sodium entry. This is accompanied by the influx of calcium, the binding of synaptic vesicles to the presynaptic membrane, and electrical changes in the postsynaptic membrane.
   TMP11 562

26. (C) Sectioning of the anterolateral spinal cord at T-6 on the left side should interrupt ascending pain signals from the ascending colon that have entered on the right side at levels below the lesion.
   TMP11 602

27. (A) The periaqueductal gray in the midbrain contains neurons that contribute to the descending pain suppression system.
   TMP11 603

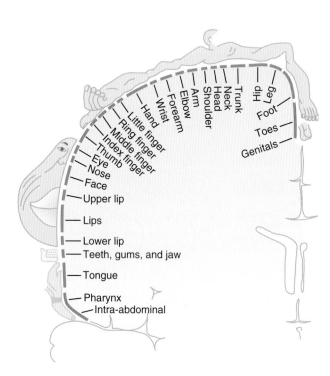

28. (B) The lower limb is represented in the superior and medial portion of the postcentral gyrus (see the figure above; from Penfield W, Rasmussen T: Cerebral Cortex of Man: A Clinical Study of Localization of Function. New York: Hafner, 1968).
   TMP11 589, 590

29. (B) Neurons in the nucleus raphe magnus use serotonin as a transmitter agent.
   TMP11 602

30. (B) As the receptor potential increases above threshold, action potential frequency increases.
   TMP11 575

31. (C) A spinal cord interneuron in the dorsal horn uses enkephalin as a transmitter agent that effectively inhibits pain signaling.
   TMP11 603

32. (C) The Brodmann number designation for the primary somatosensory cortex is 3, 1, 2.
   TMP11 589

33. (B) Tactile cutaneous stimulation involving type Aβ fibers can lead to pain suppression.
   TMP11 603

34. (B) The size of the representation of various body parts in the primary somatosensory cortex is correlated with the density of cutaneous receptors in that body part.
   TMP11 590

35. (D) Layer IV of the somatosensory cortex receives the bulk of the input from the somatosensory nuclei of the thalamus.
   TMP11 590

36. (E) At rest, the intracellular potassium concentration is higher than its extracellular concentration, and potassium tends to move out of the cell. At the same time, extracellular sodium and chloride concentrations are greater than their respective intracellular concentrations.
   TMP11 565

37. (D) Visceral pain fibers can provide input to anterolateral tract cells that also receive somatic pain signals from the skin surface. The convergence of these two types of pain signals onto single spinal cord neurons is thought to be the basis for referred pain.
   TMP11 603, 604

38. (A) The cells in the six layers of the primary somatosensory cortex are functionally organized into vertical columns extending from the white matter to the pial surface.
   TMP11 591

39. (C) When stimulated repeatedly in a short period, sensory receptors exhibit some degree of adaptation. They are not immediately inactivated, nor do they continuously respond or increase their permeability to calcium.
   TMP11 575, 576

40. (A) Visceral pain signals from structures in the abdomen and thorax travel toward the spinal cord in association with fibers of the sympathetic system.
   TMP11 603, 604

41. (E) Herpes zoster is characterized by excessive pain in a dermatomal distribution that results from a viral infection of a dorsal root ganglion.
   TMP11 605

42. (D) Brown-Séquard syndrome is characterized by the loss of pain sensation on one side of the body, coupled with a loss of discriminative sensations,

such as proprioception and vibratory sensation, on the opposite side of the body.
TMP11 606

43. (D) The lateral medullary syndrome exhibits one of the most characteristic patterns of sensory loss in clinical neurology—pain sensation is lost over one side of the body from feet to neck and on the opposite side of the face. The side of facial pain loss indicates the side of the lesion.
TMP11 606

44. (A) Opening of ligand-gated chloride channels and movement of chloride ions into the cell lead to hyperpolarization of the membrane. Neither an increased extracellular sodium concentration nor the movement of potassium into the cell leads to hyperpolarization of the membrane.
TMP11 566, 567

45. (E) Paralysis of the contralateral arm and leg is a motor deficit, which typically would not be observed following damage to the primary somatosensory cortex.
TMP11 591, 592

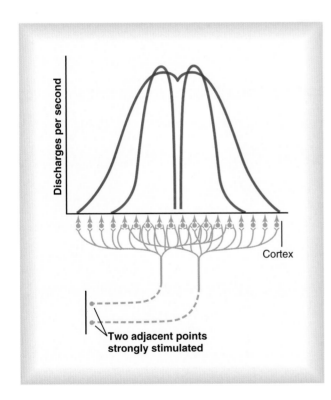

46. (B) The process of lateral inhibition, illustrated in the figure above, underlies the ability to discriminate two points simultaneously applied.
TMP11 592, 593

47. (A) Touching or pulling on the postcentral gyrus is least likely to evoke a painful sensation because brain tissue lacks pain receptors.
TMP11 606

48. (C) High-frequency repetitive stimulation (indentation or pressure) of the skin is sensed by pacinian corpuscles.
TMP11 586

49. (D) G proteins can activate gene transcription and generally do not close ion channels or inactivate cAMP or cGMP. Their action can be influenced by the influx of calcium, and they typically produce slow postsynaptic potentials.
TMP11 562

50. (B) Glycine typically evokes inhibitory responses. Norepinephrine is associated with the locus ceruleus, and serotonin with the raphe nuclei.
TMP11 563, 564

51. (B) In spatial summation, increasing signal strength is transmitted by using greater numbers of sensory fibers.
TMP11 578

52. (C) The range of stimulus intensity detected by the somatosensory system is equivalent to that of other sensory systems such as vision and audition.
TMP11 593, 594

53. (D) Vasospasm and eventually ischemia in a sensory area of cortex are thought to be the basis for the prodromal symptoms experienced by patients with migraines.
TMP11 607

54. (D) The action potential is described as an "all or none" process. Once initiated, the action potential runs its course to completion.
TMP11 566

55. (C) Proprioceptive sensation is dependent on tactile and joint capsule receptors.
TMP11 594, 595

56. (B) Warm receptors transmit signals mainly along relatively slow conducting type C fibers.
TMP11 608

57. (A) Descending cortical modulation of somatosensation involves an increase or decrease in the perception of signal intensity.
TMP11 597

58. (C) Both warm and cold receptors are able to respond to steady-state temperatures as well as changes in temperature.
TMP11 608

59. (E) Although dendrites do not possess the membrane machinery to initiate and conduct action potentials, they are able to support electrotonic spread of an electrical charge for variable distances over their membranes.
TMP11 568, 569

60. (D) Divergence occurs when input signals are sent to multiple neurons in a pool, and each neuron then initiates a signal in its own output channel.
TMP11 580

The Nervous System: Special Senses

1. Which of the following statements regarding the lateral geniculate nucleus is correct?
   (A) Layer I is called a parvocellular layer
   (B) Layer I receives signals from the lateral half of the retina
   (C) Layer I receives signals that originate from rods
   (D) Layer IV receives signals from the ipsilateral retina
   (E) Layer IV receives signals from Y ganglion cells

2. Which of the following substances elicits the sensation of sour taste?
   (A) Aldehydes
   (B) Alkaloids
   (C) Amino acids
   (D) Hydrogen ions
   (E) Ketones

3. Which of the following statements regarding the refraction of light is correct?
   (A) Light waves have a longer wavelength in transparent solids than in air
   (B) Light waves travel at a higher velocity through transparent solids than through air
   (C) The refractive index of a transparent solid is the ratio of the velocity of light in air to the velocity of light in the substance
   (D) The refractive index of air is zero
   (E) When light waves strike a transparent solid, they always reflect away from the solid rather than travel through the solid

4. When comparing the fovea with the periphery of the retina, which of the following statements is correct?
   (A) The fovea contains a greater proportion of cones
   (B) The fovea contains a greater proportion of ganglion cells
   (C) The fovea contains a greater proportion of horizontal cells
   (D) The fovea contains a greater proportion of rods
   (E) The fovea is more vascular

5. Which of the following is the middle ear ossicle that is attached to the tympanic membrane?
   (A) Columella
   (B) Incus
   (C) Malleus
   (D) Modiolus
   (E) Stapes

6. Light entering the eye passes through which retinal layer first?
   (A) Inner nuclear layer
   (B) Outer nuclear layer
   (C) Outer plexiform layer
   (D) Photoreceptor layer
   (E) Retinal ganglion layer

7. Which of the following statements regarding the primary visual cortex is correct?
   (A) It contains regions for form, motion, visual detail, and color
   (B) It is also called Brodmann's area 18
   (C) It is also called V-2
   (D) It lies adjacent to the calcarine fissure of the occipital lobe
   (E) It is typically located in the temporal lobe

8. The optic radiation terminates mainly in which layer of primary visual cortex?
   (A) Layer I
   (B) Layer II
   (C) Layer III
   (D) Layer IV
   (E) Layer V

9. When parallel light rays pass through a concave lens, which of the following occurs?
   (A) They converge toward each other
   (B) They diverge away from each other
   (C) They maintain their parallel relationship
   (D) They reflect back in the direction from which they came
   (E) They refract to one focal point

10. Which of the following statements regarding the attenuation reflex is correct?
    (A) It can increase the intensity of low-frequency sound transmission by 30 to 40 decibels
    (B) It increases the rigidity of the ossicular system, thereby reducing conduction of low-frequency sounds
    (C) It masks high-frequency sounds in a loud environment so that lower-frequency sounds are more easily heard
    (D) It occurs following a latent period of 4 to 8 seconds after a loud sound
    (E) It protects the cochlea from the damaging vibrations of relatively quiet but high-frequency sounds

11. Which of the following substances elicits the sensation of bitter taste?
    (A) Aldehydes
    (B) Alkaloids
    (C) Amino acids
    (D) Hydrogen ions
    (E) Ketones

12. Which of the following arteries provides the blood supply for the internal layers of the retina?
    (A) Anterior choroidal artery
    (B) Central retinal artery
    (C) Choroid branches of ciliary artery
    (D) Lenticulostriate artery
    (E) Thalamogeniculate artery

13. Which of the following statements regarding the focal length of a convex lens is correct?
    (A) Converging light rays passing through a convex lens converge at a focal point farther away than the focal length of that lens
    (B) Diverging light rays passing through a convex lens converge at a focal point closer than the focal length of that lens
    (C) Parallel light rays passing through a convex lens converge at a focal point equal to the focal length of that lens
    (D) The image produced by a convex lens is right side up, but its two lateral sides are reversed with respect to the object
    (E) The lens with the greatest convexity has the longest focal length

14. If a convex lens has a focal length of 1 centimeter (0.01 meter), what is the refractive power of that lens in diopters?
    (A) +0.01
    (B) +0.10
    (C) +1
    (D) +10
    (E) +100

15. Which of the following statements regarding events in the primary visual cortex is correct?
    (A) "Color blobs" are interspersed among primary visual columns and are the primary areas for deciphering color
    (B) Primary visual columns contain signals from both eyes, with adjacent columns also receiving signals from both eyes
    (C) Rapidly changing black-and-white visual signals are transmitted by parvocellular neurons of the lateral geniculate nucleus to the primary visual cortex
    (D) Visual signals are transmitted by X ganglion cells, the majority of which form synapses in layer V of the primary visual cortex
    (E) Visual signals of accurate detail and color are transmitted from the retina by Y ganglion cells

16. Which of the following taste sensations is the most sensitive (i.e., has the lowest stimulation threshold)?
    (A) Acid
    (B) Bitter
    (C) Salty
    (D) Sour
    (E) Sweet

17. Which of the following statements regarding the basilar membrane is correct?
    (A) It vibrates best at high frequency near the base of the cochlea, whereas it vibrates best at low frequency at the apex of the cochlea
    (B) The spiral ganglion lies on its surface
    (C) It contains basilar fibers whose diameter increases from the base of the cochlea to the apex of the cochlea
    (D) It contains basilar fibers whose length decreases from the base of the cochlea to the apex of the cochlea
    (E) It separates the scala media from the scala vestibuli

18. Which primary taste stimulus is correctly paired with its primary location on the tongue?
    (A) Bitter—anterior tongue
    (B) Salty—lateral tongue
    (C) Salty—posterior tongue
    (D) Sour—posterior tongue
    (E) Sweet—anterior tongue

19. Analysis of visual detail occurs in which secondary visual area?
    (A) Brodmann's area 18
    (B) Inferior ventral and medial regions of the occipital and temporal cortex
    (C) Frontal lobe
    (D) Occipitoparietal cortex
    (E) Posterior midtemporal area

20. Which of the following neural elements is responsible for the accommodation of the lens when the eye is focused on an object that is moving closer?
    (A) Parasympathetic nerve fibers in the abducens nerve
    (B) Parasympathetic nerve fibers in the oculomotor nerve
    (C) Parasympathetic nerve fibers in the trochlear nerve
    (D) Sympathetic nerve fibers in the abducens nerve
    (E) Sympathetic nerve fibers in the oculomotor nerve

21. Which of the following pairs of molecules combine to form rhodopsin?
    (A) Bathorhodopsin and 11-*cis* retinal
    (B) Bathorhodopsin and all-*trans* retinal
    (C) Bathorhodopsin and scotopsin
    (D) Scotopsin and 11-*cis* retinal
    (E) Scotopsin and all-*trans* retinal

22. A deficiency of which vitamin prevents the formation of an adequate quantity of retinal, eventually leading to night blindness?
    (A) Vitamin A
    (B) Vitamin C
    (C) Vitamin D
    (D) Vitamin E
    (E) Vitamin K

23. What is the name of the condition in which the lens of the eye becomes almost totally unaccommodating in persons older than 70 years?
    (A) Amblyopia
    (B) Emmetropia
    (C) Hyperopia
    (D) Myopia
    (E) Presbyopia

24. Which compartment of the cochlea contains the organ of Corti?
    (A) Ampulla
    (B) Saccule
    (C) Scala media
    (D) Scala tympani
    (E) Scala vestibuli

25. Which of the following statements regarding the transmission of taste information from the tongue to the cerebral cortex is correct?
    (A) The majority of thalamic neurons in the taste pathway synapse in the occipital lobe
    (B) The nerve fibers carrying taste information from the tongue have no synapse in the brain stem
    (C) The nerve fibers carrying taste information from the tongue synapse in the solitary nucleus
    (D) The thalamic nucleus involved in the taste pathway is the dorsal medial nucleus
    (E) The thalamic nucleus involved in the taste pathway is the ventral posterolateral nucleus

26. Which cells in layer IV of the primary visual cortex detect orientation of lines and borders?
    (A) Border cells
    (B) Complex cells
    (C) Ganglion cells
    (D) Hypercomplex cells
    (E) Simple cells

27. Which of the following best describes the transmission of sound waves in the cochlea?
    (A) The foot of the stapes moves inward against the oval window, and the round window bulges outward
    (B) The foot of the stapes moves inward against the round window, and the oval window bulges outward
    (C) The head of the malleus moves inward against the oval window, and the round window bulges outward
    (D) The incus moves inward against the oval window, and the round window bulges outward
    (E) The incus moves inward against the round window, and the oval window bulges outward

28. Which of the following events causes rods to hyperpolarize in response to light?
    (A) Decrease in sodium conductance into the outer segment
    (B) Decrease in sodium pump activity at the inner segment
    (C) Increase in potassium conductance into the outer segment
    (D) Increase in sodium conductance into the outer segment
    (E) Increase in sodium pump activity at the inner segment

29. Which of the following statements regarding the cranial nerve innervation of the tongue is correct?
    (A) Taste information from the anterior two thirds of the tongue is transmitted to the solitary nucleus by the glossopharyngeal nerve
    (B) Taste information from the pharynx is transmitted to the solitary nucleus by the facial nerve
    (C) Taste information from the posterior third of the tongue is transmitted to the solitary nucleus by the glossopharyngeal nerve
    (D) Taste information from the posterior third of the tongue initially travels with the lingual nerve
    (E) Taste information from the posterior third of the tongue initially travels with the chorda tympani nerve

30. Olfactory receptor cells belong to which of the following groups of cells?
    (A) Bipolar neurons
    (B) Fibroblasts
    (C) Modified epithelial cells
    (D) Multipolar neurons
    (E) Pseudounipolar neurons

31. Which of the following statements regarding hair cells is correct?
    (A) Hair cells depolarize when their stereocilia are bent toward the shortest stereocilium
    (B) Nerve fibers stimulated by hair cells have their cell bodies in the cochlear nuclei of the brain stem
    (C) The stereocilia are longer on the side of the hair cell nearest the modiolus
    (D) There are more inner hair cells than outer hair cells in the organ of Corti
    (E) Transmission of auditory signals is performed mainly by inner hair cells rather than outer hair cells

32. Which of the following occurs in conjunction with a very small pupil?
    (A) Aqueous humor production increases
    (B) Sympathetic nerve fibers are activated
    (C) The pupillary dilator muscle contracts
    (D) There is excellent depth of focus
    (E) Vision in conditions of poor illumination is optimized

33. Which of the following events occurs in photoreceptors during phototransduction in response to light?
    (A) Phosphodiesterase activity decreases
    (B) Transducin activity decreases
    (C) Hydrolysis of cGMP increases
    (D) Neurotransmitter release increases
    (E) Number of open voltage-gated calcium channels increases

34. Which of the following conditions is caused by a lesion of the optic chiasm?
    (A) Bitemporal hemianopsia
    (B) Blindness in both eyes
    (C) Heteronymous hemianopsia
    (D) Homonymous hemianopsia
    (E) Scotomata

35. Which of the following statements regarding astigmatism is correct?
    (A) Light rays do not come to a common focal point
    (B) Light rays being emitted from distant objects are focused behind the retina
    (C) Light rays being emitted from distant objects are focused in front of the retina
    (D) Light rays being emitted from distant objects are in sharp focus on the retina
    (E) There is a cloudy or opaque area or areas in the lens

36. The stereocilia of hair cells are embedded in which membrane?
    (A) Basilar
    (B) Reissner's
    (C) Tectorial
    (D) Tympanic
    (E) Vestibular

37. Which of the following cranial nerves is correctly paired with the extraocular muscle it innervates?
    (A) Abducens nerve—medial rectus
    (B) Oculomotor nerve—inferior oblique
    (C) Oculomotor nerve—lateral rectus
    (D) Oculomotor nerve—superior oblique
    (E) Trochlear nerve—superior rectus

38. After olfactory receptor cells bind odor molecules, a sequence of intracellular events occurs that culminates in the entrance of specific ions that depolarize the olfactory receptor cell. Which of the following ions is involved?
    (A) Calcium ions
    (B) Chloride ions
    (C) Hydrogen ions
    (D) Potassium ions
    (E) Sodium ions

39. For the eye to adapt to intense light, which of the following may occur?
    (A) Bipolar cells continuously transmit signals at the maximum rate possible
    (B) Photochemicals in both rods and cones are reduced to retinal and opsins
    (C) Levels of rhodopsin are very high
    (D) Pupil size increases
    (E) Vitamin A converts into retinal

40. Which of the following is considered to be an advantage of wearing contact lenses?
    (A) They amplify the refraction that normally occurs at the anterior surface of the cornea
    (B) They are permanent and never need to be replaced
    (C) They magnify the size of the object
    (D) They minimize refraction errors for individuals with abnormally shaped corneas
    (E) They move as the eye moves to give a broader field of clear vision

41. Which lobe of the cerebral cortex contains the small bilateral cortical area that controls voluntary fixation movements?
    (A) Frontal
    (B) Limbic
    (C) Occipital
    (D) Parietal
    (E) Temporal

42. Which of the following sensory systems has the smallest range of intensity discrimination?
    (A) Auditory
    (B) Gustatory
    (C) Olfactory
    (D) Somatosensory
    (E) Visual

43. Which of the following molecules moves from the endolymph into the stereocilia and depolarizes the hair cell?
    (A) Calcium ions
    (B) Chloride ions
    (C) Hydrogen ions
    (D) Potassium ions
    (E) Sodium ions

44. Which of the following events prompts the auditory system to interpret a sound as loud?
    (A) Fewer inner hair cells become stimulated
    (B) Fewer outer hair cells become stimulated
    (C) Hair cells excite nerve endings at a diminished rate
    (D) Amplitude of vibration of the basilar membrane decreases
    (E) Amplitude of vibration of the basilar membrane increases

45. Sometimes there is a lack of fusion of the eyes in one or more of the visual coordinates, and both eyes are not fixed on the object of attention at the same time. Which of the following could be responsible for this condition?
    (A) Opticokinetic movements
    (B) Pursuit movements
    (C) Saccades
    (D) Stereopsis
    (E) Strabismus

46. Which of the following statements regarding visual acuity is correct?
    (A) Normal visual acuity allows two bright spots of light to be distinguished from 10 meters away as long as the spots are at least 2 millimeters apart
    (B) Visual acuity is optimized near the periphery of the retina
    (C) Visual acuity is optimized when light from a distant point source is focused on a large area of retina
    (D) Visual acuity is optimized where many rods and cones are associated with one optic nerve fiber
    (E) A person with 20/20 vision can see letters at 200 feet that should be able to be seen at 20 feet

47. Which of the following statements regarding the olfactory bulb is correct?
    (A) Each glomerulus in the olfactory bulb responds to a variety of odors
    (B) Each glomerulus receives input from only one olfactory receptor cell
    (C) Mitral and tufted cells all project to the orbitofrontal cortex
    (D) Olfactory receptor cells synapse on mitral and tufted cells in the olfactory bulb
    (E) Olfactory receptor cells reach the olfactory bulb by passing around the cribriform plate

48. Which of the following statements regarding the transmission of auditory information from the ear to the cerebral cortex is correct?
    (A) Inferior colliculus neurons synapse in the cochlear nuclei of the brain stem
    (B) Neurons with cell bodies in the spiral ganglion of Corti synapse in the inferior colliculus
    (C) The majority of neurons from the cochlear nuclei synapse in the contralateral superior olivary nucleus
    (D) There is no crossing over of information between the right and left auditory pathways in the brain stem
    (E) Trapezoid neurons synapse in the cochlear nuclei of the brain stem

49. Which of the following statements regarding color vision is correct?
    (A) Green is perceived when only green cones are stimulated
    (B) The stimulation ratio of the three types of cones allows specific color perception
    (C) The wavelength of light corresponding to white is shorter than that corresponding to blue
    (D) When there is no stimulation of red, green, or blue cones, there is the sensation of seeing white
    (E) Yellow is perceived when green and blue cones are stimulated equally

50. Which of the following functions remains intact with complete bilateral destruction of the primary auditory cortex?
    (A) Ability to detect the direction from which a sound comes
    (B) Ability to discriminate different patterns of sound
    (C) Ability to discriminate different pitches of sound
    (D) Ability to react in a relatively nonspecific manner to a sound
    (E) Ability to recognize a combination or sequence of tones

51. Which of the following muscles is contracted as part of the pupillary light reflex?
    (A) Ciliary muscle
    (B) Pupillary dilator muscle
    (C) Pupillary sphincter muscle
    (D) Radial fibers of the iris
    (E) Superior oblique muscle

52. Which of the following allows the visual apparatus to accurately determine the distance of an object from the eye (depth perception)?
    (A) Monocular vision
    (B) Location of the retinal image on the retina
    (C) Phenomenon of stationary parallax
    (D) Phenomenon of stereopsis
    (E) Size of the retinal image if the object is of unknown size

53. Which of the following is the most common cause of glaucoma?
    (A) Drugs that reduce the secretion of aqueous humor
    (B) Increased resistance to fluid outflow through trabecular spaces into the canal of Schlemm
    (C) Normal function of phagocytes on the surface of trabeculae
    (D) Phagocytosis of proteins and small particles by the epithelium of the iris
    (E) Activation of reticuloendothelial cells in the interstitial gel outside the canal of Schlemm

54. Which of the following statements regarding the two types of deafness is correct?
    (A) An audiogram of a person with conduction deafness shows much greater loss of air conduction than bone conduction of sound
    (B) An audiogram of a person with nerve deafness shows much greater loss of bone conduction than air conduction of sound
    (C) Conduction deafness occurs when the cochlea or cochlear nerve is impaired
    (D) Nerve deafness occurs when the physical structures that conduct the sound into the cochlea are impaired
    (E) Prolonged exposure to very loud sounds is more likely to cause deafness for high-frequency sounds than for low-frequency sounds

55. Which of the following statements regarding color blindness is correct?
    (A) Blue weakness is a genetically inherited state in which blue cones are overrepresented
    (B) Ishihara charts can help determine whether a person has blue weakness
    (C) Red-green color blindness is inherited from the father
    (D) Red-green color blindness occurs if a person is missing either red cones or green cones
    (E) Red-green color blindness occurs more often in females than in males

56. Horner's syndrome occurs when sympathetic nerve fibers to the eye are interrupted, leading to which of the following symptoms on the affected side of the face?
    (A) Persistent constriction of blood vessels of the face
    (B) Profuse sweating
    (C) Superior eyelid maintained in an open position
    (D) Overproduction of lacrimal gland fluid
    (E) Persistent constriction of the pupil to a smaller diameter than in the opposite eye

57. Which of the following neurotransmitters is released by both rods and cones at their synapses with bipolar cells?
    (A) Acetylcholine
    (B) Dopamine
    (C) Glutamate
    (D) Glycine
    (E) Serotonin

58. Olfactory information transmitted to the orbitofrontal cortex passes through which thalamic nucleus?
    (A) Dorsomedial
    (B) Lateral geniculate
    (C) Medial geniculate
    (D) Ventral posterolateral
    (E) Ventral posteromedial

59. Which of the following provides about two thirds of the 59 diopters of refractive power of the eye?
    (A) Anterior surface of the cornea
    (B) Anterior surface of the lens
    (C) Iris
    (D) Posterior surface of the cornea
    (E) Posterior surface of the lens

60. Transmission of visual signals to the primary visual cortex from the retina includes a synapse in which structure?
    (A) Lateral geniculate nucleus
    (B) Medial geniculate nucleus
    (C) Pretectal nucleus
    (D) Superior colliculus
    (E) Suprachiasmatic nucleus

61. Which of the following statements regarding retinal ganglion cells is correct?
    (A) One W ganglion cell from the periphery of the retina typically transmits information from one rod
    (B) One X ganglion cell from the fovea typically transmits information from as many as 200 cones
    (C) W ganglion cells respond best to directional movement or vision under very bright conditions
    (D) X ganglion cells respond best to color images and are the most numerous of the three types of ganglion cells
    (E) Y ganglion cells respond best to rapid changes in the visual image and are the most numerous of the three types of ganglion cells

62. Auditory information is relayed through which thalamic nucleus?
    (A) Dorsomedial
    (B) Lateral geniculate
    (C) Medial geniculate
    (D) Ventral posterolateral
    (E) Ventral posteromedial

63. Olfactory pathways use medial or lateral olfactory areas. Which of the following pathways is correctly paired with another structure in that pathway?
    (A) Lateral olfactory area—hippocampus
    (B) Lateral olfactory area—septal nuclei
    (C) Medial olfactory area—amygdala
    (D) Medial olfactory area—dorsomedial thalamic nucleus
    (E) Medial olfactory area—pyriform cortex

64. Which of the following photoreceptors responds to the longest wavelengths of light?
    (A) Blue cones
    (B) Green cones
    (C) Pigment layer cells
    (D) Red cones
    (E) Rods

65. Which of the following structures secretes the intraocular fluid of the eye?
    (A) Ciliary process
    (B) Cornea
    (C) Iris
    (D) Lens
    (E) Trabecula

66. Which type of papillae is located in the posterior part of the tongue?
    (A) Circumvallate
    (B) Foliate
    (C) Fungiform
    (D) Fungiform and circumvallate
    (E) Papilla of Vater

67. Which structure functions to ensure that each of the three sets of extraocular muscles is reciprocally innervated so that one muscle of the pair relaxes while the other contracts?
    (A) Edinger-Westphal nucleus
    (B) Medial longitudinal fasciculus
    (C) Pretectal nucleus
    (D) Superior colliculus
    (E) Suprachiasmatic nucleus

68. Which of the following retinal cells has action potentials?
    (A) Amacrine cells
    (B) Bipolar cells
    (C) Ganglion cells
    (D) Horizontal cells
    (E) Photoreceptors

69. Which type of papillae is located in the folds along the lateral surfaces of the tongue?
    (A) Circumvallate
    (B) Foliate
    (C) Fungiform
    (D) Fungiform and circumvallate
    (E) Papilla of Vater

70. The primary auditory cortex lies primarily in which lobe of the cerebral cortex?
    (A) Frontal lobe
    (B) Limbic lobe
    (C) Occipital lobe
    (D) Parietal lobe
    (E) Temporal lobe

71. The intraocular fluid of the eye flows from the canal of Schlemm into which of the following locations?
    (A) Anterior chamber
    (B) Aqueous veins
    (C) Lens
    (D) Posterior chamber
    (E) Trabeculae

72. Which type of papillae is most responsible for salty taste?
    (A) Circumvallate
    (B) Foliate
    (C) Fungiform
    (D) Fungiform and circumvallate
    (E) Papilla of Vater

73. Which brain stem structure plays a major role in determining the direction from which a sound originates?
    (A) Cochlear nucleus
    (B) Inferior colliculus
    (C) Lateral lemniscus
    (D) Superior olivary nucleus
    (E) Trapezoid

74. Visual contrast is enhanced due to lateral inhibition by which retinal cells?
    (A) Amacrine cells
    (B) Bipolar cells
    (C) Ganglion cells
    (D) Horizontal cells
    (E) Photoreceptors

75. Destruction of which structure could impair the involuntary fixation mechanism for holding the eyes firmly on an object once it has been found?
    (A) Edinger-Westphal nucleus
    (B) Lateral geniculate nucleus
    (C) Medial longitudinal fasciculus
    (D) Superior colliculus
    (E) Suprachiasmatic nucleus

Answers

1. (C) Layers I and II of the lateral geniculate nucleus are called magnocellular layers and receive rod input from Y retinal ganglion cells. Layers III to VI are called parvocellular layers and receive cone input from X retinal ganglion cells.
   TMP11 640, 641

2. (D) The taste sensation of sour is proportional to the logarithm of the hydrogen ion concentration caused by acids. Sweet is caused by a long list of chemicals, including sugars, alcohols, aldehydes, ketones, and amino acids.
   TMP11 663, 664

3. (C) Light rays travel through air at a velocity of about 300,000 km/sec; they travel much slower through transparent solids. Thus, the refractive index of air is 1.00, and the refractive index of any transparent solid is greater than 1.00.
   TMP11 613

4. (A) The fovea is composed almost entirely of cones. Blood vessels, ganglion cells, and other layers of cells are all displaced to one side, which allows light to pass unimpeded to the cones.
   TMP11 626

5. (C) The malleus is attached to the tympanic membrane, and the stapes is attached to the oval window. The incus has articulations with both these bones.
   TMP11 651, 652

6. (E) Light passes through the eye to the retina in the posterior portion of the eye. The most anterior layer of the retina, through which light passes first, is the retinal ganglion layer. Light then passes through the other cell layers until it reaches the photoreceptors in the posterior region of the retina.
   TMP11 626, 627

7. (D) The primary visual cortex of the occipital lobe lies superior and inferior to the calcarine fissure, so that visual information from the superior visual field ends up inferior to the calcarine fissure, and visual information from the inferior visual field ends up superior to the calcarine fissure.
   TMP11 641, 642

8. (D) Similar to most of the cerebral cortex, the primary visual cortex has six distinct layers. As is true of other sensory systems, the sensory projection to the cortex (optic radiation, in this case) terminates mainly in layer IV.
   TMP11 642

9. (B) A concave lens diverges light rays; in contrast, a convex lens converges light rays toward each other. If a convex lens has the appropriate curvature, parallel light rays will be bent so that all pass through a single point called the focal point.
   TMP11 613, 614

10. (B) The tensor tympani muscle pulls the handle of the malleus inward, whereas the stapedius muscle pulls the stapes outward. These two forces oppose each other and thereby cause the entire ossicular system to become more rigid, reducing the intensity of low-frequency sounds by 30 to 40 decibels.
    TMP11 652

11. (B) The sensation of bitter is caused by many nitrogen-containing organics, as well as by alkaloids.
    TMP11 664

12. (B) The central retinal artery enters the eyeball through the center of the optic nerve and then divides to supply the internal layers of the retina with nutrients. However, the outer layers of the retina, especially the photoreceptors, depend mainly on blood vessels of the choroid, which are located between the retina and the sclera.
    TMP11 628

13. (C) The distance beyond a convex lens at which parallel rays converge to a common focal point is called the focal length of the lens. Thus, the focal point is equal to the focal length for a convex lens. Also, the greater the curvature of the convex lens, the shorter the focal length where these parallel rays converge.
    TMP11 615, 616

14. (E) The more that a convex lens bends parallel light rays, the greater its refractive power, measured in diopters. By definition, a convex lens with a focal length of 1 meter has a refractive power of +1 diopter. If a convex lens can bend parallel light rays twice as much, it is said to have twice the refractive power, or +2 diopters, and a focal length of 0.5 meter. Thus, there is an inverse relationship between the focal length and the refractive power. In this case, the convex lens has a focal length of 1 centimeter (0.01 meter) and therefore has 100 times the refractive power, or 100 diopters.
    TMP11 616, 617

15. (A) Similar to other sensory areas of cerebral cortex, the primary visual cortex contains vertical neuronal columns called primary visual columns.

"Color blobs" are special column-like areas of primary visual cortex that receive lateral signals from the adjacent primary visual columns and are activated specifically by color signals.
TMP11 642, 643

16. (B) The bitter taste sense is much more sensitive than the others because it provides an important protective function against many dangerous toxins in food.
TMP11 664

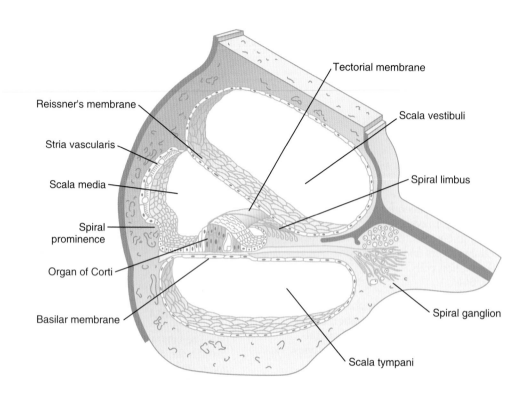

17. (A) The basilar membrane (pictured above) contains basilar fibers whose length increases progressively from the base of the cochlea to the apex, whereas the overall stiffness of the basilar fibers decreases. As a result, the stiff fibers near the cochlea vibrate best at high frequency, and the less stiff fibers near the apex vibrate best at low frequency. (Figure drawn by Sylvia Colard Keene, from Fawcett DW: Bloom & Fawcett: A Textbook of Histology, 11th ed. Philadelphia: WB Saunders, 1986.)
TMP11 653

18. (E) The sweet and salty taste senses are located principally on the tip of the tongue, the sour taste sense on the two lateral sides of the tongue, and the bitter taste sense on the posterior tongue and soft palate.
TMP11 665

19. (B) Visual information from the primary visual cortex (Brodmann's area 17) is relayed to Brodmann's area 18 and then into other areas of cerebral cortex for further processing. Analysis of three-dimensional position, gross form, and motion of objects occurs in the posterior midtemporal area and occipitoparietal cortex. Analysis of visual detail and color occurs in the inferior ventral and medial regions of the occipital and temporal cortex.
TMP11 643

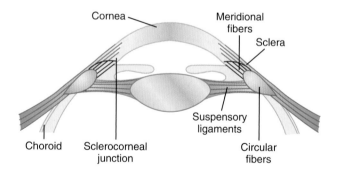

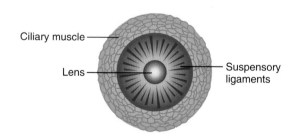

20. (B) The parasympathetic nerve fibers stimulate the ciliary muscle, which relaxes the suspensory ligaments of the lens, thus allowing the lens to become thicker and increase its refractive power (see the figure above). This increase in refractive power

allows the eye to focus on objects that are closer, because refractive power is inversely correlated with focal length.

TMP11 617, 618

21. (D) Rhodopsin is the light-sensitive chemical in rods. Scotopsin and all-*trans* retinal are the breakdown products of rhodopsin, which has absorbed light energy. The all-*trans* retinal is converted into 11-*cis* retinal, which can recombine with scotopsin to form rhodopsin.

TMP11 629

22. (A) One form of vitamin A is all-*trans* retinol, which is converted through two different pathways into 11-*cis* retinal, which then combines with scotopsin to form rhodopsin. Vitamin A is stored in large quantities in the liver. However, many months of a diet deficient in vitamin A can lead to night blindness, because rhodopsin is crucial for rod function.

TMP11 629

23. (E) In presbyopia, each eye remains focused permanently at an almost constant distance. The eyes can no longer accommodate for both near and far vision. Hyperopia and myopia refer to farsightedness and nearsightedness, respectively. Emmetropia is normal vision. Amblyopia has several causes that result in either an absence or a loss of binocular vision.

TMP11 618

24. (C) The ampulla and saccule are part of the vestibular apparatus, not the cochlear apparatus. The cochlea has three main compartments, with fluid movement occurring in the scala vestibuli and scala media in response to sound vibrations. The organ of Corti is contained within the scala media.

TMP11 652, 653

25. (C) All taste fibers synapse in the solitary nucleus and send second-order neurons to the ventral posteromedial nucleus of the thalamus. Third-order neurons project to the lower tip of the postcentral gyrus in the parietal cortex.

TMP11 665, 666

26. (E) The simple cells of the primary visual cortex detect orientation of lines and borders, whereas the complex cells detect lines oriented in the same direction but are not position specific. That is, the line can be displaced moderate distances laterally or vertically, and the same few neurons will be stimulated as long as the line is oriented in the same direction.

TMP11 643, 644

27. (A) The malleus is connected to the tympanic membrane, the incus articulates with the malleus and stapes, and the stapes is connected to the oval window.

TMP11 654

28. (A) The inner segment of a rod continually pumps sodium from inside the rod to the outside. However, the outer segment of the rod is very leaky to sodium

ions, so sodium ions continually leak back to the inside of the rod. When rhodopsin decomposes, it decreases the rod membrane conductance for sodium ions into the outer segment. This decrease in the movement of positive ions into the rod hyperpolarizes the rod.

TMP11 629, 630

29. (C) Taste impulses from the anterior two thirds of the tongue pass first into the lingual nerve, then through the chorda tympani into the facial nerve, and finally to the solitary nucleus. Taste sensations from the posterior third of the tongue are transmitted through the glossopharyngeal nerve to the solitary nucleus. Taste signals from the pharyngeal region are transmitted via the vagus nerve.

TMP11 665, 666

30. (A) The receptor cells for the smell sensation are bipolar nerve cells derived originally from the central nervous system itself.

TMP11 667

31. (E) Although there are three to four times as many outer hair cells as inner hair cells, about 90 per cent of the auditory nerve fibers are stimulated by the inner hair cells.

TMP11 655, 656

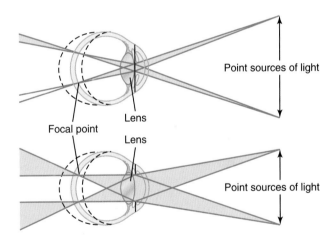

32. (D) The greatest possible depth of focus occurs when the pupil is extremely small, because all light rays pass nearly through the center of the lens, and light rays passing through the center of a lens are always in focus (see the figure above). In this situation, retinal displacement away from the focal point has minimal impact on the image focus.

TMP11 618, 619

33. (C) In the dark state, cyclic guanosine monophosphate (cGMP) helps maintain the open state of the sodium channels in the outer membrane of the rod. Hydrolysis of cGMP by light causes these sodium channels to close. Less sodium is able to enter the rod outer segment, thus hyperpolarizing the rod.

TMP11 630, 631

34. (A) Bitemporal hemianopsia occurs when the temporal half of each visual field has been lost, colloquially called "tunnel vision." The retinal ganglion cells from the nasal retina convey information from temporal visual fields through the optic chiasm to the contralateral lateral geniculate nucleus. Thus, a lesion of the optic chiasm affects vision from both retinas—specifically, information from the temporal visual fields.
   TMP11 644, 645

35. (A) Astigmatism most often results when the curvature of the cornea is too great in one of its planes. Because the curvature of the astigmatic lens along one plane is less than the curvature along the other plane, light rays striking the two planes will be bent to different degrees. Thus, light rays passing through an astigmatic lens do not come to a common focal point.
   TMP11 620

36. (C) The scala media is bordered by the basilar membrane and Reissner's membrane and contains a tectorial membrane. The apical border of hair cells has stereocilia that are embedded in the tectorial membrane.
   TMP11 655

37. (B) The abducens nerve innervates the lateral rectus muscle. The trochlear nerve innervates the superior oblique muscle. The oculomotor nerve innervates the medial rectus, inferior oblique, superior rectus, and inferior rectus muscles.
   TMP11 645

38. (E) Even the minutest concentration of a specific odorant initiates a cascading effect that opens extremely large numbers of sodium channels. This accounts for the exquisite sensitivity of the olfactory neurons to even the slightest amount of odorant.
   TMP11 667, 668

39. (B) The reduction of rhodopsin and cone pigments by light decreases the concentrations of photosensitive chemicals in rods and cones. Thus, the sensitivity of the eye to light is correspondingly reduced. This is called light adaptation.
   TMP11 631, 632

40. (E) The advantage of wearing contact lenses is that contact lenses cover the entire eye and rotate with the eye; glasses are best used to see objects directly in front of the person.
   TMP11 620, 621

41. (A) A bilateral premotor cortical region of the frontal lobes controls voluntary fixation movements. A lesion of this region makes it difficult for a person to "unlock" the eyes from one point of fixation and move them to another point.
   TMP11 645, 646

42. (C) Concentrations that are only 10 to 50 times above threshold values evoke maximum intensity of smell, which is in contrast to most other sensory systems of the body, in which the range of intensity discrimination may reach 1 trillion to 1.This might be explained by the fact that smell is concerned more with detecting the presence or absence of odors than with quantifying their intensity.
   TMP11 668, 669

43. (D) Although most cells in the nervous system depolarize in response to sodium entry, hair cells depolarize in response to potassium entry.
   TMP11 656

44. (E) There are at least three ways in which the auditory system determines loudness. First, the amplitude of vibration of the basilar membrane increases so that hair cells excite nerve endings at more rapid rates. Second, more and more hair cells on the fringes of the resonating portion of the basilar membrane become stimulated. Third, outer hair cells become recruited at a significant rate.
   TMP11 656, 657

45. (E) There are three types of strabismus (horizontal, torsional, and vertical), and they often occur in combination. This condition is often caused by an abnormal "set" of the fusion mechanism of the visual system.
   TMP11 648

46. (A) Visual acuity is optimized at the fovea, especially when light is focused on a small area of retina. The fovea contains cones, each of which associates with one or a small number of optic nerve fibers.
   TMP11 621

47. (D) Olfactory receptor cells reach the olfactory bulb by passing through the cribriform plate. Each bulb contains several thousand glomeruli, each of which is the terminus for about 25,000 axons of olfactory receptor cells. These glomeruli are composed of mitral and tufted cells, and each glomerulus responds preferentially to a different odor signal. The mitral and tufted cells project to several locations in the brain.
   TMP11 669

48. (C) Neurons with cell bodies in the spiral ganglion of Corti synapse in the cochlear nuclei. The majority of the cochlear nuclei neurons synapse in the contralateral superior olivary nucleus. Crossing over occurs in at least three places in the pathway, and a preponderance of auditory transmission is in the contralateral pathway. From the superior olivary nucleus, the auditory pathway passes upward through the lateral lemniscus, with most auditory fibers terminating at the inferior colliculus. From there, the pathway continues on to the medial geniculate nucleus and then the primary auditory cortex.
   TMP11 657, 658

49. (B) Research has shown that the nervous system perceives the sensation of a specific color by interpreting the set of ratios of stimulation of the three

types of cones. Investigators used only red, green, and blue monochromatic lights mixed in different combinations. All gradations of colors that the human eye can see were detected using just these three colors.
TMP11 632, 633

50. (D) Destruction of the primary auditory cortex on one side only slightly reduces hearing in the opposite ear because of the many crossover connections in the neural pathway. However, destruction of both primary auditory cortices greatly reduces or abolishes the ability to discriminate different sound pitches and patterns of sound, as well as causing an inability to detect the direction from which a sound comes. The ability to react in a relatively nonspecific manner to a sound remains intact in cases of bilateral destruction.
TMP11 659

51. (C) In a normal individual, shining a light in either eye results in both pupils constricting due to contraction of the pupillary sphincter muscles. In contrast, the pupillary dilator muscle dilates the pupil. The ciliary muscle is involved in focusing the eye (accommodation).
TMP11 649

52. (D) Because one eye is a little more than 2 inches to the side of the other eye, the images on the two retinas differ from each other. This binocular parallax (stereopsis) means that a person with two eyes has a far greater ability to judge relative distances when objects are nearby than does a person with only one eye.
TMP11 622

53. (B) Glaucoma is a disease of the eye in which the intraocular pressure becomes pathologically high, sometimes rising acutely to 60 to 70 mm Hg. Pressures above 30 mm Hg for long periods can lead to loss of vision. The most common cause of this higher intraocular pressure is the obstruction of fluid outflow into the canal of Schlemm.
TMP11 623-625

54. (A) With nerve deafness, there is damage to the cochlea, auditory nerve, or neural pathway. The ability to hear sound as tested by both air conduction and bone conduction is greatly reduced or lost with nerve deafness. However, with conduction deafness, the person retains the ability to hear sound by bone conduction, but not by air conduction.
TMP11 660, 661

55. (D) If either the red cones or the green cones are missing, a person cannot distinguish colors between the wavelengths of 525 and 675 nanometers (green, yellow, orange, and red). This is especially true for distinguishing red from green. Red-green color blindness is a genetic disorder that occurs almost exclusively in males, because the genes for the various cones are on the X chromosome.
TMP11 633

56. (E) Horner's syndrome typically occurs when the sympathetic nerve fibers that originated from thoracic spinal cord are interrupted in the cervical sympathetic chain on their way to the eye.
TMP11 650

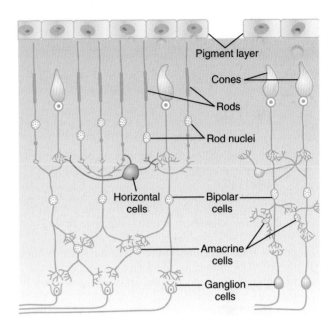

57. (C) At least eight types of neurotransmitter substances have been identified for amacrine cells. The neurotransmitters used for bipolar and horizontal cells are unclear, but it is well established that rods and cones release glutamate at their synapses with bipolar cells (pictured above).
TMP11 635

58. (A) A newer olfactory pathway projects to the dorsomedial thalamic nucleus and then to the orbitofrontal cortex. However, the older olfactory pathways bypass the thalamus to reach the cortex, in contrast to other sensory systems, which have thalamic relays.
TMP11 669, 670

59. (A) The principal reason why the anterior surface of the cornea provides most of the refractive power of the eye is that the refractive index of the cornea is markedly different from that of air.
TMP11 617

60. (A) Retinal ganglion cells synapse in several locations, but those conveying information that ultimately ends up in the primary visual cortex synapse in the lateral geniculate nucleus. From there, neurons project to the primary visual cortex.
TMP11 640

61. (D) There are three distinct groups of retinal ganglion cells, designated as W, X, and Y cells. W cells transmit rod visual signals. Y cells are the least numerous and transmit information about rapid changes in the visual image. X cells are the most

numerous and receive input from cones regarding the visual image and color vision.
TMP11 637

62. (C) The medial geniculate nucleus is the thalamic nucleus that conveys auditory information from the brain stem to the primary auditory cortex.
TMP11 657

63. (A) Olfactory pathways using the medial olfactory area are associated with the septal nuclei, and those using the lateral olfactory area are associated with the pyriform cortex, the amygdala, and the hippocampus.
TMP11 669

64. (D) Blue cones respond to the shortest wavelengths of light, followed by rods and then green cones; red cones respond to the longest wavelengths of light.
TMP11 631

65. (A) Ciliary processes secrete all the aqueous humor of the intraocular fluid, at an average rate of 2 to 3 µl/min. These processes are linear folds that project from the ciliary muscle into the space behind the iris. The intraocular fluid flows from behind the iris through the pupil into the anterior chamber of the eye.
TMP11 623

66. (A) Circumvallate papillae are located in the posterior part of the tongue, fungiform papillae in the anterior part of the tongue, and foliate papillae in the lateral part of the tongue. The papilla of Vater empties pancreatic secretions and bile into the duodenum.
TMP11 665

67. (B) The medial longitudinal fasciculus is a pathway for nerve fibers entering and leaving the oculomotor, trochlear, and abducens nuclei of the brain stem. This allows communication to coordinate the contraction of the various extraocular eye muscles.
TMP11 645

68. (C) Only ganglion cells have action potentials. Photoreceptors, bipolar cells, amacrine cells, and horizontal cells all appear to operate through graded potentials.
TMP11 635

69. (B) Foliate papillae are located in the folds along the lateral surfaces of the tongue, fungiform papillae are located in the anterior part of the tongue, and circumvallate papillae are located in the posterior part of the tongue. The papilla of Vater empties pancreatic secretions and bile into the duodenum.
TMP11 665

70. (E) Most of the primary auditory cortex is in the temporal lobe, but the association auditory cortices extend over much of the insular lobe and even onto the lateral portion of the parietal lobe.
TMP11 658

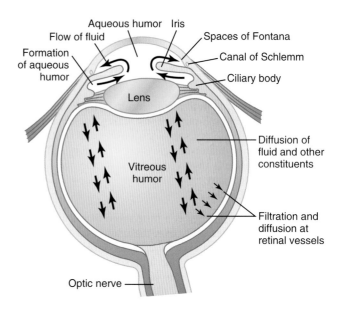

71. (B) Intraocular fluid flows from the anterior chamber of the eye, between the cornea and the iris through a meshwork of trabeculae into the canal of Schlemm, which empties into extraocular aqueous veins (see the figure above).
TMP11 623, 624

72. (C) Fungiform papillae are most responsible for salty and sweet tastes, foliate papillae for sour tastes, and circumvallate papillae for bitter tastes. The papilla of Vater empties pancreatic secretions and bile into the duodenum and is not involved in taste differentiation.
TMP11 665

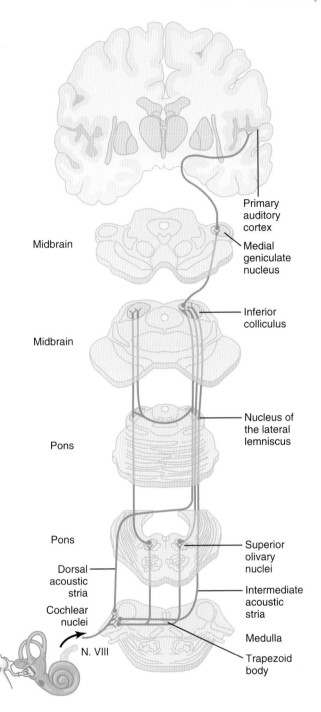

Midbrain

Primary
auditory
cortex

Medial
geniculate
nucleus

Midbrain

Inferior
colliculus

Pons

Nucleus of
the lateral
lemniscus

Pons

Dorsal
acoustic
stria

Cochlear
nuclei

N. VIII

Superior
olivary
nuclei

Intermediate
acoustic
stria

Medulla

Trapezoid
body

73. (D) The superior olivary nuclei (pictured left) receive auditory information from both ears and begin the process of detecting the direction from which a sound comes. The lateral part of the superior olivary nucleus does so by comparing the different intensities of sound reaching the two ears, whereas the medial part of the superior olivary nucleus detects the time lag between signals entering both ears.
   TMP11 660

74. (D) There appear to be many types of amacrine cells and at least six types of functions. In a sense, amacrine cells begin the analysis of visual signals before they leave the retina. However, horizontal cells, which are always inhibitory, have lateral connections between photoreceptors and bipolar cells. This lateral connection provides the same phenomenon of lateral inhibition that is important in all other sensory systems, helping to ensure transmission of visual contrast.
   TMP11 635-637

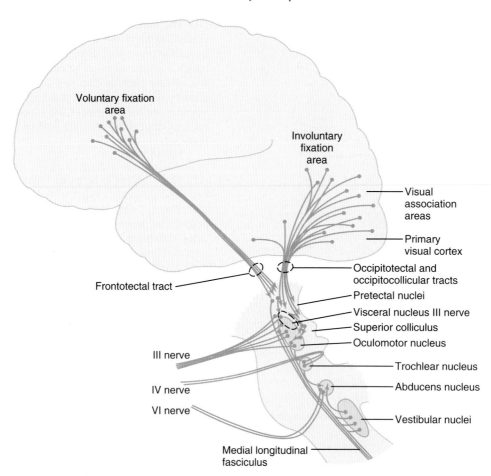

75. (D) The involuntary fixation capability is lost
(for the most part) when the superior colliculi are
destroyed. After signals for fixation originate in the
visual fixation areas of the occipital cortex, they pass
to the superior colliculi, then on to the reticular
areas, and finally into the motor nuclei (see the
figure above).
      TMP11 645, 646

The Nervous System: Motor and Integrative Neurophysiology

1. The phylogenetically new cerebral cortex, the neo-cortex, is composed of six layers tangential to the pial surface of the hemisphere. Which of the following statements concerning the organization of these six layers is correct?
   (A) The neurons in layers I, II, and III perform most of the thalamocortical connections within the same hemisphere
   (B) The neurons in layers II and III form connections with the basal ganglia
   (C) Specific incoming signals from the cerebellum terminate primarily in layer IV
   (D) The neurons in layer V have axons that extend beyond layer V to subcortical regions and the spinal cord
   (E) The neurons in layer VI send their axons to the hippocampus

2. As they leave the spinal cord and course peripherally to skeletal muscle, the axons of motor neurons must pass through which of the following structures?
   (A) Posterior column
   (B) Posterior root
   (C) Ventral white commissure
   (D) Posterior horn
   (E) Anterior root

3. Which of the following is the type of neuron whose axon forms synaptic junctions with the skeletal muscle cells (extrafusal fibers) that constitute the major part of a muscle?
   (A) Alpha motor neurons
   (B) Pyramidal neurons
   (C) Gamma motor neurons
   (D) Granule cells
   (E) Purkinje cells

4. Ascending fibers from the excitatory elements of the reticular activating system reach the intralaminar nuclei of the thalamus and from there are distributed to which of the following locations?
   (A) They project to the somatosensory nuclei of the thalamus
   (B) They extend widely throughout many areas of cortex
   (C) The reach the motor nuclei of the thalamus
   (D) They course primarily to the precentral gyrus
   (E) They extend primarily to the postcentral gyrus

5. Which of the following statements concerning the general functional role of the cerebellum is correct?
   (A) The cerebellum directly stimulates motor neurons required to make a movement
   (B) The cerebellum is unable to make corrective adjustments to a movement once it is performed
   (C) The cerebellum does not receive feedback from muscles that execute the actual movement
   (D) The cerebellum is not involved in the planning of a movement, only its execution
   (E) The cerebellum plays an active role in the coordination of the muscles required to make a movement

6. Which of the following spinal cord levels contains the entire population of preganglionic sympathetic neurons?
   (A) C-5 to T-1
   (B) C-3 to C-5
   (C) S-2 to S-4
   (D) T-1 to L-2
   (E) T-6 to L-1

7. Which of the following statements best describes a functional role for the lateral hemispheres of the cerebellum?
   (A) Control and coordinate movements of the axial muscles as well as the shoulder and hip
   (B) Control movements that involve distal limb musculature
   (C) Function with the cerebral cortex to plan movements
   (D) Stimulate motor neurons through connections to the spinal cord

8. Which of the following would produce an increase in cerebral blood flow?
   (A) Increase in carbon dioxide concentration
   (B) Increase in oxygen concentration
   (C) Decrease in the activity of cerebral cortex neurons
   (D) Decrease in carbon dioxide concentration
   (E) Decrease in arterial blood pressure from 120 to 90 mm Hg

9. Which of the following is the correct Brodmann number for the primary motor cortex?
   (A) 6
   (B) 5
   (C) 4
   (D) 3
   (E) 1

10. Which of the following body parts is represented most laterally and inferiorly within the primary motor cortex?
    (A) Face
    (B) Hand
    (C) Neck
    (D) Abdomen
    (E) Lower limb

11. Which of the following is the type of neuron whose axon forms synaptic junctions with skeletal muscle cells (intrafusal fibers) within the muscle spindles?
    (A) Alpha motor neurons
    (B) Pyramidal neurons
    (C) Gamma motor neurons
    (D) Granule cells
    (E) Purkinje cells

12. Preganglionic sympathetic axons pass through which of the following structures?
    (A) Dorsal root
    (B) Dorsal primary ramus
    (C) White ramus
    (D) Gray ramus
    (E) Ventral primary ramus

13. Which of the following statements best describes a functional role for the cerebellar vermis?
    (A) Controls and coordinates movements of the axial muscles as well as the shoulder and hip
    (B) Controls movements that involve distal limb musculature
    (C) Functions with the cerebral cortex to plan movements
    (D) Stimulates motor neurons through its connections to the spinal cord

14. Which of the following statements about sleep is correct?
    (A) Although fast-wave sleep is frequently referred to as "dreamless sleep," dreams and even nightmares can occur at this time
    (B) Individuals rarely awake spontaneously from rapid eye movement (REM) sleep
    (C) Muscle tone throughout the body is markedly suppressed during REM sleep
    (D) Heart rate and respiratory rate typically become very regular during REM sleep

15. Which of the following statements concerning intrinsic spinal cord circuitry is correct?
    (A) Motor neurons greatly outnumber spinal cord interneurons
    (B) Most incoming sensory fibers from the periphery synapse with motor neurons and not interneurons
    (C) Most descending supraspinal motor system axons synapse directly with motor neurons
    (D) Spinal cord interneurons are localized solely within the anterior horn
    (E) Both excitatory and inhibitory interneurons are found in the spinal cord

16. Which of the following statements best describes a functional role for the intermediate zone of the cerebellum?
    (A) Controls and coordinates movements of the axial muscles as well as the shoulder and hip
    (B) Controls movements that involve distal limb musculature
    (C) Functions with the cerebral cortex to plan movements
    (D) Stimulates motor neurons through its connections to the spinal cord

17. Under which of the following conditions would the sympathetic nervous system play the most important role in regulating cerebral blood flow?
    (A) Increase of 50 per cent in cerebral arterial pressure occurring over 1 hour
    (B) Doubling of cerebral carbon dioxide concentration
    (C) Increase of 70 per cent in cerebral arterial pressure occurring over 2 minutes
    (D) Decrease of 50 per cent in oxygen concentration
    (E) 50 per cent increase in the firing rate of cerebral neurons

18. A large portion of the cerebral cortex does not fit into the conventional definition of motor or sensory cortex. Which of the following terms is used to refer to the type of cortex that receives input primarily from several other regions of the cerebral cortex?
    (A) Cortex that is agranular
    (B) Secondary somatosensory cortex
    (C) Association cortex
    (D) Supplementary motor cortex
    (E) Secondary visual cortex

19. Which statement concerning the premotor cortex is correct?
    (A) The premotor cortex is located just posterior to the primary motor cortex
    (B) The lateral-to-medial sequence in the somatotopic organization of the premotor cortex is the reverse of that seen in the primary motor cortex
    (C) Stimulation of a small, discrete group of neurons in the premotor cortex produces contraction of an individual muscle
    (D) Stimulation of the premotor cortex does not lead to any muscle activation
    (E) The premotor cortex sets the specific posture required for the limb to produce the desired movement

20. Which of the following features is characteristic of the supplementary motor cortex?
    (A) It has no somatotopic representation of the body
    (B) Stimulation of the supplementary motor cortex leads to bilateral movements, typically involving both hands
    (C) It is located just anterior to the premotor cortex on the lateral surface of the hemisphere
    (D) Like the premotor cortex, stimulation of the supplementary motor cortex leads to discrete movement of individual muscles
    (E) The supplementary cortex functions totally independent of the premotor and primary motor cortices

21. Administration of a drug that blocks serotonin production has which of the following effects on sleep?
    (A) Sleep induction is almost immediate
    (B) Rapid eye movement (REM) sleep is blocked
    (C) Sleep induction is significantly prolonged or blocked
    (D) REM sleep is induced immediately

22. Recurrent branches of motor neuron axons contact which of the following structures within the spinal cord gray matter?
    (A) Renshaw cell
    (B) Motor unit
    (C) Propriospinal connections
    (D) Skeletal muscle fibers

23. Which of the following projection systems is contained in the superior cerebellar peduncle?
    (A) Pontocerebellar projections
    (B) Cerebellothalamic projections
    (C) Posterior spinocerebellar projections
    (D) Corticospinal projections

24. Which of the following terms applies to the combination of a motor neuron and all the skeletal muscle fibers contacted by that motor neuron?
    (A) Golgi tendon organ
    (B) Motor unit
    (C) Propriospinal neurons
    (D) Skeletal muscle fibers

Questions 25-28

    (A) Parieto-occipital association cortex in nondominant hemisphere
    (B) Wernicke's area
    (C) Visual association cortex in dominant hemisphere
    (D) Broca's area
    (E) Ventral portion of medial occipitotemporal association cortex

Match the cortical functions described in the questions below with the correct region from the list above.

25. Lesions in this cortical region cause prosophenosia (or prosopagnosia), the inability to recognize faces. ( )

26. A cortical region that provides the neural circuitry for word formation or the motor aspects of language. ( )

27. A cortical region that provides the analysis of the spatial coordinates of the body in space as well as the environment surrounding the body. ( )

28. A cortical region that provides the processing of information necessary for reading. ( )

29. Broca's area is a specialized portion of motor cortex. Which of the following conditions best describes the deficit resulting from damage to Broca's area?
    (A) Spastic paralysis of the contralateral hand
    (B) Paralysis of the muscles of the larynx and pharynx
    (C) Inability to use the two hands to grasp an object
    (D) Inability to direct the two eyes to the contralateral side
    (E) Inability to speak whole words correctly

30. A stroke involving the middle cerebral artery on the left side is likely to cause which of the following symptoms?
    (A) Paralysis of left side of face and left upper extremity
    (B) Paralysis of left lower extremity
    (C) Complete loss of vision in both eyes
    (D) Loss of ability to comprehend speech
    (E) Loss of vision in left half of both eyes

31. The fibers of the corticospinal tract pass through which of the following structures?
    (A) Medial lemniscus
    (B) Medullary pyramid
    (C) Posterior funiculus
    (D) Medial longitudinal fasciculus
    (E) Anterior roots

32. Administration of a cholinergic antagonist has which of the following effects on sleep?
    (A) Sleep induction is almost immediate
    (B) Rapid eye movement (REM) sleep is blocked
    (C) Sleep induction is significantly prolonged or blocked
    (D) REM sleep is induced immediately

33. Which of the following statements concerning muscle spindles is correct?
    (A) Intrafusal muscle fibers are innervated by alpha motor neurons
    (B) The nuclei of nuclear bag fibers are aligned in a single row in the central region of the fiber
    (C) The primary sensory ending (Ia) is linked to an intermediate-sized, relatively slow-conducting fiber
    (D) Nuclear chain–type muscle fibers signal the rate of change in muscle length
    (E) Type II, flower-spray endings are related to nuclear chain fibers

34. The peripheral sensory input that activates the ascending excitatory elements of the reticular formation comes mainly from which of the following?
    (A) Pain signals
    (B) Proprioceptive sensory information
    (C) Corticospinal system
    (D) Medial lemniscus
    (E) Input from pacinian corpuscles

35. Signals from motor areas of the cortex reach the contralateral cerebellum after first passing through which of the following structures?
    (A) Thalamus
    (B) Caudate nucleus
    (C) Red nucleus
    (D) Basilar pontine nuclei
    (E) Dorsal column nuclei

36. Cells of the adrenal medulla receive synaptic input from which of the following types of neurons?
    (A) Preganglionic sympathetic neurons
    (B) Postganglionic sympathetic neurons
    (C) Preganglionic parasympathetic neurons
    (D) Postsynaptic parasympathetic neurons
    (E) Presynaptic parasympathetic neurons

37. Which of the following statements about muscle and passive stretch of muscle spindles is true?
    (A) Primary (Ia) sensory fibers increase their firing rate
    (B) Secondary sensory fibers decrease their firing rate
    (C) Alpha motor neurons are inhibited
    (D) Gamma motor neurons are stimulated
    (E) Muscle spindles go completely slack

38. Which of the following statements concerning electroencephalogram activity is correct?
    (A) Beta waves occur in normal adults who are awake but in a quiet, resting state
    (B) Alpha waves occur at 14 to 80 cycles per second during periods of heightened, excited activity or high tension
    (C) Theta waves are commonly seen in children but also occur in adults during emotional disappointment or in degenerative brain states
    (D) Delta waves are characteristic of slow-wave sleep

39. Which of the following projection systems is contained in the middle cerebellar peduncle?
    (A) Pontocerebellar projections
    (B) Cerebellothalamic projections
    (C) Posterior spinocerebellar projections
    (D) Corticospinal projections

40. Which of the following projection systems is contained in the inferior cerebellar peduncle?
    (A) Pontocerebellar projections
    (B) Cerebellothalamic projections
    (C) Posterior spinocerebellar projections
    (D) Corticospinal projections

41. Cerebrospinal fluid (CSF) provides a cushioning effect both inside and outside the brain. Which of the following spaces lies outside the brain or spinal cord and contains CSF?
    (A) Lateral ventricle
    (B) Third ventricle
    (C) Cisterna magna
    (D) Epidural space
    (E) Aqueduct of Sylvius

42. Which of the following types of neurons innervates nuclear bag intrafusal fibers that signal a change in muscle length?
    (A) Static gamma motor neuron
    (B) Alpha motor neuron
    (C) Dynamic gamma motor neuron
    (D) Corticospinal neuron
    (E) Renshaw cell

43. Projections from the fastigial nucleus reach which of the following cerebellar cortical zones?
    (A) Vermis
    (B) Intermediate zone
    (C) Lateral hemisphere

44. Preganglionic parasympathetic neurons that contribute to the innervation of the descending colon and rectum are found in which of the following structures?
    (A) Superior cervical ganglion
    (B) Dorsal motor nucleus of the vagus
    (C) Superior mesenteric ganglion
    (D) Ciliary ganglion
    (E) Spinal cord levels S-2 and S-3

45. Stimulation in which of the following brain regions is thought to lead to the induction of alpha waves?
    (A) Intralaminar nuclei of the thalamus
    (B) Ventrolateral nucleus of the thalamus
    (C) Raphe nuclei
    (D) Nucleus accumbens septi

46. Which of the following types of neurons innervates nuclear bag intrafusal fibers that signal the rate of change in muscle length?
    (A) Static gamma motor neuron
    (B) Alpha motor neuron
    (C) Dynamic gamma motor neuron
    (D) Corticospinal neuron
    (E) Renshaw cell

47. Which of the following structures serves as an "alternative pathway" for signals from the motor cortex to the spinal cord?
    (A) Red nucleus
    (B) Basilar pontine nuclei
    (C) Caudate nucleus
    (D) Thalamus
    (E) Dorsal column nuclei

48. A reticular area that inhibits the ascending reticular activating system is located at which of the following levels?
    (A) Caudal midbrain
    (B) Lateral thalamus
    (C) Postcentral gyrus
    (D) Rostral pons
    (E) Medial medulla

49. Like the primary visual cortex, the primary motor cortex is organized into vertical columns composed of cells linked together throughout the six layers of the cortex. The cells that contribute axons to the corticospinal tract are concentrated in which cortical layer?
    (A) Layer I
    (B) Layer II
    (C) Layer III
    (D) Layer IV
    (E) Layer V

50. When a muscle is suddenly stretched, a signal is transmitted over Ia sensory fibers from muscle spindles. Which of the following statements best describes the response elicited by these spindle afferent signals?
    (A) Contraction of the muscle in which the active spindles are located
    (B) Relaxation of the muscle in which the active spindles are located
    (C) Contraction of muscles antagonistic to those in which the active spindles are located
    (D) Relaxation of intrafusal fibers in the active spindles
    (E) Direct synaptic activation of gamma motor neurons

51. Which of the following allows cerebrospinal fluid to pass directly from the ventricular system into the subarachnoid space?
    (A) Foramen of Magendie
    (B) Aqueduct of Sylvius
    (C) Third ventricle
    (D) Lateral ventricle
    (E) Arachnoid villi

52. There is an area in the dominant hemisphere that, when damaged, might leave the sense of hearing intact but not allow words to be arranged into a comprehensive thought. Which of the following terms is used to identify this portion of the cortex?
    (A) Primary auditory cortex
    (B) Wernicke's area
    (C) Broca's area
    (D) Angular gyrus
    (E) Limbic association cortex

53. Projections from the interposed nucleus reach which of the following cerebellar cortical zones?
    (A) Vermis
    (B) Intermediate zone
    (C) Lateral hemisphere

54. Projections from the dentate nucleus reach which of the following cerebellar cortical zones?
    (A) Vermis
    (B) Intermediate zone
    (C) Lateral hemisphere

55. Motor cortex neurons receive feedback from muscles activated by the corticospinal system. This feedback arises from which of the following structures?
    (A) Red nucleus
    (B) Spinocerebellar tracts
    (C) Skin surface of fingers used to grasp an object
    (D) Muscle spindles in muscles antagonistic to those used to make a movement
    (E) Vestibular nuclei

56. Which of the following symptoms is typically associated with the epileptic condition that involves a postseizure depression period lasting from a few minutes to several hours?
    (A) Tonic-clonic seizure
    (B) Brain wave pattern described as spike and dome
    (C) Jacksonian march

57. The sweat glands and piloerector muscles of hairy skin are innervated by which of the following fiber types?
    (A) Cholinergic postganglionic parasympathetic fibers
    (B) Cholinergic postganglionic sympathetic fibers
    (C) Adrenergic preganglionic parasympathetic fibers
    (D) Adrenergic postganglionic sympathetic fibers
    (E) Adrenergic preganglionic sympathetic fibers

58. In controlling the fine muscles of the hands and fingers, corticospinal axons can synapse primarily with which of the following?
    (A) Posterior horn neurons
    (B) Spinal cord interneurons
    (C) Spinal cord motor neurons
    (D) Purkinje cells
    (E) Renshaw cells

59. Which of the following statements concerning spinal cord motor circuits is correct?
    (A) Dynamic gamma motor neurons innervate static nuclear bag fibers
    (B) Descending supraspinal axons synapse with either alpha or gamma motor neurons
    (C) Clonus is caused by a hyperactive stretch reflex
    (D) The contractile elements of intrafusal fibers are found at the central (nuclear) region of the fiber
    (E) Both types of sensory fibers in a muscle spindle are mechanoreceptors that signal stretch of the two polar, noncontractile ends of the intrafusal fiber

60. Which of the following cells receives direct synaptic input from Golgi tendon organs?
    (A) Type Ia inhibitory interneurons
    (B) Dynamic gamma motor neurons
    (C) Alpha motor neurons
    (D) Type Ib inhibitory interneurons
    (E) Type II excitatory interneurons

61. Which of the following neurotransmitters is used by the axons of the locus ceruleus neurons, which are distributed throughout much of the brain?
    (A) Norepinephrine
    (B) Dopamine
    (C) Serotonin
    (D) Acetylcholine

62. Which of the following statements concerning mossy and climbing fibers is correct?
    (A) Mossy fibers provide direct excitatory input to Purkinje cells
    (B) Climbing fibers evoke simple spikes in Purkinje cells
    (C) All spinocerebellar axons terminate as mossy fibers in the cerebellar cortex
    (D) All pontocerebellar axons terminate as climbing fibers in the cerebellar cortex
    (E) All climbing fibers originate in the red nucleus

63. In addition to influencing the function of muscles, the corticospinal system regulates movement by its involvement with which of the following?
    (A) Spinal reflex circuits, such as those involved in the stretch reflex
    (B) Control of pain processing in the intralaminar thalamic nuclei
    (C) Vestibulo-ocular reflex
    (D) Brain stem preganglionic parasympathetic neurons
    (E) Memory circuits in the hippocampus

64. The perivascular space (Virchow-Robin space) in the brain is formed between the wall of small penetrating vessels and which of the following structures?
    (A) Dura mater
    (B) Arachnoid membrane
    (C) Pia mater
    (D) Choroid plexus
    (E) Ependymal cells

65. Focal epilepsy may result from a localized area of brain degeneration or glial scar formation; subsequently, a wave of abnormal brain electrical activity spreads in an orderly manner away from the initial site of origin. Which of the following symptoms is typically associated with this epileptic condition?
    (A) Tonic-clonic seizure
    (B) Spike and dome brain wave pattern
    (C) Jacksonian march

66. The excitatory or inhibitory effect of a postganglionic sympathetic fiber is determined by which of the following features or structures?
    (A) The function of the postsynaptic receptor to which it binds
    (B) The specific organ innervated
    (C) The ganglion where the postganglionic fiber originates
    (D) The ganglion containing the preganglionic fiber
    (E) The emotional state of the individual

67. Which of the following neurotransmitters is used by the axons of substantia nigra neurons, which project to the caudate and putamen?
    (A) Norepinephrine
    (B) Dopamine
    (C) Serotonin
    (D) Acetylcholine

68. Which of the following statements concerning the function of cerebellar neurons is correct?
    (A) Basket cells evoke excitatory responses in Purkinje cells
    (B) Granule cells evoke excitatory responses in Purkinje cells
    (C) Golgi cells evoke excitatory responses in basket cells
    (D) Purkinje cells evoke excitatory responses in cerebellar nuclear cells
    (E) Stellate cells evoke excitatory responses in basket cells

69. Which of the following correctly describes the relationship of cerebrospinal fluid pressure to venous pressure in the superior sagittal sinus?
    (A) A few millimeters higher
    (B) A few millimeters lower
    (C) Equal to
    (D) Twice the value
    (E) Half the value

70. A vascular lesion that causes degeneration of corticospinal axons in the basilar pons is likely to lead to which of the following conditions?
    (A) Paralysis involving primarily the muscles around the contralateral shoulder and hip joints
    (B) Paralysis of the muscles of mastication
    (C) Loss of voluntary control of discrete movements of the contralateral hand and fingers
    (D) Inability to speak clearly
    (E) Inability to convert short-term memory to long-term memory

71. Which statement best describes a characteristic functional difference between a Golgi tendon organ and a muscle spindle?
    (A) Output signals of a Golgi tendon organ lead to inactivation of the muscle associated with the active tendon organ
    (B) Golgi tendon organs do not function in the course of voluntary movements that require a normal level of tension development in the associated muscle
    (C) Signals arising from a Golgi tendon organ do not contribute to conscious proprioception
    (D) Signals arising from a Golgi tendon organ are synaptically linked directly to an alpha motor neuron
    (E) Signals from a Golgi tendon organ are conducted along sensory fibers that conduct more rapidly than those of a muscle spindle

72. The cerebellum is sometimes described as a "timing device." Which of the following statements best describes the basis for this function?
    (A) The cerebellum receives visual input that enables it to determine any point in the 24-hour light-dark cycle
    (B) The cerebellum computes the exact time used to excite adjacent Purkinje cells
    (C) The cerebellar circuitry determines only the duration or end point of each movement
    (D) The cerebellar circuitry enhances the turn-on and turn-off times for each movement by delivering an excitatory signal followed by a precisely timed inhibitory signal
    (E) The cerebellar circuitry determines only the precise timing of the turn-on signal, and the turn-off signal begins when the cerebellum ceases to function

73. Output signals from Golgi tendon organs are transmitted to which of the following higher centers?
    (A) Inferior colliculus
    (B) Globus pallidus
    (C) Cerebellum
    (D) Red nucleus
    (E) Substantia nigra

74. Which type of cholinergic receptor is found at synapses between preganglionic and postganglionic neurons of the sympathetic system?
    (A) Muscarinic
    (B) Nicotinic
    (C) Alpha
    (D) Beta$_1$
    (E) Beta$_2$

75. Damage limited to the primary motor cortex (area 4) is thought to cause hypotonia in the affected muscles. However, most cortical lesions, particularly those caused by vascular infarcts, involve primary motor cortex in addition to surrounding areas of cortex or cortical efferent axons. The latter type of cortical lesion causes which of the following?
    (A) Spastic muscle paralysis
    (B) Flaccid muscle paralysis
    (C) No paralysis, but jerky, fast movements
    (D) Complete blindness in the contralateral eye
    (E) Loss of sensation in the contralateral foot

76. The term "limbic cortex" includes the orbitofrontal cortex, subcallosal gyrus, cingulate gyrus, and which of the following areas?
    (A) Supplementary motor cortex
    (B) Postcentral gyrus
    (C) Lingual gyrus
    (D) Parahippocampal gyrus
    (E) Paracentral lobule

77. The cerebellum participates in the learning of motor skills, and the climbing fibers' input to Purkinje cells is thought to be important to this process. Which of the following statements concerning this process is correct?
    (A) Under resting conditions, climbing fibers evoke complex spikes in Purkinje cells at a very rapid rate
    (B) When a novel movement is performed, the actual movement may not match the intended movement, which tends to decrease the firing rate of climbing fiber–initiated simple spikes
    (C) The decrease in climbing fiber input decreases the overall sensitivity (excitability) of the Purkinje cells
    (D) On the first trial of a new movement, the Purkinje cell adopts a new, relatively long-term level of excitability
    (E) Neurons in the inferior olivary complex and their axons projecting to the cerebellum are important contributors to the process

78. Occlusion of which of the following structures leads to communicating hydrocephalus?
    (A) Aqueduct of Sylvius
    (B) Lateral ventricle
    (C) Foramen of Luschka
    (D) Foramen of Magendie
    (E) Arachnoid villi

79. Evaluation of a patient reveals the following deficits: decreased aggressiveness and ambition and inappropriate social responses, inability to process sequential thoughts in order to solve a problem, and inability to process multiple bits of information that could then be recalled instantaneously to complete a thought or solve a problem. Damage to which of the following brain regions might be responsible for such deficits?
    (A) Premotor cortex
    (B) Parieto-occipital cortex in nondominant hemisphere
    (C) Broca's area
    (D) Limbic association cortex
    (E) Prefrontal association cortex

80. The withdrawal reflex is initiated by stimulation delivered to which of the following receptors?
    (A) Muscle spindle
    (B) Joint capsule receptor
    (C) Cutaneous free nerve ending
    (D) Golgi tendon organ
    (E) Pacinian corpuscle

81. Which substance activates alpha- and beta-adrenergic receptors equally well?
    (A) Acetylcholine
    (B) Norepinephrine
    (C) Epinephrine
    (D) Serotonin
    (E) Dopamine

82. The posterior and lateral hypothalamus, in combination with the preoptic area, is involved in the control of which of the following functions?
    (A) Cardiovascular functions involving blood pressure and heart rate
    (B) Regulation of thirst and water intake
    (C) Stimulation of uterine contractility and milk ejection from the breast
    (D) Signaling that food intake is sufficient (satiety)
    (E) Secretion of hormones from the anterior lobe of the pituitary gland

83. Which of the following statements concerning the reticulospinal system is correct?
    (A) Reticulospinal neurons do not receive input from motor areas of the cerebral cortex
    (B) Medullary reticulospinal fibers excite motor neurons that activate extensor muscles
    (C) Pontine reticulospinal fibers course in the spinal cord posterior funiculus
    (D) Medullary reticulospinal fibers course in the medial part of the ventral funiculus of the spinal cord
    (E) Pontine reticulospinal fibers excite spinal cord motor neurons that activate limb extensor muscles

84. Which of the following statements concerning the vestibulocerebellum is correct?
    (A) Deficits associated with lesions in vestibulo-cerebellar circuits are far more debilitating when the patient tries to perform slow types of movement
    (B) The vestibulocerebellum depends on linkages involving the vestibular nerve and nuclei, the vermis of the cerebellar cortex, and the inter-posed nuclei
    (C) Because the neural elements involved in vestibulocerebellar circuits are among the most rapidly conducting pathways in the brain, even with rapid movement there is always sufficient time to allow the cerebellum to correct errors based on the actual parameters of the ongoing movement
    (D) Vestibulocerebellar circuits use the speed and direction of a movement to determine the parameters of the movement after it is performed
    (E) Vestibulocerebellar circuits use the vestibu-lospinal system to make adjustments to a movement

85. In the patellar tendon reflex, which of the following synapses directly on alpha motor neurons that innervate the muscle being stretched?
    (A) Ia sensory fiber
    (B) Ib sensory fiber
    (C) Excitatory interneurons
    (D) Gamma motor neurons
    (E) Inhibitory interneurons

86. Which of the following statements best describes the functional role played by the pontine reticu-lospinal fibers in comparison to the medullary retic-ulospinal system?
    (A) The pontine system works in concert with the medullary system, with each providing excita-tory influence to extensor muscles
    (B) The pontine system essentially functions in an opposing manner to the medullary system
    (C) The pontine system provides an initial slow excitatory influence, which is followed by rapid excitation from the medullary system
    (D) The medullary system provides slow excitation to extensor motor neurons, whereas the pontine system provides slow excitation of flexor motor neurons
    (E) The medullary system provides excitation to upper limb extensor motor neurons, whereas the pontine system provides excitation to lower limb extensor motor neurons

87. Which of the following reflexes is correctly paired with the sensory structure that mediates the reflex?
    (A) Autogenic inhibition—muscle spindle
    (B) Reciprocal inhibition—Golgi tendon organ
    (C) Reciprocal inhibition—pacinian corpuscle
    (D) Stretch reflex—muscle spindle
    (E) Golgi tendon reflex—Meissner's corpuscle

88. Which of the following represents the structural basis of the blood–cerebrospinal fluid barrier?
    (A) Tight junctions between the ependymal cells forming the ventricular walls
    (B) Arachnoid villi
    (C) Tight junctions between adjacent choroid plexus cells
    (D) Astrocyte foot processes
    (E) Tight junctions between adjacent endothelial cells of brain capillaries

89. Which of the following disorders is characterized by the inability to comprehend spoken language or speak fluently with meaning?
    (A) Broca's aphasia
    (B) Wernicke's aphasia
    (C) Global aphasia

90. Which of the following statements concerning the withdrawal reflex is correct?
    (A) The withdrawal reflex involves direct synaptic linkage between the incoming sensory signal and the alpha motor neurons that specify the muscles to be activated
    (B) The withdrawal reflex, through its pro-priospinal intersegmental connections, can initiate the movement of all four limbs if so required
    (C) The withdrawal reflex circuits are active only when a flexor muscle is required to respond to a painful stimulus
    (D) Inhibitory interneurons are not involved in the withdrawal reflex circuits
    (E) The withdrawal reflex is easily modified by descending supraspinal pathways

91. Nasal, lacrimal, salivary, and gastrointestinal glands are stimulated by which of the following substances?
    (A) Acetylcholine
    (B) Norepinephrine
    (C) Epinephrine
    (D) Serotonin
    (E) Dopamine

92. Which of the following reflexes best describes incoming pain signals that elicit movements per-formed by antagonistic muscle groups on either side of the body?
    (A) Crossed extensor reflex
    (B) Withdrawal reflex
    (C) Reciprocal inhibition
    (D) Autogenic inhibition

93. The spinocerebellum is involved in the control of ballistic movements, which are entirely preplanned, in that the initiation, trajectory, and end point are programmed by the cerebellum. With regard to patients with cerebellar lesions that interfere with ballistic movements, which of the following state-ments is correct?
    (A) Movements are slow to be initiated
    (B) Speed of the movement is faster than desired
    (C) Movement turn-off is reached more quickly
    (D) Spastic paralysis appears in the affected muscle group
    (E) Resting tremor develops in the affected limbs

94. Decerebrate rigidity results from which of the following situations?
    (A) Damage to the brain stem systems that control flexor motor neurons
    (B) Overactivity in the medullary reticulospinal system, which leads to hyperactivity in limb extensor muscles
    (C) Imbalance in the activity of the medullary and pontine reticulospinal systems, such that excitation of extensor motor neurons is the end result
    (D) Interruption of the medullary reticulospinal axons
    (E) Interruption of the pontine reticulospinal axons

95. Brain edema is a serious complication of altered fluid dynamics in the brain. Continued progression of brain edema may lead to which of the following situations?
    (A) Relaxation of the smooth muscle vasculature and decreased blood flow
    (B) Increased blood flow, leading to increased oxygen concentration
    (C) Vasoconstriction and decreased edema
    (D) Relaxation of the smooth muscle vasculature and increased blood flow
    (E) Compression of blood vessels, leading to ischemia and compensatory capillary dilatation

96. Which portion of the cerebellum functions in the planning of sequential movement?
    (A) Vermis and fastigial nucleus
    (B) Intermediate zone and fastigial nucleus
    (C) Lateral hemisphere and interposed nucleus
    (D) Cerebrocerebellum and dentate nucleus
    (E) Spinocerebellum and interposed nucleus

97. Bilateral lesions involving the ventromedial hypothalamus lead to which of the following deficits?
    (A) Decreased eating and drinking
    (B) Loss of sexual drive
    (C) Excessive eating, rage and aggression, and hyperactivity
    (D) Uterine contractility and mammary gland enlargement
    (E) Obsessive-compulsive disorder

98. Which of the following reflexes best describes signals from Ia sensory fibers that stimulate muscle activation in the ipsilateral limb and at the same time inhibit antagonistic muscles in the contralateral limb?
    (A) Crossed extensor reflex
    (B) Withdrawal reflex
    (C) Reciprocal inhibition
    (D) Autogenic inhibition

99. Which of the following terms best describes the cerebellar deficit in which there is a failure to perform rapid alternating movements, indicating a failure of "progression" from one part of the movement to the next?
    (A) Past pointing
    (B) Intention tremor
    (C) Dysarthria
    (D) Cerebellar nystagmus
    (E) Dysdiadochokinesia

100. The function of which of the following is dominated by the sympathetic nervous system?
    (A) Systemic blood vessels
    (B) Heart
    (C) Gastrointestinal gland secretion
    (D) Salivary glands
    (E) Gastrointestinal motility

101. Which of the following structures is maximally sensitive to linear head movement in the horizontal plane?
    (A) Macula of the utricle
    (B) Macula of the saccule
    (C) Crista ampullaris of the anterior semicircular duct
    (D) Crista ampullaris of the horizontal semicircular duct

102. A patient seems to be able to comprehend spoken language but is unable to speak the appropriate words or form sounds into words. The patient has no problem swallowing. Which of the following terms best describes this patient's condition?
    (A) Broca's aphasia
    (B) Wernicke's aphasia
    (C) Global aphasia

103. Schizophrenia is thought to be caused in part by excessive production and release of which of the following neurotransmitter agents?
    (A) Norepinephrine
    (B) Serotonin
    (C) Acetylcholine
    (D) Substance P
    (E) Dopamine

104. Which sequence below accurately describes the flow of signals linking the basal ganglia to other parts of the brain?
    (A) Globus pallidus → putamen → cerebral cortex → thalamus
    (B) Thalamus → putamen → cerebral cortex → globus pallidus
    (C) Cerebral cortex → caudate → globus pallidus → thalamus
    (D) Cerebral cortex → thalamus → caudate → globus pallidus
    (E) Putamen → caudate → thalamus → cerebral cortex → globus pallidus

105. Which of the following structures is maximally sensitive to horizontal rotation of the head?
    (A) Crista ampullaris of the posterior semicircular duct
    (B) Macula of the saccule
    (C) Crista ampullaris of the anterior semicircular duct
    (D) Crista ampullaris of the horizontal semicircular duct

106. Under awake, resting conditions, brain metabolism accounts for about 15 per cent of the total metabolism of the body, which is among the highest metabolic rates of all tissues in the body. Which of the following cellular populations of the nervous system contributes most substantially to this high rate of metabolism?
    (A) Astrocytes
    (B) Neurons
    (C) Ependymal cells
    (D) Choroid plexus cells
    (E) Brain endothelial cells

107. The concept of "autonomic tone" is quite advantageous because it allows the nervous system to have fine control over the function of an organ or organ system. This is exemplified in the control of systemic arterioles. Which of the following actions would lead to vasodilatation of systemic arterioles?
    (A) Increased activity of preganglionic parasympathetic neurons
    (B) Decreased activity of postganglionic parasympathetic neurons
    (C) Increased activity of postganglionic sympathetic neurons
    (D) Decreased activity of postganglionic sympathetic neurons
    (E) Increased activity of preganglionic sympathetic neurons

108. Which of the following terms best describes the sudden jerky or flailing limb movements observed in a patient with a vascular infarct involving the subthalamic nucleus?
    (A) Athetosis
    (B) Choreiform movements
    (C) Resting tremor
    (D) Hemiballism

109. Which of the following statements concerning memory processing in the brain is correct?
    (A) The brain forms positive memory through the facilitation of synaptic circuits but is unable to form negative memory by learning to ignore irrelevant information
    (B) Short-term memory is considered to be a list of 7 to 10 discrete facts that can be recalled within a period of several hours
    (C) It appears that rehearsal and repetition of information are not advantageous in converting short-term memory to long-term memory
    (D) Lesions involving the hippocampus cause a profound deficit in short-term memory
    (E) No morphological or structural changes occur in the process of long-term memory formation

110. Which of the following structures is maximally sensitive to linear head movement in the vertical plane?
    (A) Macula of the utricle
    (B) Macula of the saccule
    (C) Crista ampullaris of the anterior semicircular duct
    (D) Crista ampullaris of the horizontal semicircular duct

111. Retrograde amnesia is the inability to recall long-term memories from the past. Damage to which of the following brain regions leads to retrograde amnesia?
    (A) Hippocampus
    (B) Dentate gyrus
    (C) Amygdaloid complex
    (D) Thalamus
    (E) Mammillary nuclei of the hypothalamus

112. Which of the following terms best describes the rapid, jerky movements, usually of the upper limb, observed in a patient who is not attempting to make any voluntary movement?
    (A) Intention tremor
    (B) Spasticity
    (C) Choreiform movements
    (D) Akinesia

113. Although the sympathetic nervous system is often activated in such a way that it leads to mass activation of sympathetic responses throughout the body, it can also be activated to produce relatively discrete responses. Which of the following is an example of a local or discrete sympathetic action?
    (A) Heating of a patch of skin causes relatively restricted vasodilatation in the heated region
    (B) Food in the mouth causes salivation
    (C) Emptying of the bladder causes reflexive emptying of the bowel
    (D) Dust particle in the eye causes increased tear fluid release
    (E) Bright light introduced into one eye causes pupillary constriction in both eyes

114. Which of the following statements concerning the transduction mechanism in vestibular hair cells is correct?
    (A) Movement that bends the stereocilia away from the kinocilium has a depolarizing influence on the hair cell
    (B) Attachment of the stereocilia to the kinocilium activates voltage-gated sodium channels in the membrane of the kinocilium
    (C) Depolarization of the hair cell is achieved by inward movement of sodium from the endolymph
    (D) Deflection of the cupula such that stereocilia move toward the kinocilium causes the hair cell to depolarize
    (E) Inward movement of potassium through voltage-gated potassium channels in the stereocilia membrane has a depolarizing influence on the hair cell

115. When an experimental animal is given the choice of eating especially appetizing food or having the reward center stimulated, the animal most often chooses reward center stimulation rather than food. Which of the following cell groups is considered the reward center?
    (A) Lateral and ventromedial hypothalamic nuclei
    (B) Periventricular hypothalamus and midbrain central gray
    (C) Supraoptic nuclei of the hypothalamus
    (D) Anterior hypothalamic nucleus

116. Which of the following terms best describes the slow, writhing movements of an arm that cannot be stopped or initiated by a patient?
   (A) Athetosis
   (B) Choreiform movements
   (C) Resting tremor
   (D) Bradykinesia

117. Which component of the basal ganglia plays the major role in the control of cognitive (memory-guided) motor activity?
   (A) Globus pallidus
   (B) Substantia nigra
   (C) Caudate nucleus
   (D) Putamen
   (E) Subthalamic nucleus

118. The amount of energy used by the brain is among the highest of any organ in the body, but unfortunately, glycogen storage in the brain is minimal; thus, anaerobic glycolysis is not a significant source of energy. Considering this information about brain metabolism, which of the following statements is correct?
   (A) The brain is dependent on glucose delivery via the vascular system
   (B) Glucose delivered to the brain via the vascular system can be stored in neurons for several hours
   (C) Cessation of blood flow to the brain can be safely tolerated for up to about 10 minutes owing to brain tissue's considerable capacity for oxygen storage
   (D) Glucose delivery to neurons is vitally dependent on insulin
   (E) An overdose of insulin causes glucose to be rapidly transported into the brain at the expense of other insulin-dependent tissues

119. All the hair cells in the crista ampullaris of the horizontal semicircular duct have their stereocilia and kinocilium oriented according to which of the following patterns?
   (A) Same pattern, with a progressive increase in stereocilia length from shortest to tallest, with the tallest located adjacent to the kinocilium
   (B) Random pattern, with progression from shortest to tallest stereocilia, with the shortest located adjacent to the kinocilium
   (C) Same pattern, with a progressive decrease in stereocilia length from tallest to shortest, with the shortest located adjacent to the kinocilium
   (D) Random pattern, with progression from tallest to shortest stereocilia, with the shortest located adjacent to the kinocilium
   (E) Random pattern, with random distribution of stereocilia of various lengths

120. Stimulation of the punishment center can inhibit the reward center, demonstrating that fear and punishment can take precedence over pleasure and reward. Which of the following cell groups is considered the punishment center?
   (A) Lateral and ventromedial hypothalamic nuclei
   (B) Periventricular hypothalamus and midbrain central gray
   (C) Supraoptic nuclei of the hypothalamus
   (D) Anterior hypothalamic nucleus

121. A wide variety of neurotransmitters have been identified in the cell bodies and afferent synaptic terminals in the basal ganglia. A deficiency of which of the following transmitters is typically associated with Parkinson's disease?
   (A) Norepinephrine
   (B) Dopamine
   (C) Serotonin
   (D) GABA
   (E) Substance P

122. Drugs that stimulate specific adrenergic receptors are called sympathomimetic drugs. Which of the following is a sympathomimetic drug?
   (A) Reserpine
   (B) Phentolamine
   (C) Propranolol
   (D) L-dopa
   (E) Phenylephrine

Answers

1. (D) Neurons in layer V project into the subcortical white matter and from there to a wide variety of subcortical locations, including the basal ganglia, brain stem, and spinal cord. The cells in layer VI project to the thalamus. Cells in layers I, II, and III form intracortical connections of various types, and those in layer IV receive thalamocortical projections.
   TMP11 714

2. (E) Axons of motor neurons in the anterior horn exit the spinal cord through the anterior root. The posterior root serves as the entry point for sensory fibers coming into the posterior horn region of the spinal cord. The posterior column and ventral white commissure are fiber tracts located solely within the spinal cord.
   TMP11 673, 674

3. (A) Alpha motor neurons form direct synaptic contact with skeletal extrafusal muscle fibers, whereas gamma motor neurons form synaptic junctions with intrafusal muscle fibers. Pyramidal, granule, and Purkinje neurons are located in the central nervous system and have no direct contact with skeletal muscle.
   TMP11 673, 674

4. (B) A characteristic feature of the reticular activating system is that it produces widespread activation of many cortical regions. This is achieved through

diffuse projections from the intralaminar nuclei of the thalamus.
TMP11 728, 729

5. (E) The output of the cerebellum is quite removed from motor neurons and the activation of muscle, particularly in the case of limb or paraxial musculature. Although the output of the cerebellum clearly influences muscle activity, it does so by very indirect means. The cerebellar nuclei project to the motor nuclei of the thalamus and to the red nucleus and thus can influence activity in the corticospinal and rubrospinal tracts.
TMP11 700, 701

6. (D) All preganglionic sympathetic neurons are located in the intermediolateral cell column (lateral horn), and this cell group extends from T-1 to L-2.
TMP11 748, 749

7. (C) The lateral cerebellar hemispheres function with the cerebral cortex in the planning of complex movements.
TMP11 705, 706

8. (A) The most potent stimulator of cerebral blood flow is a local increase in carbon dioxide concentration, followed in order by a decrease in oxygen concentration and an increase in local neuronal activity.
TMP11 761, 762

9. (C) The primary motor cortex corresponds to Brodmann's area 4 and is located within the precentral gyrus. Area 6 is the premotor cortex, area 5 is part of the superior parietal lobule, and areas 3 and 1 form part of the primary somatosensory cortex in the postcentral gyrus.
TMP11 685, 686

10. (A) The face region of the motor cortex is most inferior and lateral in the territory of the middle cerebral artery, whereas the lower limb is in the paracentral lobule in the territory of the anterior cerebral artery.
TMP11 686

11. (C) Gamma motor neurons form direct synaptic contact with the skeletal muscle fibers known as intrafusal fibers. Extrafusal muscle fibers are innervated by alpha motor neurons, whereas Purkinje, granule, and pyramidal neurons have no synaptic contact with muscles in the periphery.
TMP11 673, 674

12. (C) Preganglionic sympathetic axons pass through the white communicating rami to enter the sympathetic trunk. Postganglionic sympathetic axons course through gray rami and might be found in dorsal and ventral primary rami.
TMP11 748, 749

13. (A) The cerebellar vermis is involved with the control of axial muscles as well as proximal limb muscles in the shoulder and hip.
TMP11 699, 700

14. (C) Although some bodily movements, in addition to eye movements, may occur during rapid eye movement (REM) sleep, there is a significant overall reduction in muscle tone during the REM period. Slow-wave sleep sometimes includes dreaming. Individuals often awake spontaneously from REM sleep, and heart and respiratory rates become irregular during REM sleep.
TMP11 739, 740

15. (E) There are two populations of spinal cord interneurons—one capable of producing excitation, and the other capable of producing inhibition in their postsynaptic target neurons. All other statements are false.
TMP11 674, 675

16. (B) The intermediate zone of the cerebellum influences the function of distal limb muscles.
TMP11 699, 700

17. (C) The only situation in which the sympathetic innervation of cerebral blood vessels might play a major role in controlling blood flow is a substantial increase in blood pressure that occurs very rapidly.
TMP11 762, 763

18. (C) The association cortex is defined by the fact that it receives multiple inputs from a wide variety of sensory areas of cortex. It is the true multimodal cortex.
TMP11 716

19. (E) The postural set necessary to initiate limb movements is controlled by the premotor cortex.
TMP11 686

20. (B) A characteristic feature of the supplementary motor cortex is that stimulation on one side produces bilateral limb movements, usually involving both hands.
TMP11 686

21. (C) Stimulation of the raphe nuclei in the caudal pons and medulla causes a very strong induction of sleep.
TMP11 740

22. (A) Recurrent branches of motor neuron axons form synaptic contact with Renshaw cells.
TMP11 674, 675

23. (B) Cerebellothalamic projections are contained in the superior cerebellar peduncle.
TMP11 701

24. (B) The combination of a motor neuron and all the muscle fibers innervated by that motor neuron is called a motor unit.
TMP11 673

25. (E) The ventromedial portion of the occipitotemporal association cortex is known to be the facial recognition cortex.
TMP11 717, 718

26. (D) Broca's area is known to be the control center for the motor aspects of language.
    TMP11 717

27. (A) The parieto-occipital association cortex in the nondominant hemisphere is known to control the analysis of three-dimensional space for the individual's own body as well as the surrounding environment.
    TMP11 716

28. (C) The visual association cortex (angular gyrus) in the dominant hemisphere serves as the processing and analysis center for reading.
    TMP11 716

29. (E) Broca's aphasia typically involves an inability to speak words correctly in the absence of any true paralysis of the laryngeal or pharyngeal musculature.
    TMP11 721, 722

30. (D) A stroke involving the left middle cerebral artery is likely to cause an aphasic syndrome that might involve the loss of speech comprehension or the loss of the ability to produce speech sounds. Any paralysis resulting from the lesion would affect the right side of the body; similarly, any visual field deficits would affect the right visual field of each eye.
    TMP11 721

31. (B) Corticospinal fibers pass through the medullary pyramid.
    TMP11 687

32. (B) Cholinergic neurons in the dorsolateral pons are considered to be rapid eye movement (REM)–generating cells. Consequently, if a cholinergic antagonist is administered, these cells will not be capable of inducing REM sleep.
    TMP11 740, 741

33. (E) Type II "flower-spray" endings are related to nuclear chain–type intrafusal fibers. Intrafusal fibers are innervated by gamma motor neurons. The nuclei of nuclear bag fibers form a cluster in the central nuclear region of the cell. The primary sensory (type Ia) fibers are among the fastest conducting fibers in the nervous system. Nuclear chain fibers signal only the change in muscle length.
    TMP11 675, 676

34. (A) Pain signals traveling through the anterolateral system, but not any of the discriminative sensations coursing through the medial lemniscal system, provide input to the cells in the reticular formation that give rise to ascending projections to the intralaminar nuclei of the thalamus.
    TMP11 728, 729

35. (D) The main pathway linking the cerebral cortex and the cerebellum involves cortical projections to the ipsilateral basilar pontine nuclei, the cells of which then project to the contralateral cerebellum.
    TMP11 688

36. (A) Preganglionic sympathetic axons synapse on cells in the adrenal medulla that function as postganglionic sympathetic neurons.
    TMP11 749, 750

37. (A) When a muscle and its spindles are passively stretched, the Ia sensory fibers increase their firing rate. The firing of type II sensory fibers is largely unaffected, whereas alpha motor neurons can be stimulated and gamma motor neurons are unaffected.
    TMP11 675, 676

38. (D) Delta waves exhibit the highest voltage and lowest frequency among the commonly described electroencephalogram waves. Alpha waves are seen in the quiet, waking state; beta waves are seen in a heightened state of alertness; and theta waves are not commonly seen in children.
    TMP11 741, 742

39. (A) Pontocerebellar axons are contained in the middle cerebellar peduncle.
    TMP11 700

40. (C) Posterior spinocerebellar fibers pass through the inferior cerebellar peduncle.
    TMP11 700, 701

41. (C) The cerebrospinal fluid outside the brain and spinal cord is located within the subarachnoid space. Dilated regions of the subarachnoid space are identified as cisterns. The cisterna magna is one of the largest cisterns and is positioned at the caudal end of the fourth ventricle between the cerebellum and the posterior surface of the medulla.
    TMP11 764

42. (A) Static motor neurons innervate static nuclear bag fibers that sense only the change in muscle length.
    TMP11 676

43. (A) Projections from the fastigial nucleus reach the cerebellar vermis.
    TMP11 701

44. (E) Preganglionic parasympathetic neurons that contribute to the innervation of the descending colon and rectum are found at S-2 and S-3 levels of the spinal cord.
    TMP11 750

45. (A) Stimulation of the intralaminar nuclei of the thalamus leads to the induction of the widespread cortical activity that underlies the appearance of alpha waves.
    TMP11 742

46. (C) Dynamic motor neurons innervate dynamic nuclear bag fibers that sense the rate of change in muscle length.
    TMP11 676

47. (A) Cortical projections to the red nucleus provide an alternative pathway for the cerebral cortex to control flexor muscles through the rubrospinal tract.
TMP11 688, 689

48. (E) Portions of the ventral and medial medulla provide inhibitory control over cells of the ascending reticular activating system.
TMP11 729

49. (E) Corticospinal axons originate from cell bodies (pyramidal neurons) in layer V of the motor areas of the cortex.
TMP11 687, 688

50. (A) When a muscle is stretched, signals traveling over Ia sensory fibers lead to contraction of the muscle in which the active spindles are located. At the same time, the antagonist muscles are inactivated. The intrafusal fibers in the spindle do not go slack due to the tonic activation of gamma motor neurons by supraspinal systems. They are not influenced by signals carried on Ia sensory fibers.
TMP11 678

51. (A) The foramen of Magendie and the two lateral foramina of Luschka form the communication channels between the ventricular system within the brain and the subarachnoid space that lies outside the brain and spinal cord.
TMP11 764

52. (B) Wernicke's area in the dominant hemisphere is responsible for interpreting spoken language. Damage to Wernicke's area eliminates comprehension of spoken language.
TMP11 718

53. (B) Projections from the interposed nucleus reach the cerebellar intermediate zone.
TMP11 701

54. (C) Projections from the dentate nucleus reach the lateral hemisphere.
TMP11 701

55. (C) The palmar (volar) surfaces of the skin contain receptors that project through the medial lemniscal system to the primary somatosensory cortex. When these fingers are flexed and grasp an object, the cutaneous receptors send signals to the primary somatosensory cortex. These cortical neurons then project to the adjacent motor cortex and the pyramidal neurons that sent the original message down the corticospinal tract to cause contraction of the finger flexors. The motor cortex neurons are then said to be "informed" of the muscle contractions they originally specified.
TMP11 690

56. (A) Grand mal epilepsy is associated with the appearance of tonic-clonic seizure activity.
TMP11 743, 744

57. (B) Sweat glands and the piloerector smooth muscle of hairy skin are innervated by the population of cholinergic postganglionic sympathetic neurons.
TMP11 750, 751

58. (C) Although the majority of corticospinal axons synapse with the pool of spinal cord interneurons, some synapse directly with the motor neurons that innervate muscles controlling the wrist and finger flexors.
TMP11 690

59. (C) Clonus is caused by hyperactive stretch reflexes. All the other statements are incorrect.
TMP11 679

60. (D) Golgi tendon organs provide direct synaptic input to type Ib inhibitory interneurons. Type Ia interneurons and alpha motor neurons receive input from muscle spindle afferents, whereas dynamic gamma motor neurons and excitatory interneurons receive their input from supraspinal systems.
TMP11 679

61. (A) Neurons in the locus ceruleus use the neurotransmitter norepinephrine in their widespread projections throughout the brain.
TMP11 730

62. (C) All spinocerebellar axons terminate as mossy fibers; only the axons that arise in the inferior olivary nucleus form climbing fibers.
TMP11 701, 702

63. (A) In addition to influencing the activation of muscles, the corticospinal tract can increase the gain of certain spinal cord reflex pathways, such that some reflexes are enhanced and others are inhibited.
TMP11 691

64. (C) The perivascular space (also known as the Virchow-Robin space) is formed between the outer wall of small vessels penetrating into the brain and the pia mater, which lines the outer surface of the brain and is only loosely attached to the brain.
TMP11 765

65. (C) Often a focal epileptic seizure spreads progressively and sequentially into neighboring cortical regions to produce the so-called jacksonian march. For example, seizure activity begins in the face and spreads along the motor cortex to sequentially involve the forelimb and eventually the hindlimb.
TMP11 743, 744

66. (A) The excitatory or inhibitory effect of a postganglionic sympathetic fiber is determined solely by the type of receptor to which it binds.
TMP11 752

67. (B) Cells in the pars compacta portion of the substantia nigra use the neurotransmitter dopamine in their projections to the caudate and putamen.
TMP11 730, 731

68. (B) Granule cell axons have branches that form the parallel fiber system in the molecular layer, where they provide excitatory input to Purkinje cell dendrites.
    TMP11 702

69. (A) Cerebrospinal fluid (CSF) flows across the valvelike arachnoid villi when the CSF pressure is only a few millimeters higher than the pressure within the superior sagittal sinus.
    TMP11 765

70. (C) The most characteristic deficit following damage to corticospinal tract neurons involves discrete voluntary movement of the contralateral hand and fingers.
    TMP11 691

71. (A) Signals from Golgi tendon organs lead to inhibition of the associated muscle, whereas muscle spindle activity leads to excitation of the muscles associated with the active spindle. Golgi tendon organs, similar to muscle spindles, function in the course of normal movement. Golgi tendon organ afferents conduct more slowly than spindle afferents do, and tendon organs provide input to interneurons and not to motor neurons, similar to the muscle spindles.
    TMP11 679

72. (D) Cerebellar circuitry enhances the turn-on and turn-off times for each movement. This provides the precise timing for the start and end of each movement.
    TMP11 702, 703

73. (C) Golgi tendon organs provide input to the cerebellum. They do not provide input to the inferior colliculus, globus pallidus, red nucleus, or substantia nigra.
    TMP11 679

74. (B) Nicotinic cholinergic receptors are found at synapses between preganglionic and postganglionic sympathetic neurons.
    TMP11 752

75. (A) Lesions that damage primary motor cortex and other surrounding motor cortical areas lead to spastic paralysis in the affected muscles.
    TMP11 691

76. (D) The parahippocampal gyrus is an important component of the limbic cortex or limbic lobe.
    TMP11 731

77. (E) The climbing fiber (inferior olivary) input to a Purkinje cell is thought to alter the excitability of the Purkinje cell, making it more or less responsive to granule cell input.
    TMP11 703

78. (E) Noncommunicating hydrocephalus results when a blockage of cerebrospinal fluid flow occurs within the ventricular system or at the sites of communication between the ventricular system and the subarachnoid space. Communicating hydrocephalus occurs when a blockage occurs either within the subarachnoid space or at the arachnoid villi, thus preventing communication between the subarachnoid space and the superior sagittal sinus.
    TMP11 766

79. (E) Behavioral deficits, changes in personality, and diminished problem-solving ability are all signs of damage to the prefrontal association cortex.
    TMP11 719, 720

80. (C) The withdrawal reflex is activated by stimuli from free nerve endings. Muscle spindles provide the afferent signals for the stretch reflex, and Golgi tendon organs are the source of stimuli for the inverse myotatic reflex.
    TMP11 680, 681

81. (C) Epinephrine activates alpha- and beta-adrenergic receptors equally well. Norepinephrine excites both types of receptors but has a markedly greater effect on alpha receptors.
    TMP11 752

82. (A) The posterior and lateral hypothalamus, in combination with the preoptic hypothalamus, is an important group of cells controlling cardiovascular functions such as heart rate and blood pressure.
    TMP11 733

83. (E) Pontine reticulospinal fibers excite motor neurons supplying extensor muscles. In contrast, medullary reticulospinal fibers lead to inhibition of extensor motor neurons.
    TMP11 692

84. (E) The vestibulocerebellum provides output signals to the ascending portion of the medial longitudinal fasciculus (MLF) for adjustments to the extraocular muscles, and it provides signals to the descending MLF and the vestibulospinal tract for the control of axial and limb musculature. The vestibulocerebellar circuits do not provide significant output to the thalamus and cortex that might then influence the corticospinal system.
    TMP11 704

85. (A) Ia sensory fibers synapse directly with alpha motor neurons, whereas Ib sensory fibers synapse with inhibitory interneurons. Excitatory interneurons play an important role in the withdrawal reflex. Gamma motor neurons receive input primarily from supraspinal systems.
    TMP11 676, 677

86. (B) The pontine and medullary reticulospinal systems function in an opposing manner to influence the motor neurons that control axial and limb extensor muscles.
    TMP11 692

87. (D) The stretch reflex is mediated by muscle spindles. Autogenic inhibition involves Golgi tendon

organs. Reciprocal inhibition is also related to muscle spindles.
TMP11 677

88. (C) The tight junctions formed between adjacent choroid epithelial cells represent the structural basis of the blood–cerebrospinal fluid barrier. The blood-brain barrier is formed by the tight junctions between adjacent endothelial cells of brain capillaries.
TMP11 766

89. (C) A patient who is unable to speak fluently and who is unable to understand spoken language has a large lesion involving most of the central speech areas. This disorder is referred to as global aphasia.
TMP11 720, 721

90. (B) The withdrawal reflex is dependent on cutaneous sensory input to alpha motor neurons and can involve flexors or extensors as required to remove the limb from the painful stimulus. The withdrawal reflex generally involves excitatory interneurons and is subject to very little modification through supraspinal systems.
TMP11 680, 681

91. (A) The nasal, lacrimal, salivary, and gastrointestinal glands are stimulated by cholinergic postganglionic parasympathetic neurons.
TMP11 754

92. (A) The crossed extensor reflex is dependent on incoming pain signals distributed to both sides of the spinal cord via excitatory interneurons.
TMP11 681

93. (A) Both the initiation and the execution of ballistic-type movements are slowed dramatically with lesions that involve the spinocerebellum.
TMP11 705

94. (C) In decerebrate rigidity, the cortical projections that normally activate the inhibitory reticulospinal system are lost. Although cortical activation of the excitatory pontine reticulospinal system is also lost, the latter system continues to be activated by intact ascending somatosensory (pain) pathways. This leads to activation of extensor motor neurons without the inhibitory influence of the medullary reticulospinal fibers.
TMP11 692

95. (E) Brain edema leads to compression of brain vasculature, decreased blood flow, ischemia, and compensatory vasodilatation. This ultimately leads to an even further increase in edema.
TMP11 766, 767

96. (D) The cerebrocerebellum and the dentate nucleus are involved with the thalamus and cortex in the planning of complex movements.
TMP11 706

97. (C) Lesions involving the ventromedial hypothalamus lead to excessive eating (hyperphagia), excessive drinking, rage and aggression, and hyperactivity.
TMP11 735

98. (C) Reciprocal inhibition involves the activation of one muscle via Ia sensory input to an alpha motor neuron and collateral input from that sensory fiber to an inhibitory interneuron that inactivates an antagonist muscle.
TMP11 681, 682

99. (E) Dysdiadochokinesia is a cerebellar deficit that involves a failure of progression from one part of a movement to the next. Consequently, movements that include rapid alternation between flexion and extension are most severely affected.
TMP11 707

100. (A) The innervation and function of systemic blood vessels are influenced primarily, if not exclusively, by the sympathetic nervous system.
TMP11 754, 755

101. (A) The hair cells in the macula of the utricle are maximally sensitive to linear head movement in the horizontal plane.
TMP11 693

102. (A) A patient who is able to comprehend spoken language but who has difficulty forming sounds into appropriate words exhibits the signs of Broca's aphasia.
TMP11 721, 722

103. (E) Schizophrenia is thought to be caused in part by excessive release of dopamine. Occasionally, patients with Parkinson's disease exhibit schizophrenic symptoms due to an inability to control L-dopa therapy and the subsequent production of dopamine.
TMP11 745, 746

104. (C) The flow of signals proceeds from the cerebral cortex to the caudate (or putamen), globus pallidus, thalamus, and finally back to the cerebral cortex. Such a loop is characteristic of the flow of information from several different regions of the cortex to the basal ganglia and then back to the cortex via the thalamus.
TMP11 708, 709

105. (D) Hair cells in the crista ampullaris of the horizontal semicircular duct are maximally sensitive to rotational head movement in the horizontal plane.
TMP11 694

106. (B) The high metabolic rate in the nervous system is primarily due to the high metabolic activity in neurons, even in the resting state.
TMP11 767

107. (D) Decreased activity of postganglionic sympathetic neurons leads to vasodilatation of systemic arterioles. In contrast, increased activity in postganglionic sympathetics results in vasoconstriction.
TMP11 756

108. (D) Lesions that involve the subthalamic nucleus result in rapid flailing movements of a limb, which are referred to as hemiballism.
TMP11 709

109. (D) Hippocampal lesions interfere with the formation of short-term memory and its conversion to long-term memory. These patients retain previously formed long-term memory but are unable to form new long-term memory and are said to exhibit anterograde amnesia. The brain is able to form both positive and negative memories. The duration of short-term memory is a matter of seconds to minutes. Rehearsal and repetition are helpful in forming long-term memories. Certain structural changes in neurons and synaptic boutons may contribute to long-term memory formation and storage.
TMP11 724

110. (B) Hair cells in the macula of the saccule are maximally sensitive to linear head movement in the vertical plane.
TMP11 693

111. (D) Lesions involving the thalamus lead to retrograde amnesia because they are believed to interfere with the process of retrieving long-term memory stored in other portions of the brain.
TMP11 726

112. (C) Rapid, jerky involuntary movements of the limbs are termed choreiform movements.
TMP11 709

113. (A) An example of a relatively restricted or local sympathetic action is the vasodilatation or vasoconstriction of blood vessels that occurs upon the warming or cooling of a patch of skin.
TMP11 757

114. (D) When cupula deflection moves the stereocilia toward the kinocilium, mechanically gated potassium channels are opened in the kinocilium membrane, and potassium in the endolymph moves into the hair cell and causes it to be depolarized.
TMP11 694

115. (A) The reward center is localized to the lateral and ventromedial regions of the hypothalamus.
TMP11 735

116. (A) A slow, writhing type of involuntary movement observed after basal ganglia lesions is called athetosis.
TMP11 709

117. (C) The caudate nucleus is involved in the basal ganglia circuits that control memory-guided motor activity.
TMP11 709

118. (A) The brain is totally dependent on a minute-to-minute supply of glucose delivered by the vascular system, because there is no substantial storage of either glucose or glycogen by the brain. The delivery of glucose to the brain is not at all dependent on the availability of insulin.
TMP11 767

119. (A) All the hair cells in the crista ampullaris of the horizontal semicircular duct have the same orientation. The stereocilia proceed in sequence from shortest to tallest, with the tallest stereocilium located adjacent to the kinocilium.
TMP11 694

120. (B) The punishment center is primarily localized to the periventricular hypothalamus and the midbrain central gray.
TMP11 735

121. (B) Degeneration of the dopaminergic cells in the pars compacta of the substantia nigra is thought to be the primary defect in Parkinson's disease.
TMP11 711

122. (E) Phenylephrine is a sympathomimetic drug that stimulates adrenergic receptors. Reserpine, phentolamine, and propranolol are sympathetic antagonists.
TMP11 759

Gastrointestinal
Physiology

1. Under normal conditions, saliva contains a high concentration of which of the following ions?
   (A) Potassium
   (B) Chloride
   (C) Sodium
   (D) Calcium

2. Activation of which of the following is normally associated with contraction of the smooth muscle of the gastrointestinal tract?
   (A) Submucosal plexus (Meissner's plexus)
   (B) Celiac ganglia
   (C) Myenteric plexus (Auerbach's plexus)
   (D) Mesenteric ganglia

Questions 3 and 4

For questions 3 and 4, refer to the figure below.

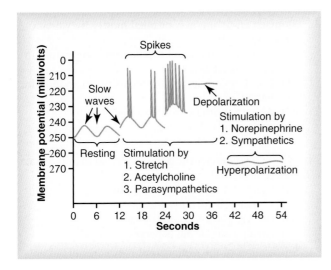

3. Which of the following is true of slow-wave electrical potentials in gastrointestinal smooth muscle?
   (A) They are similar to true action potentials and lead directly to contraction of gastrointestinal smooth muscle
   (B) They occur at the same frequency in all portions of the gastrointestinal tract
   (C) They occur as a result of calcium influx through sodium-calcium channels
   (D) They are changes in the resting membrane varying between 5 and 15 millivolts

4. Which of the following would most likely decrease the number of spike potentials generated in gastrointestinal smooth muscle?
   (A) Sympathetic stimulation
   (B) Stretching of the muscle
   (C) Acetylcholine
   (D) Stimulation of the vagus nerve

5. The basic process of digestion involves which of the following chemical reactions?
   (A) Hydrolysis
   (B) Condensation
   (C) Reduction
   (D) Oxidation

6. In which of the following food substances is chewing essential for digestion?
   (A) Fruits and vegetables
   (B) Cheese
   (C) Meat
   (D) Eggs

7. The pathophysiologic basis of which of the following conditions is associated with damage to the myenteric plexus?
   (A) Sprue
   (B) Acute pancreatitis
   (C) Achalasia
   (D) Chronic gastritis

8. Which of the following is the main digestible carbohydrate normally consumed in the human diet?
   (A) Cellulose
   (B) Maltose
   (C) Starch
   (D) Amylose

9. When salivary secretion is maximally stimulated, the salivary concentration of which of the following ions is increased?
   (A) Potassium
   (B) Chloride
   (C) Bicarbonate
   (D) Sodium

10. Which of these salivary glands secretes primarily a serous type of substance?
    (A) Sublingual
    (B) Submandibular
    (C) Buccal
    (D) Parotid

11. Chronic gastritis is often associated with which of the following?
    (A) Microcytic anemia
    (B) Hyperchlorhydria
    (C) Steatorrhea
    (D) Pernicious anemia

12. Which of the following characterizes carbohydrate digestion?
    (A) It begins when food comes in contact with saliva
    (B) It begins when food comes in contact with gastric juice
    (C) It begins when food comes in contact with pancreatic secretions
    (D) It ends when starch has been converted to maltose

13. A patient with trigeminal neurapraxia (temporary segmental demyelination of the trigeminal nerve leading to conduction difficulties) would have the greatest difficulty with which of the following activities?
    (A) Swallowing
    (B) Chewing
    (C) Receptive relaxation of the upper esophageal sphincter
    (D) Secondary peristalsis in the esophagus

14. Which of the following has the most powerful stimulatory effect on salivary secretion under normal conditions?
    (A) Sympathetic stimulation
    (B) Gritty material
    (C) Sour taste stimulus
    (D) Trigeminal stimulation

15. During which stage of swallowing is respiration inhibited?
    (A) Voluntary stage
    (B) Pharyngeal stage
    (C) Esophageal stage
    (D) Postprandial stage

16. Inhibition of the myenteric plexus leads to which of the following conditions?
    (A) Increased secretion of secretin from the duodenal mucosa
    (B) Decrease in gut motility
    (C) Hyperacidity in the stomach
    (D) Diarrhea

17. A 45-year-old woman presents to her local physician with complaints of a dry mouth. She indicates that this condition has been bothering her for at least 10 years. Following examination and diagnostic testing, she is diagnosed with idiopathic xerostomia. A patient with this diagnosis is most likely to be predisposed to which of the following conditions?
    (A) Dental caries
    (B) Malabsorption syndrome
    (C) Iron deficiency
    (D) Gastritis

18. Which of the following best describes how infection with *Helicobacter pylori* can lead to ulcer formation?
    (A) Bacterial enzymes degrade the protective mucous layer, exposing the gastric mucosa to acidic secretions
    (B) Bacterial cell wall products cause local inflammation of the gastric mucosa
    (C) A specific toxin produced by the bacteria causes hypersecretion of acid by the parietal cells
    (D) The bacterial cell wall antigen activates an immune response against the cells that produce mucus, inhibiting its production

19. A 55-year-old man with a history of chronic alcohol consumption presents to his local physician with nonspecific complaints of dyspepsia. Examination and diagnostic testing reveal that this individual has selective destruction of the gastric glands of the stomach. This condition would predispose the patient to which of the following?
    (A) Steatorrhea
    (B) Gastric hypomotility
    (C) Gastric ulcer
    (D) Anemia

20. A 40-year-old man presents with symptoms of upper gastrointestinal discomfort, dysphagia, and a nonspecific feeling of pressure or aching in his chest. Radiographic findings indicate distention of the lower esophagus most likely caused by a failure of receptive relaxation of the gastroesophageal sphincter. Which of the following conditions best fits this description?
    (A) Gastroesophageal reflux
    (B) Barrett's esophagus
    (C) Gastritis
    (D) Achalasia

21. Lack of adequate acid secretion by the gastric glands of the stomach has the greatest effect on the digestion of which of the following?
    (A) Meats
    (B) Grains
    (C) Fats
    (D) Fruits and vegetables

22. Stomach emptying is controlled mostly by which of the following?
    (A) Local neurohumoral mechanisms originating in the stomach itself
    (B) Local neurohumoral mechanisms originating in the duodenum
    (C) Activity of the small intestine
    (D) Vasovagal reflexes that reduce the tone in the muscle wall of the body of the stomach

23. The proenzyme pepsinogen is secreted mainly from which of the following structures?
    (A) Epithelial cells of the duodenum
    (B) Acinar cells of the pancreas
    (C) Gastric glands of the stomach
    (D) Ductal cells of the pancreas

24. Stimulation of the submucosal plexus results in an increase in which of the following?
    (A) Motility of the gut
    (B) Secretion of the gut
    (C) Sphincter tone
    (D) Stomach pH

25. Acid secretion in ulcer disease can be reduced by which of the following interventions?
    (A) Blockade of secretin secretion
    (B) Blockade of histamine H_2 receptors
    (C) Blockade of the action of pepsin
    (D) Treatment with antibiotics

26. Digestion of which of the following occurs almost entirely in the small intestine?
    (A) Protein
    (B) Fat
    (C) Starch
    (D) Fruits and vegetables

27. Inhibition of vagal function has the greatest effect on which segment of the alimentary tract?
    (A) Stomach
    (B) Descending colon
    (C) Rectum
    (D) Anal sphincter

28. The volume of food in the stomach has which of the following effects on stomach emptying?
    (A) As the volume of food in the stomach increases, the rate of emptying increases
    (B) As the volume of food in the stomach increases, the rate of emptying decreases
    (C) As the volume of food in the stomach decreases, the rate of emptying increases
    (D) The volume of food in the stomach has little if any effect of the rate of stomach emptying

29. In the condition of gastritis, which of the following describes the absorption of food products from the stomach?
    (A) Decreased as a result of inflammation of the gastric mucosa
    (B) Increased as a result of inflammation of the gastric mucosa
    (C) Within normal limits except for the absorption of lipids
    (D) Within normal limits except for the absorption of carbohydrates

30. Which of the following cell types found in the intestinal tract secretes hydrochloric acid?
    (A) Parietal cells
    (B) Peptic cells
    (C) Acinar cells
    (D) Mucous neck cells

31. The enterogastric reflex can be elicited by which of the following?
    (A) Distention of the duodenum
    (B) Acidic chyme in the duodenum
    (C) Hyperosmotic chyme in the duodenum
    (D) All of the above

32. Which of the following components of bile is critical for fat digestion?
    (A) Calcium salts
    (B) Lecithin
    (C) Bilirubin
    (D) Bicarbonate

33. Maximum activation of the proteolytic precursor pepsinogen to the active enzyme pepsin requires which of the following?
    (A) pH of 5 or greater
    (B) Contact with previously formed pepsin and pH of 5 or greater
    (C) Contact with intrinsic factor
    (D) Contact with previously formed pepsin and pH of 3.5 or less

34. A high level of sympathetic stimulation is most likely to cause which of the following effects on gastrointestinal function?
    (A) Increase in gastric acid secretion
    (B) Increase in mucus secretion
    (C) Decrease in stomach pH
    (D) Decrease in motility

35. Which of the following substances stimulates the motor activity of the stomach?
    (A) Gastrin
    (B) Secretin
    (C) Norepinephrine
    (D) Cholecystokinin

36. A 39-year-old man presents at the emergency department with a dull, boring pain in his midepigastric region, along with nausea and vomiting. He has a mild fever and mild tachycardia and is hypotensive. There is a marked tenderness to deep palpation of the left upper abdomen, and bowel sounds are diminished. His blood chemistry reveals an elevated serum amylase activity. On taking his medical history, it is noted that the pain, nausea, and vomiting began after he had a meal following a binge of drinking alcohol. It is further noted that this individual consumes, on average, about a liter of alcoholic spirits per day. Which of the following is a possible preliminary diagnosis?
    (A) Acute gastritis
    (B) Gastroesophageal reflux
    (C) Ulcerative colitis
    (D) Pancreatitis

37. Absorption of water in the small intestine occurs by which of the following?
    (A) Passive diffusion
    (B) Active transport
    (C) Solvent drag
    (D) Couple transport with glucose

Questions 38 and 39

For questions 38 and 39, refer to the figure below.

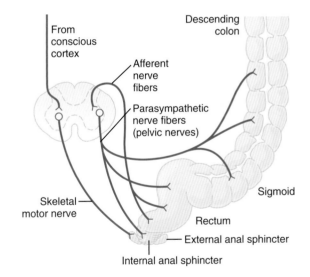

38. Which of the following describes the external anal sphincter?
    (A) It is composed of striated muscle and is under voluntary control
    (B) It is composed of intestinal smooth muscle and is under involuntary control
    (C) It automatically relaxes when a peristaltic wave approaches the anus
    (D) It is innervated by sympathetic fibers

39. Damage to the pelvic nerves does which of the following?
    (A) Has little, if any, effect on the defecation reflex
    (B) Attenuates the defecation reflex
    (C) Increases the strength of the defecation reflex
    (D) Results in a continuous urge to defecate (rectal urgency)

40. Which of the following substances is released from the mucosa of the duodenum in response to acidic gastric juice?
    (A) Cholecystokinin
    (B) Substance P
    (C) Secretin
    (D) Gastric inhibitory peptide

41. Which of the following is true of the gastroenteric reflex?
    (A) It stimulates contractions of the colon
    (B) It increases peristaltic activity of the stomach
    (C) It leads to defecation
    (D) It leads to increased peristaltic activity in the small intestine

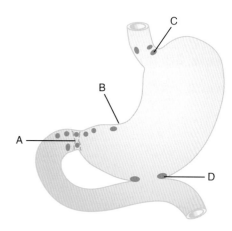

42. The most common site of peptic ulcer formation is shown at which point on the figure above?
    (A) Point A
    (B) Point B
    (C) Point C
    (D) Point D

43. Sodium transport through the brush border of the intestinal epithelial cells occurs by which of the following mechanisms?
    (A) Active transport
    (B) Passive diffusion
    (C) Co-transport with hydrogen ions
    (D) Facilitated diffusion

44. A 45-year-old man is found to have a condition in which the parietal cells of his stomach have been destroyed by an autoimmune mechanism. His diagnosis is chronic autoimmune gastritis. This condition is often associated with which of the following?
    (A) Pernicious anemia
    (B) Gastric ulceration
    (C) Steatorrhea
    (D) Protein deficiency

45. Hypochlorhydria is a condition in which acid secretion by the stomach is greatly reduced. How does this condition affect the digestion and absorption of food?
    (A) Digestion and absorption of all food substances are nearly normal
    (B) Digestion and absorption of all foods substances are markedly reduced
    (C) Digestion and absorption of carbohydrates are greatly affected by this condition
    (D) Digestion and absorption of fats are greatly affected by this condition

46. How does gastrin stimulate hydrochloric acid secretion by the parietal cells of the gastric gland?
    (A) Indirectly through a cyclic guanosine monophosphate (cGMP)-mediated pathway
    (B) Indirectly via stimulation of histamine release from enterochromaffin cells
    (C) Directly by acting on a gastrin receptor located on the parietal cell
    (D) Indirectly through a cyclic adenosine monophosphate (cAMP)-mediated pathway

47. Congenital absence of the myenteric plexus would most likely lead to which of the following derangements in gastrointestinal function?
    (A) Sluggish peristalsis in the segment of the gastrointestinal tract involved
    (B) Hypersecretion of acid by the stomach
    (C) Chronic diarrhea
    (D) Intolerance to fatty foods

48. Psychological stress is often associated with peptic ulcer disease. Which of the following is thought to be a contributing factor in stress-induced ulcer disease?
    (A) Sympathetic stimulation decreases gastric acid secretion
    (B) Sympathetic stimulation increases peristalsis, which decreases the transit time of ingested food
    (C) Psychological stress increases mucous secretion
    (D) Sympathetic stimulation decreases the alkaline mucous secretions of Brunner's glands located in the first few centimeters of the duodenal wall

49. Which of the following substances can inhibit small intestinal motility?
    (A) Secretin
    (B) Gastrin
    (C) Cholecystokinin
    (D) Insulin

50. Inhibition of which of the following enzymes has the greatest effect on digestion?
    (A) Chymotrypsin
    (B) Enterokinase
    (C) Pancreatic amylase
    (D) Ptyalin

51. A 22-year-old woman visits her physician with complaints of abdominal pain, blood-streaked stools, and bouts of diarrhea. The patient indicates that she first began to experience these symptoms 6 months previously. She describes periods of relatively normal bowel function for about a week at a time, interspersed with periods of abdominal discomfort and diarrhea since the symptoms first began. Over the last month, the abdominal pain and diarrhea have been more frequent, which has caused her to seek medical attention. The pathophysiology of the diarrhea is most likely related to which of the following?
    (A) Malabsorption syndrome
    (B) Emotional stimulation of the parasympathetic nervous system
    (C) Inflammatory bowel process
    (D) Overuse of laxatives

52. Which of the following decreases blood flow to the villi of the small intestine?
    (A) Adenosine
    (B) Bradykinin
    (C) Norepinephrine
    (D) Gastrin

53. Which of the following normally prevents the activation of pancreatic enzymes?
    (A) Storage at an acidic pH within the acinar cells
    (B) Storage at a neutral pH within the acinar cells
    (C) Tonic secretion of sodium bicarbonate
    (D) Secretion of trypsin inhibitor by the acinar cells

54. Which of the following type of motor activity in the small intestine is stimulated by local irritation of the intestinal mucosa?
    (A) Haustration
    (B) Segmentation movement
    (C) Peristaltic rush
    (D) Secondary peristalsis

55. Which of the following is the most potent stimulator of pancreatic secretion?
    (A) Secretin
    (B) Serotonin
    (C) Histamine
    (D) Cholecystokinin

Questions 56 and 57

Use the following information to answer questions 56 and 57:

A 24-year-old man received a knife wound to the abdomen that severed the superior mesenteric artery. The patient was admitted to the emergency department. Upon examination, it was determined that the patient was in circulatory shock as a result of blood loss.

56. Which of the following structures in the gastrointestinal tract is most at risk in this patient as a consequence of the circulatory shock?
    (A) Submucosal glands
    (B) Brunner's glands
    (C) Tips of the villi
    (D) Sphincter muscles

57. In this patient, which of the following describes the peristaltic activity of the gut?
    (A). Decreased in all areas
    (B) Increased in all areas
    (C) Increased in the esophagus, stomach, and small intestine
    (D) Increased in the colon

58. Inhibition of the active transport of sodium through the basolateral membrane of the small intestinal epithelial cells does which of the following?
    (A) Facilitates glucose uptake from the small intestine
    (B) Attenuates glucose uptake from the small intestine
    (C) Facilitates the absorption of water
    (D) Attenuates the absorption of fructose

59. Which of the following is not normally found in abundance in the portal blood?
    (A) Glucose
    (B) Triglycerides
    (C) Short-chain fatty acids
    (D) Amino acids

Questions 60-62

Use the following figure to answer questions 60 to 62.

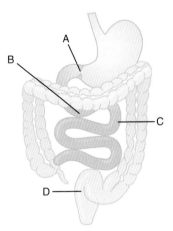

60. A 56-year-old man presents to the emergency room with vomiting that his relatives indicate has lasted for 3 days. The patient is admitted to the hospital, and initial tests reveal that he is expelling an acidic vomitus and his blood pH is slightly alkaline. An intestinal obstruction is suspected. Based on this limited information, where would one suspect the obstruction to be located?
    (A) Point A
    (B) Point B
    (C) Point C
    (D) Point D

61. A 76-year-old woman presents to her physician with complaints of constipation and abdominal discomfort that have been persistent for the last 2 weeks but had a gradual onset over the past 6 weeks. Because of her history, the physician suspects that an abdominal obstruction may be the cause of her constipation. Based on this information, where would one suspect the obstruction to be located?
    (A) Point A
    (B) Point B
    (C) Point C
    (D) Point D

62. A 66-year-old woman presents to a local clinic with a 4-day history of nausea and vomiting. She indicates that she might have "eaten something bad." She is very weak and has symptoms of severe dehydration. She reports that she has not had a bowel movements since the episodes of vomiting began. While her immediate medical history is being taken, she vomits; on testing, it is determined that the vomitus is slightly alkaline. The examining physician suspects an intestinal obstruction. Based on this information, where would one suspect the obstruction to be located?
    (A) Point A
    (B) Point B
    (C) Point C
    (D) Point D

63. A 45-year-old woman was diagnosed with chronic, progressive ulcerative colitis at age 32. The medical treatment options for her condition have been exhausted, and she is referred to a surgeon for total colectomy. This treatment can predispose a patient to which of the following?
    (A) Dehydration
    (B) Protein deficiency
    (C) Bleeding tendencies
    (D) Pernicious anemia

64. Which of the following normally stimulates the release of digestive enzymes from the acinar cells of the pancreas?
    (A) Histamine
    (B) Cholecystokinin
    (C) Secretin
    (D) Gastrin

65. Ganglionic blockade has the greatest effect on which of the following gastrointestinal reflexes?
    (A) Gastrocolic reflex
    (B) Enterogastric reflex
    (C) Gastroenteric reflex
    (D) Myenteric reflex

66. Which of the following are paired correctly?
    (A) Cholecystokinin—gallbladder relaxation
    (B) Secretin—relaxation of the sphincter of Oddi
    (C) Secretin—stimulation of enzymatic release from the pancreatic acinar cells
    (D) Cholecystokinin—relaxation of the sphincter of Oddi

67. Which of the following is not normally associated with activation the peristaltic reflex?
    (A) Distention of the gut wall
    (B) Sympathetic stimulation
    (C) Presence in the gut of a hypertonic solution
    (D) Irritation of the epithelium of the gut

68. Which of the following describes how bicarbonate ions are absorbed from the small intestine?
    (A) Directly via facilitated diffusion
    (B) Indirectly via active transport
    (C) Directly via simple diffusion
    (D) Indirectly in the form of carbon dioxide and water

69. The secretion of bile is important for the proper digestion of which of the following?
    (A) Complex carbohydrates
    (B) Lipids
    (C) Proteins
    (D) Monosaccharides

70. Inhibition of sodium transport has the least effect on absorption of which of the following?
    (A) Glucose
    (B) Dipeptides
    (C) Galactose
    (D) Monoglycerides

71. Which of the following is true of mass movements?
    (A) They normally move colonic contents from the cecum to the transverse colon
    (B) They are strong peristaltic contractions of the small intestine in response to mucosal irritation
    (C) They normally occur approximately 9 to 12 times per minute
    (D) They are a modified type of peristalsis that occurs in the large intestine

72. Which of the following may predispose an individual to peptic ulcers?
    (A) Inhibition of Brunner's glands
    (B) Inhibition of potassium-hydrogen exchange in the cell wall of the parietal cell
    (C) Inhibition of gastrin
    (D) Excessive stimulation of bicarbonate secretion by the pancreas

73. A 46-year-old woman presents with a history of dyspepsia and nonspecific upper right quadrant pain. She notes that the color of her stool has "faded" over the last several weeks. Ultrasonic examination of the liver discovers numerous objects in the gallbladder and what appears to be a dilation of the common bile duct. Absorption of which of the following substances is likely to be affected in this patient?
    (A) Vitamin B_{12}
    (B) Proteins
    (C) Fats
    (D) Carbohydrates

74. Which of the following best characterizes the secretions of the small intestine?
    (A) Hypotonic and slightly acidic
    (B) Hypotonic and slightly alkaline
    (C) Isotonic and slightly alkaline
    (D) Isotonic and slightly acidic

75. A 60-year-old man is being treated for persistent diverticulitis with a prolonged course of antibiotic therapy. The antibiotic being used has broad-spectrum activity and over time has caused sterilization of the gut in this patient. Which of the following sequelae is likely to be observed in this patient?
    (A) Vitamin B_{12} deficiency
    (B) Steatorrhea
    (C) Vitamin K deficiency
    (D) Bloating due to excess gas formation

76. Which of the following best characterizes the secretions of the large intestine?
    (A) They contain enzymes for the final digestion of food
    (B) They are mostly mucus
    (C) They contain large quantities of bicarbonate ions
    (D) They consist mostly of trapped bacteria from the crypts of Lieberkühn

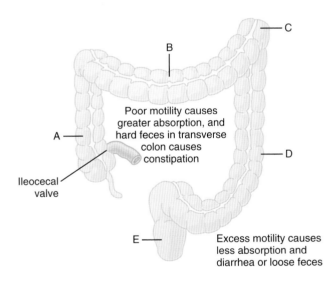

77. Which point in the figure above indicates the place in the colon where the colonic chyme is fluid?
    (A) Point A
    (B) Point B
    (C) Point C
    (D) Point D
    (E) Point E

Answers

1. (A) Under normal conditions, sodium ions are actively reabsorbed from all the salivary ducts, and potassium ions are actively secreted in exchange for the sodium. This greatly reduces the sodium concentration of the saliva and increases the potassium concentration to as much as seven times that in the plasma.
   TMP11 794

2. (C) The myenteric plexus is located between the longitudinal and circular muscle layers in the gut wall. It mainly controls motor activity along the length of the gut. When stimulated, its principal effects are to increase tonic contractions, or "tone," of the gut wall; to increase the intensity of rhythmic contractions; and to increase the velocity of conduction of excitatory waves along the gut wall, causing more rapid movement of the peristaltic waves.
   TMP11 772, 774, 775

3. (D) The rhythmic contraction of gastrointestinal smooth muscle is determined by the frequency of slow-wave potentials. Slow-wave potentials are undulating changes in the resting membrane potential usually varying from 5 to 15 millivolts in intensity. Although these slow waves do not cause contraction of gastrointestinal smooth muscle directly, they control the appearance of spike potentials, and it is these spike potentials that lead to contraction.
   TMP11 772, 773

4. (A) Spike potentials are similar to action potentials in nerves and lead to contraction of gastrointestinal smooth muscle. Any factor that causes depolarization of gastrointestinal smooth muscle will lead to an increase in the number of spike potentials. Parasympathetic stimulation that results in the release of acetylcholine or stretch of the gastrointestinal smooth muscle depolarizes the smooth muscle membrane and leads to an increase in the number of spike potentials. Sympathetic stimulation, in contrast, leads to hyperpolarization of the smooth muscle membrane and a decrease in the number of spike potentials.
   TMP11 773

5. (A) Almost all the carbohydrates, fats, and proteins in the diet are combinations of smaller subunits bound together by the chemical process of condensation. The process of condensation removes a hydrogen ion from one subunit and a hydroxyl ion from another subunit to bind the two subunits together. The hydrogen and hydroxyl ions then bind together to form water (thus the term *condensation*). Digestion is simply the reverse of the condensation process—a hydrogen ion is added to one subunit, and a hydroxyl ion is added to the adjacent subunit. This process is called hydrolysis, and in essence, it adds water back to the complex structure and breaks it into its component parts.
   TMP11 808

6. (A) Chewing is important for the digestion of all solid foods. It is especially important for most fruits and vegetables because these foods have an indigestible cellulose membrane surrounding the nutrient

portion that must be broken to allow contact with digestive enzymes.
TMP11 781

7. (C) Achalasia is a condition in which the lower esophageal sphincter fails to relax during swallowing. Pathophysiological studies have shown damage in the neural network of the myenteric plexus of the lower two thirds of the esophagus, which causes spasticity of the musculature of the lower esophagus. As a result, the lower portion of the esophagus fails to undergo receptive relaxation as the bolus of food approaches this area after swallowing.
TMP11 819

8. (C) Only three major sources of carbohydrates exist in the normal human diet: sucrose from cane sugar, lactose from milk, and a wide variety of large polysaccharides collectively known as starches. Although some diets may contain a large quantity of cellulose, this substance cannot be digested by the human gut and is not considered a food. Maltose is a product of the digestion of starch but is not consumed in large quantities in the human diet.
TMP11 809

9. (D) During maximal salivation, the ionic concentration of the saliva changes considerably. This occurs because the rate of formation of the primary secretion by the acini can increase by as much as 20-fold. This increased volume of primary secretion flows through the ducts so rapidly that the sodium cannot be reabsorbed at the normal rate. Therefore, under conditions of maximal salivation, the concentration of sodium in saliva can rise to five times normal.
TMP11 794

10. (D) The parotid gland secretes a serous solution that contains ptyalin, an enzyme that begins the digestion of starches. The sublingual and submandibular glands also secrete a serous type of solution, but they secrete a mucous substance that provides lubrication and serves a protective purpose as well. The buccal glands secrete only the mucous substance.
TMP11 793

11. (D) Pernicious anemia results from an insufficient amount of vitamin B_{12}. Without an adequate amount of vitamin B_{12}, newly forming red blood cells fail to mature while they are still in the bone marrow. Chronic gastritis often leads to gastric atrophy, which reduces gastric secretions. Normal gastric secretions contain a glycoprotein called *intrinsic factor* that is secreted by the same parietal cells that secrete hydrochloric acid. Intrinsic factor combines with vitamin B_{12} in the stomach and protects it from being digested and destroyed as it passes into the small intestine. Without intrinsic factor, there is inadequate absorption of vitamin B_{12} from the ileum.
TMP11 820

12. (A) Saliva contains the enzyme ptyalin, which hydrolyzes starch into the disaccharide maltose and other small polymers of glucose. Under normal conditions, food does not stay in the mouth for a long time. However, starch digestion continues as the food is passed from the mouth through the esophagus and into the stomach. Before the acidic environment of the stomach inactivates ptyalin, as much as 40 per cent of the starch in food substances is converted to maltose. Therefore, carbohydrate digestion begins when food comes in contact with saliva.
TMP11 809

13. (B) The muscles of mastication are controlled by the trigeminal nerve. Therefore, damage to the trigeminal nerve would have the greatest effect on chewing.
TMP11 781

14. (C) Many taste stimuli can affect salivary secretion, but one of the most powerful stimulators is sour taste. In contrast, the presence of a rough object or a gritty substance (such as sand or dirt) can decrease salivary secretion. Under certain conditions, sympathetic stimulation can increase salivary secretion, but this effect is relatively weak and is not as powerful as parasympathetic stimulation.
TMP11 794

15. (B) Swallowing is principally a reflex act initiated by the voluntary movement of a bolus of food toward the pharynx. It is during the pharyngeal stage of swallowing that respiration is inhibited.
TMP11 783

16. (B) The myenteric plexus functions mainly to control motor activity along the length of the gut. When it is stimulated, the principal effects are an increase in the tone of the gut wall, an increased intensity of rhythmic contractions, an increase in the rate of rhythmic contractions, and an increase in the velocity of conduction of excitatory waves along the gut wall. Therefore, inhibition of the myenteric plexus decreases motility of the gut.
TMP11 774

17. (A) Saliva is important for normal oral health. It contains proteolytic enzymes that attack bacteria and food particles that provide nutrition for the bacteria. Therefore, lack of saliva can contribute to poor oral health, including dental caries.
TMP11 794

18. (A) More than three quarters of patients with peptic ulcer have been found to have a chronic infection with the bacterium *Helicobacter pylori*. This bacterium releases a digestive enzyme that liquefies the protective mucous barrier and exposes the underlying epithelium to the corrosive actions of the acid secreted by the stomach.
TMP11 821

19. (D) In addition to secreting hydrochloric acid, pepsinogen, and mucus, the gastric glands secrete intrinsic factor. Intrinsic factor is secreted by the parietal cells of the gastric gland, the same cells that secrete hydrochloric acid. Intrinsic factor binds to vitamin B_{12} and protects it from digestion until it can

be absorbed in the terminal ileum. Without intrinsic factor, only about 2 per cent of the vitamin B_{12} is absorbed. Lack of vitamin B_{12} causes failure of maturation of red blood cells, which leads to pernicious anemia.
TMP11 797

20. (D) Failure of receptive relaxation of the gastroesophageal sphincter leads to an impairment of food passage from the esophagus into the stomach. This causes dilation of the lower portion of the esophagus, a condition called achalasia.
TMP11 819

21. (A) Pepsin is an important proteolytic enzyme secreted in precursor form by the gastric glands of the stomach. This enzyme is most active at a pH of 2 to 3. Therefore, an acidic environment is essential for maximal activation of pepsin. Pepsin has an almost unique ability to digest collagen, which is the major constituent of the connective tissue of meats. Digestion of collagen allows the other proteolytic enzymes of the digestive tract to penetrate into the substance of the meat and digest the cellular proteins.
TMP11 810

22. (B) By far the most powerful regulators of stomach emptying are the local signals that originate in the duodenum. The emptying of chyme into the duodenum occurs at a rate no greater than can be processed, digested, and absorbed by the small intestine.
TMP11 785, 786

23. (C) Pepsinogen is the precursor of the enzyme pepsin. Pepsinogen is secreted from the peptic or chief cells of the gastric gland. To be converted from the precursor form to the active form (pepsin), pepsinogen must come in contact with hydrochloric acid or pepsin itself. Pepsin is a proteolytic enzyme that digests collagen and other types of connective tissue in meats.
TMP11 797

24. (B) The submucosal plexus, in contrast to the myenteric plexus, is concerned with controlling the function of the inner wall of the intestine. The submucosal plexus helps control local secretory function, local absorption, and local blood flow to each minute segment of the intestine. Stimulation of the submucosal plexus would most likely lead to an increase in secretion from the stomach; this would result in a decrease in pH because of the increased secretion of hydrochloric acid.
TMP11 774, 775

25. (B) Blockade of H_2 receptors has been shown to be an effective way of inhibiting acid secretion in ulcer disease. Although antibiotics are effective in treating ulcer disease, they do not inhibit acid secretion.
TMP11 821

26. (B) The vast majority of fat digestion occurs in the small intestine. Little, if any, quantitative digestion

of fat occurs in other parts of the gastrointestinal tract. In contrast, carbohydrate digestion begins when food comes in contact with saliva, and protein digestion begins in the stomach through the action of pepsin.
TMP11 811

27. (A) The vagus nerve supplies parasympathetic innervation to the proximal portion of the alimentary tract. The distal portion of the colon, the rectum, and the anus receive parasympathetic input from the sacral portion of the spinal cord. Therefore, inhibition of vagal function would affect the upper portions of the alimentary tract more so than the distal portions.
TMP11 775

28. (A) In general, as the volume of food in the stomach increases, the rate of stomach emptying increases. Stretching of the stomach wall elicits local myenteric reflexes that result in intense peristaltic, ringlike constrictions that push food toward the pylorus. When pyloric tone is normal, each contraction forces several milliliters of chyme into the duodenum.
TMP11 785

29. (B) Paradoxically, absorption from the stomach is increased as a result of gastritis. This results from a breakdown of the gastric barrier that normally limits absorption in a healthy stomach. The gastric barrier is composed of a thick layer of mucus and tight junctions between adjacent epithelial cells. This combination normally limits the diffusion of ions and other food substances.
TMP11 819, 820

30. (A) Hydrochloric acid is secreted by the parietal cells of the gastric gland. Inside the parietal cell, water dissociates into hydrogen ions and hydroxyl ions in the cytoplasm. The hydrogen ions are then actively secreted into the canaliculus of the gastric gland in exchange for potassium ions through an active process that is catalyzed by H^+, K^+-ATPase. Chloride ions are then secreted into the canaliculus to complete the formation of hydrochloric acid.
TMP11 797

31. (D) The enterogastric reflex slows stomach emptying. Signals from the duodenum in response to volume, acidity, concentration, and the presence of certain breakdown products of proteins and fats decrease the pumping of chyme through the pylorus into the duodenum. These signals decrease the propulsive contractions of the stomach and increase the tone of the pyloric sphincter, thus decreasing the expulsion of chyme into the duodenum.
TMP11 785, 786

32. (B) The main function of bile in digestion is to assist in the digestion of fat. It does so by breaking fat globules into smaller sizes so that the water-soluble digestive enzymes can act on the globules'

surfaces. This breakdown of globules is called emulsification. Lecithin is especially important in the emulsification process. The nonpolar portion of the lecithin molecule dissolves in the surface layer of the globule, while the polar portion projects outward, allowing the combination to become miscible in the surrounding watery fluids.
TMP11 811

33. (D) Maximal activation of the enzyme pepsin from the precursor pepsinogen requires contact with previously formed pepsin and an acid pH. The optimal activity of pepsin occurs at a pH between 1.8 and 3.5. Pepsin is inactive above a pH of 5. Therefore, a highly acidic environment and activated pepsin are necessary for protein digestion.
TMP11 797

34. (D) In general, sympathetic stimulation causes a decrease in activity and function of the gastrointestinal tract. Strong stimulation of the sympathetic system can greatly inhibit motor movements of the gut. In contrast, stimulation of the parasympathetic system increases the activity and movement of the gastrointestinal tract.
TMP11 775

35. (A) Gastrin is released from the mucosa of the antral region of the stomach in response to certain types of food, particularly the digestive products of meat. Gastrin stimulates the release of highly acidic gastric juice. It also stimulates the motor activity of the stomach. In contrast, secretin, norepinephrine, and cholecystokinin all inhibit the motor activity of the stomach.
TMP11 785

36. (D) Pancreatitis is an inflammation of the pancreas that can be acute or chronic. The most common cause of pancreatitis is alcohol abuse. The second most common cause is blockage of the papilla of Vater by a gallstone, which causes the pancreatic enzymes to back up in the ducts and acini of the pancreas. This results in an accumulation of the proenzymes trypsinogen, chymotrypsinogen, and procarboxypeptidase. Once trypsin is activated, it results in a vicious circle of pancreatic enzyme activation that can lead to digestion of large portions of the pancreas itself.
TMP11 821, 822

37. (A) Water is absorbed through the intestinal membrane entirely by diffusion. Water absorption by diffusion follows the usual law of osmosis, which is that water will flow from an area of lower concentration to an area of higher concentration of particles. In the case of the intestine, these particles consist of nutritional substances and the various ions absorbed by a variety of transport mechanisms.
TMP11 814

38. (A) The external anal sphincter is composed of voluntary, or at least semiconsciously, controlled striated muscle. In adults, it is usually kept continuously

constricted unless conscious signals inhibit the constriction.
TMP11 789

39. (B) For effective defecation to occur, the local myenteric reflex that stimulates contraction must be reinforced by parasympathetic signals that travel to the descending colon, sigmoid, rectum, and anus by the pelvic nerves. These parasympathetic signals intensify the peristaltic waves as well as relax the internal anal sphincter and thus convert a weak myenteric reflex to a powerful process of defecation.
TMP11 789, 790

40. (C) Secretin is released from the mucosa of the duodenum in response to acidic chyme. Cholecystokinin is released in response to fat, fatty acids, and monoglycerides. Gastric inhibitory peptide is released mainly in response to fatty acids, amino acids, and carbohydrates.
TMP11 776

41. (D) The gastroenteric reflex increases peristaltic activity in the small intestine in response to stretch or distention of the stomach. It is conducted principally through the myenteric plexus. The enhanced activity of the small intestine in response to food in the stomach prepares this segment of the intestine to receive and digest food substances.
TMP11 787

42. (A) A peptic ulcer is an excoriated area of the mucosa caused principally by the digestive action of gastric juice. The most common site of peptic ulcer occurrence is in the first few centimeters of the duodenum.
TMP11 820, 821

43. (D) Transport of sodium through the brush border of the intestinal epithelium occurs by the process of facilitated diffusion. The driving force for absorption of sodium is the active transport of sodium through the basolateral walls of the epithelial cells into the paracellular spaces. The active transport of sodium out of the cell reduces the concentration of sodium inside the cell to about one third the concentration in the chyme. This causes sodium to move down an electrochemical gradient through the brush border of the epithelial cell into the cytoplasm. However, the movement of sodium across this membrane is by facilitated diffusion, not simple diffusion. Sodium must first combine with a transport protein, which in turn must combine with a substance such as glucose.
TMP11 814

44. (A) In addition to secreting hydrochloric acid, parietal cells secrete intrinsic factor. Intrinsic factor is responsible for protecting vitamin B_{12} from destruction during passage through the upper portion of the gastrointestinal tract. Intrinsic factor binds to vitamin B_{12}, and this combination passes to the ileum. Upon reaching the ileum, the intrinsic factor–B_{12} combination binds to receptors located on the epithelial

surface of the ileum, and in this way, vitamin B_{12} is absorbed.
TMP11 820

45. (A) Although hypochlorhydria is associated with a decreased or absent digestive capacity of the stomach, the overall digestion of food in the entire gastrointestinal tract remains nearly normal. This is because trypsin and other digestive enzymes secreted by the pancreas are capable of digesting virtually all the foodstuffs.
TMP11 820

46. (B) Gastrin is a hormone secreted by the pyloric glands of the stomach. Gastrin does not stimulate the release of hydrochloric acid from the parietal cells of the gastric gland directly. Instead, it stimulates the release of histamine from enterochromaffin cells that lie adjacent to the parietal cells. It is the histamine, released in response to gastrin, that stimulates the release of hydrochloric acid from the parietal cells.
TMP11 797

47. (A) The myenteric plexus is responsible for controlling the motor activity of the gastrointestinal tract. Therefore, the absence of this plexus would lead to sluggish peristalsis in the segment of the alimentary canal involved.
TMP11 774, 775

48. (D) The usual cause of peptic ulcer disease is an imbalance between the rate of acid formation and the degree of protection afforded by the gastroduodenal mucosal barrier and the neutralization of gastric acid secretions by secretions of the pancreas. Brunner's glands, located in the wall of the upper portion of the duodenum, secrete highly alkaline mucus. This helps neutralize and protect the proximal portion of the duodenum from the acidic secretions of the stomach. Sympathetic stimulation inhibits the alkaline mucous secretions of Brunner's glands, thereby exposing the mucosa of the duodenum to the acid secretions of the stomach. Over time, this can lead to the development of peptic ulcers.
TMP11 820, 821

49. (A) Of the substances listed, only secretin can inhibit small intestinal motility. Gastrin, cholecystokinin, and insulin are all associated with an increase in the motor functions of the small bowel.
TMP11 787

50. (B) Enterokinase is an enzyme secreted by the mucosa of the duodenum in response to chyme. It is this enzyme that converts the inactive precursor of trypsin, trypsinogen, to the active form. Active trypsin can activate trypsinogen as well as the other proenzymes secreted by the pancreas—chymotrypsinogen and procarboxypeptidase.
TMP11 799, 800

51. (C) The most likely cause of diarrhea in this patient is inflammatory bowel disease (IBD).

Demographically, this patient fits the peak incidence of IBD onset in the second and third decades of life. This disorder is seen most commonly in northern European and North American peoples. IBD is rare in Central and South America, Africa, and Asia. Malabsorption syndromes, psychological stress, and overuse of laxatives are not associated with bloody stools.
TMP11 823

52. (C) In general, sympathetic stimulation by means of norepinephrine leads to a diminished activity of the gastrointestinal tract. In addition, sympathetic activation decreases blood flow to the gastrointestinal tract.
TMP11 779, 780

53. (D) Trypsin inhibitor, secreted by the acinar cells of the pancreas, inhibits the enzyme trypsin. This substance is formed in the cytoplasm of the glandular cells of the pancreas and prevents the activation of trypsin in the secretory cells of the pancreas as well as in the acini and the ductal structures. Because trypsin activates the other proteolytic enzymes of the pancreas, it is important that trypsin inhibitor be present in sufficient amounts to prevent the activation of not only trypsin but also the other enzymes.
TMP11 800

54. (C) Peristaltic rush occurs when irritating substances come in contact with the mucosa of the small bowel. Peristaltic rush consists of strong peristaltic contractions that move great distances in the small intestine. These strong peristaltic waves serve to move the irritating substances out of the small intestine.
TMP11 787

55. (A) Secretin is secreted by the mucosa of the duodenum and jejunum in response to an acidic chyme. Secretin stimulates the secretion of large quantities of sodium bicarbonate by the ductal epithelium of the pancreas. Cholecystokinin, which is also secreted from the mucosa of the duodenum and jejunum, stimulates the production of large quantities of pancreatic digestive enzymes but relatively small quantities of fluid. Without the fluid secretion, most of the enzymes remain temporarily stored in the acini and ducts until fluid is secreted. This fluid secretion, stimulated by secretin, serves to wash the enzymes into the duodenum.
TMP11 800, 801

56. (C) The arterioles and venules in the microvasculature of the villus are arranged in a parallel fashion, allowing oxygen to diffuse from the arterial side to the venous side. Under normal conditions, as much as 80 per cent of the oxygen may diffuse in this manner and not reach the tip of the villus structure. Under normal conditions, this shunting of oxygen is not harmful, but when blood flow to the gut is curtailed, the oxygen deficit at the tip of the villus can reach a point where the cells begin to die from ischemia.
TMP11 779, 780

57. (A) In shock, sympathetic activity is greatly elevated. Stimulation of the sympathetic nervous
system inhibits the activity of the gastrointestinal
tract. Therefore, peristaltic activity would be
decreased.
TMP11 775

58. (B) In the absence of sodium transport through the
intestinal membrane, glucose transport is inhibited.
Glucose absorption occurs via a co-transport mechanism with sodium. Sodium is actively transported
through the basolateral membrane of the intestinal
epithelial cell, creating an electrochemical gradient
for sodium across the brush border of the cell. Inside
the cell membrane, a carrier protein binds to the
sodium and facilitates its transport through the membrane. This protein also must combine with another
substance, such as glucose, in order to transport the
sodium. Therefore, inhibition of sodium transport
simultaneously inhibits glucose transport.
TMP11 814

59. (B) Fats are digested to monoglycerides and free
fatty acids. In this form, the end products of fat
digestion can be absorbed directly through the membrane of the intestinal epithelial cell. Once inside the
cell, the monoglycerides and the fatty acids are taken
up by the smooth endoplasmic reticulum and converted back to triglycerides. It is the triglyceride
form that is absorbed into the central lacteal and
subsequently transported in the form of lymph chy-
lomicrons. The lymph is transported in lymphatic
channels and eventually enters the circulation
through the thoracic duct, thus bypassing the portal
circulation.
TMP11 816

60. (A) The abnormal consequences of obstruction
depend on the point in the gastrointestinal tract
that becomes obstructed. If the obstruction occurs
at the pylorus, persistent vomiting of stomach
contents occurs. This produces an acidic vomitus
and can result in various degrees of whole-body
alkalosis.
TMP11 824, 825

61. (D) If the obstruction is near the distal end of the
large intestine, feces can accumulate in the colon for
several weeks. The patient develops an intense
feeling of constipation.
TMP11 824, 825

62. (C) If the obstruction is beyond the stomach,
antiperistaltic reflux from the small intestine causes
the intestinal juices to flow backward into the
stomach, and these juices are vomited along with
stomach secretions. Because the intestinal juices at
this point in the intestine consist mostly of bicarbonate secretions from the pancreas, they are slightly
alkaline. In this case, the person loses large amounts
of water and electrolytes and can become very dehydrated. However, because the amounts of acid and
base lost as a result of vomiting are nearly the same,

there is little change in body pH, and the vomitus
has a neutral or slightly alkaline character.
TMP11 824, 825

63. (C) Bacterial action in the colon is responsible for
the production of several vitamins. In particular,
colonic bacteria produce a large quantity of vitamin
K. The amount of vitamin K in the diet is usually
insufficient to maintain adequate blood coagulation.
Therefore, removal of the colon would predispose an
individual to vitamin K deficiency and resultant
bleeding tendencies.
TMP11 817

64. (B) Cholecystokinin is secreted from the mucosa of
the duodenum and jejunum in response to products
of partial protein digestion as well as long-chain
fatty acids. Cholecystokinin stimulates the secretion
of pancreatic digestive enzymes from the acinar cells
of the pancreas.
TMP11 801, 802

65. (A) The gastrocolic reflex is initiated by distention
of the stomach and duodenum after a meal. This
reflex induces peristaltic activity in the colon, resulting in what are known as mass movements. This
reflex is attenuated when the autonomic nerves to
the colon have been removed. The enterogastric,
gastroenteric, and myenteric reflexes rely on the
enteric nervous system. Therefore, autonomic ganglionic blockade would block the gastrocolic reflex
while leaving the other motor reflexes of the gastrointestinal tract relatively intact.
TMP11 789, 790

66. (D) Cholecystokinin has two major actions in stimulating the release of bile by the gallbladder: it stimulates contraction of the gallbladder and also causes
relaxation of the sphincter of Oddi. The sphincter of
Oddi guards the opening of the common bile duct
into the duodenum. Both actions of cholecystokinin
are necessary for maximal gallbladder emptying.
TMP11 803

67. (B) The usual stimulus for the peristaltic reflex and
subsequent peristalsis is distention of the gut. Chemical or physical irritation can also initiate peristaltic
activity. In general, sympathetic stimulation inhibits
peristalsis.
TMP11 776, 777

68. (D) Bicarbonate ions are secreted in large quantities
in the upper small intestine. This bicarbonate must
be reabsorbed. Bicarbonate is not absorbed directly
but rather indirectly in the following manner. When
sodium is absorbed, moderate amounts of hydrogen
ions are secreted in exchange for the sodium ions.
The hydrogen ions combine with the bicarbonate
ions to form carbonic acid (H_2CO_3). The carbonic
acid dissociates into water and carbon dioxide.
The water remains in the chyme, and the carbon
dioxide is absorbed into the blood and expired in the
lungs.
TMP11 815

69. (B) Bile is essential for proper fat digestion. The components of bile cause the emulsification of fat. Because digestion takes place in an aqueous environment, it is important that fat particles be broken down into smaller sizes so that the digestive enzymes will be able to make contact with the components of fat. The components of bile also aid in the absorption of fat. Bile induces the formation of small complexes called micelles. The micelles are soluble in the chyme and serve to ferry the lipids inside the micelles to the intestinal mucosa, where they are absorbed. Without the presence of bile, approximately 40 per cent of the ingested fat would be lost in the feces.
    TMP11 804

70. (D) The absorption of the digestive end products of both carbohydrates and proteins are transported across the intestinal epithelial membrane via a process in which sodium is co-transported along with the peptides and simple sugars. The absorption of fats is not dependent on the co-transport of sodium but occurs by direct diffusion through the lipid membranes.
    TMP11 816

71. (D) Mass movements are a form of modified peristalsis that occurs from the transverse colon to the sigmoid. They serve to force the fecal contents farther down the colon toward the rectum. When the fecal mass reaches and distends the rectum, the urge to defecate is felt.
    TMP11 789

72. (A) Brunner's glands secrete highly alkaline mucus and are located in the duodenum. The mucus secreted by these glands contains a large concentration of bicarbonate ions. This alkaline mucus serves to neutralize the acid in the gastric juice and protects the epithelium of the duodenum from excoriation by the acidic chyme that is released from the stomach. Sympathetic stimulation can inhibit the secretion of mucus by Brunner's glands. During sympathetic activation, which can occur during periods of stress, inhibition of Brunner's glands can leave the duodenum unprotected and may be a contributing factor in the development of ulcers in this area of the gastrointestinal tract.
    TMP11 805

73. (C) The symptoms described and the diagnostic evidence points to obstruction of the bile duct resulting from gallstones. Under normal conditions, the brown color of stool results from the end products of bilirubin digestion, mostly stercobilinogen and urobilin excreted in the bile. Bile is a necessary component for the digestion and absorption of fats. The bile functions to emulsify the fat that has been ingested. This process breaks the fat globules into smaller particles so that they can be acted on by digestive enzymes and absorbed more readily.
    TMP11 816

74. (C) Located over the entire surface of the small intestine are pitlike structures called crypts of Lieberkühn. Specialized cells within these crypts secrete large quantities of water and electrolytes. These secretions are similar to extracellular fluid and have a slightly alkaline pH. The volume of secretion by the small intestine is approximately 1800 ml/day. The secretion of fluid from the crypts supplies an environment in which substances from the chyme can be absorbed as they make contact with the villi of the small intestine.
    TMP11 805, 806

75. (C) Bacteria, especially bacteria of the bacilli group, are normally present in the colon. These bacteria digest small amounts of cellulose and are responsible for producing several other substances, including vitamin K, vitamin B_{12}, thiamine, riboflavin, and various gases that constitute flatus. The production of vitamin K is especially important because the normal diet provides insufficient amounts to maintain adequate blood coagulation.
    TMP11 817

76. (B) The secretions of the large intestine consist mostly of mucus. This mucus contains a moderate amount of bicarbonate and protects the wall epithelium of the large intestine from excoriation. In addition, this mucous secretion provides an adherent medium for holding the feces together.
    TMP11 806

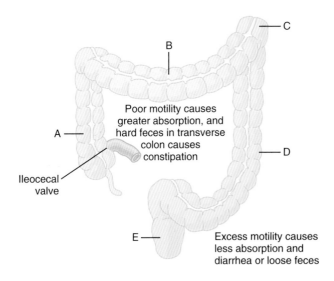

77. (A) The chyme in the ascending colon is fluid.
    TMP11 806

Metabolism and Temperature Regulation

1. The first stage in using triglycerides for energy is hydrolysis of the triglycerides to which of the following substance(s)?
   (A) Acetyl coenzyme A
   (B) Cholesterol
   (C) Glycerol 3-phosphate
   (D) Glycerol and fatty acids
   (E) Phospholipids

2. Shortly after eating a meal (after the food is eaten and begins to be digested), the respiratory exchange ratio (CO_2 production/O_2 utilization) approaches which of the following values?
   (A) 0.5
   (B) 0.6
   (C) 0.7
   (D) 0.8
   (E) 1.0
   (F) 1.2

3. An unclothed person sitting inside at normal room temperature loses the most heat by which of the following mechanisms?
   (A) Conduction to air
   (B) Conduction to objects
   (C) Convection
   (D) Evaporation
   (E) Radiation

4. After eating a meal containing a large amount of fat, which of the following changes tends to cause a feeling of satiety?
   (A) Increased levels of neuropeptide Y
   (B) Increased secretion of ghrelin by the stomach
   (C) Increased release of cholecystokinin
   (D) Decreased secretion of leptin
   (E) Decreased secretion of peptide YY from the ileum

5. A 62-year-old man has a 25-year history of alcoholism and liver disease. He visits his physician complaining of swelling in his abdomen. An increase in which of the following is the most likely cause of the ascites?
   (A) Hepatic artery pressure
   (B) Hepatic vein pressure
   (C) Hydrostatic pressure of peritoneal fluid
   (D) Plasma albumin concentration
   (E) Portal vein pressure

6. Which of the following hormones is released from adipose tissue and serves as a feedback mechanism to signal to the brain that there is increased energy storage (i.e., increased adipose tissue)?
   (A) Leptin
   (B) Peptide YY
   (C) Cholecystokinin
   (D) Neuropeptide Y
   (E) Insulin

Questions 7 and 8

Refer to the following figure to answer questions 7 and 8.

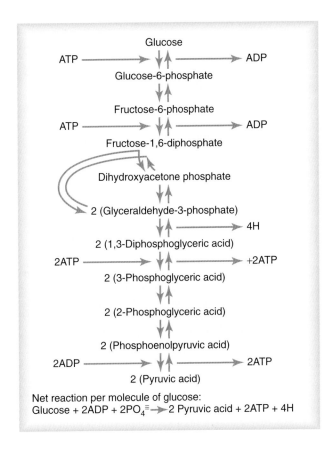

Net reaction per molecule of glucose:
Glucose + 2ADP + 2PO$_4^\equiv$ → 2 Pyruvic acid + 2ATP + 4H

7. Abundant amounts of adenosine triphosphate (ATP) in the cytoplasm of the cell inhibit which of the following steps in glycolysis?
   (A) Conversion of glucose to glucose-6-phosphate
   (B) Conversion of fructose-6-phosphate to fructose-1,6-diphosphate
   (C) Conversion of 1,3-diphosphoglyceric acid to 3-phosphoglyceric acid
   (D) Conversion of phosphoenolpyruvic acid to pyruvic acid

8. Abundant amounts of adenosine diphosphate (ADP) or adenosine monophosphate (AMP) stimulate which of the following steps in glycolysis?
   (A) Conversion of glucose to glucose-6-phosphate
   (B) Conversion of fructose-6-phosphate to fructose-1,6-diphosphate
   (C) Conversion of 1,3-diphosphoglyceric acid to 3-phosphoglyceric acid
   (D) Conversion of phosphoenolpyruvic acid to pyruvic acid

9. Approximately 95 per cent of the bile salts secreted into the small intestine are reabsorbed by the liver and reused. Which portion of the gastrointestinal tract is most important for the absorption of bile salts by an active transport process?
   (A) Colon
   (B) Duodenum
   (C) Ileum
   (D) Jejunum
   (E) Stomach

10. The fatty acid molecule is degraded in the mitochondria by the progressive release of two-carbon segments in the form of which of the following substances?
    (A) Acetyl coenzyme A
    (B) Carnitine
    (C) Glycerol
    (D) Glycerol 3-phosphate
    (E) Oxaloacetic acid

11. Cirrhosis of the liver often leads to hyperbilirubinemia (jaundice). This increase in serum bilirubin levels in patients with alcoholic cirrhosis most often results from which of the following?
    (A) Decreased excretion of bilirubin into bile
    (B) Increased uptake of bilirubin by hepatocytes
    (C) Enhanced conjugation of bilirubin
    (D) Excessive hemolysis

12. A 4-year-old boy is brought to the family physician by his parents, who report that he has a voracious appetite and is extremely obese. The boy weighs 40 kilograms and has normal blood pressure; laboratory tests reveal a very high fasting plasma insulin level. Which of the following is the most likely explanation for this boy's early-onset obesity?
    (A) Gain-of-function mutation of the cholecystokinin receptor in the hypothalamus
    (B) Mutation that prevents leptin formation by adipocytes
    (C) Decreased secretion of ghrelin
    (D) Mutation that decreases the release of neuropeptide Y in the hypothalamus
    (E) Mutation that decreases the release of agouti-related protein in the hypothalamus

13. Destruction of which of the following neuronal centers of the hypothalamus causes hyperphagia (voracious eating) and obesity?
    (A) Lateral nuclei of the hypothalamus
    (B) Ventromedial nuclei of the hypothalamus
    (C) Supraoptic nuclei of the hypothalamus
    (D) Neuropeptide Y and agouti-related peptide neurons of the arcuate nucleus

14. A 72-year-old man has a 30-year history of alcoholism and liver disease. He visits his physician complaining of swelling in his legs. A decrease in which of the following is likely to contribute to the development of edema in his legs?
    (A) Capillary hydrostatic pressure
    (B) Femoral vein pressure
    (C) Interstitial fluid hydrostatic pressure
    (D) Liver lymph flow
    (E) Plasma albumin concentration

15. A 26-year-old man is diagnosed with acquired immunodeficiency syndrome (AIDS). He has recently experienced rapid and severe weight loss. Which of the following is the most likely explanation for his weight loss?
    (A) Anorexia caused by excessive worry and loss of appetite
    (B) Cachexia due to increased release of inflammatory cytokines
    (C) Decreased activity of the melanocortin system in the hypothalamus
    (D) Excessive activation of ghrelin
    (E) Increased levels of endorphins in the hypothalamus

16. A 27-year-old man with chronic hemolytic disease develops gallstones. Which of the following is the most likely primary constituent of his gallstones?
    (A) Bilirubin
    (B) Calcium
    (C) Cholesterol
    (D) Lecithin
    (E) Triglyceride

17. A 45-year-old man is stranded in a desolate area with no food but plenty of fresh water to drink. Which of the following changes would be expected after 1 week of starvation?
    (A) Greater than 90 per cent reduction in carbohydrate stores
    (B) Greater than 20 per cent reduction in protein stores
    (C) Greater than 50 per cent reduction in fat stores
    (D) Severe vitamin A deficiency

18. The transport of glucose through the membranes of most tissue cells occurs by which of the following processes?
    (A) Facilitated diffusion
    (B) Primary active transport
    (C) Secondary active co-transport
    (D) Secondary active counter-transport
    (E) Simple diffusion

19. A scuba diver explores an underwater lava flow where the water temperature is 102°F. Which of the following profiles describes the mechanisms of heat loss that are effective in this man?

	Evaporation	Radiation	Convection	Conduction
(A)	No	No	No	Yes
(B)	No	No	No	No
(C)	Yes	Yes	No	Yes
(D)	No	Yes	No	Yes
(E)	Yes	Yes	Yes	Yes

20. About 75 per cent of the blood flowing through the liver is from the portal vein, and the remainder is from the hepatic artery during resting conditions. Which of the following best describes the liver circulation in terms of resistance, pressure, and flow?

	Resistance	Pressure	Flow
(A)	High	High	High
(B)	High	Low	High
(C)	Low	High	Low
(D)	Low	Low	High
(E)	Low	Low	Low

21. A 57-year-old obese woman on hormone replacement therapy develops gallstones. Her gallstones are most likely composed of which of the following substances?
    (A) Bile salts
    (B) Bilirubin
    (C) Calcium salts
    (D) Cholesterol
    (E) Free fatty acids

22. Deamination means removal of the amino groups from the amino acids. Which of the following substances is produced when deamination occurs by transamination?
    (A) Acetyl coenzyme A
    (B) Ammonia
    (C) Citrulline
    (D) Ornithine
    (E) α-Ketoglutaric acid

23. A 58-year-old man is admitted to the emergency department after he was found lying in the street in an inebriated state. He is markedly pale with icteric (jaundiced) conjunctivae and skin. His abdomen is distended, and there is shifting dullness, indicating ascites. The liver is enlarged about 5 centimeters below the right costal margin and tender. The spleen cannot be palpated. There is bilateral edema of his legs and feet. Which of the following values of conjugated and unconjugated bilirubin (in mg/dl) are most likely to be present in this man's plasma?

	Conjugated	Unconjugated
(A)	1.0	1.3
(B)	2.3	2.4
(C)	5.0	1.7
(D)	1.8	6.4
(E)	6.8	7.5

24. Which of the following mechanisms causes heat loss from a normal person when the environmental temperature is 106°F and the relative humidity is less than 10 per cent?
    (A) Conduction
    (B) Convection
    (C) Evaporation
    (D) Radiation

25. The hypothalamic set-point temperature normally averages about 98.6°F. Which of the following profiles describes the factors that can alter the set-point level for core temperature control?

	Skin Temperature	Pyrogens	Antipyretics	Thyroxin
(A)	No	Yes	Yes	No
(B)	No	Yes	Yes	Yes
(C)	Yes	Yes	Yes	Yes
(D)	Yes	No	No	Yes
(E)	Yes	Yes	Yes	No

26. Scurvy, which is characterized by failure of wounds to heal, petechial hemorrhages beneath the skin, and fragile blood vessels, is caused by a deficiency of which of the following vitamins?
    (A) Vitamin D
    (B) Vitamin E
    (C) Vitamin C
    (D) Vitamin K
    (E) Vitamin B_{12}

27. Deficiency of which of the following vitamins causes "night blindness" (impaired vision at nighttime)?
    (A) Thiamine (vitamin B_1)
    (B) Niacin
    (C) Riboflavin (vitamin B_2)
    (D) Vitamin B_{12}
    (E) Vitamin A

Questions 28-30

Use the figure below to answer questions 28 to 30. The diagram shows the effects of changing the set-point of the hypothalamic temperature controller. The red line indicates the body temperature, and the blue line represents the hypothalamic set-point temperature.

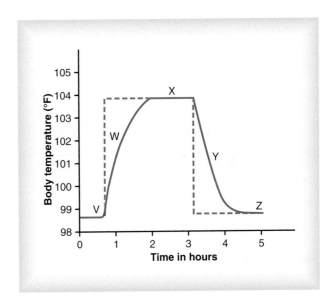

28. Which of the following sets of changes occurs at point W, compared with point V?

	Shivering	Sweating	Vasoconstriction	Vasodilation
(A)	No	No	No	No
(B)	No	Yes	No	Yes
(C)	No	Yes	Yes	No
(D)	Yes	No	No	Yes
(E)	Yes	No	Yes	No
(F)	Yes	Yes	Yes	Yes

29. Which of the following sets of changes occurs at point Y, compared with point V?

	Shivering	Sweating	Vasoconstriction	Vasodilation
(A)	No	No	No	No
(B)	No	Yes	No	Yes
(C)	No	Yes	Yes	No
(D)	Yes	No	No	Yes
(E)	Yes	No	Yes	No
(F)	Yes	Yes	Yes	Yes

30. Which of the following sets of changes occurs at point X, compared with point V?

	Shivering	Sweating	Vasoconstriction	Vasodilation
(A)	No	No	No	No
(B)	No	Yes	No	Yes
(C)	No	Yes	Yes	No
(D)	Yes	No	No	Yes
(E)	Yes	No	Yes	No
(F)	Yes	Yes	Yes	Yes

31. Deficiency of which of the following vitamins is the main cause of beriberi?
    (A) Vitamin A
    (B) Thiamine (vitamin B_1)
    (C) Riboflavin (vitamin B_2)
    (D) Vitamin B_{12}
    (E) Pyridoxine (vitamin B_6)

32. Most of the energy released from the glucose molecule occurs by which of the following processes?
    (A) Citric acid cycle
    (B) Glycogenesis
    (C) Glycogenolysis
    (D) Glycolysis
    (E) Oxidative phosphorylation

33. Deficiency of which of the following vitamins is the main cause of pellagra?
    (A) Vitamin A
    (B) Thiamine (vitamin B_1)
    (C) Niacin
    (D) Riboflavin (vitamin B_2)
    (E) Vitamin B_{12}

34. As part of an experiment examining anaerobic exercise conditioning, a 30-year-old man is asked to run on an inclined treadmill until near exhaustion. Which of the following statements concerning the conversion of pyruvic acid to lactic under anaerobic conditions is false?
    (A) Conversion of pyruvic acid to lactic acid provides a sinkhole into which the end products of glycolysis can disappear
    (B) Pyruvic acid combines with NAD^+ to produce lactic acid and NADH
    (C) The NAD^+ produced by the conversion of pyruvic acid to lactic acid can combine with two hydrogen atoms and allow glycolysis to continue
    (D) Under the above conditions, the heart can use lactic acid as an energy source

35. Which of the following is the most abundant source of high-energy phosphate bonds in the cells?
    (A) Adenosine triphosphate (ATP)
    (B) Phosphocreatine
    (C) Adenosine diphosphate (ADP)
    (D) Creatine

36. A 74-year-old man is admitted to the emergency department of a university hospital. He was found lying in his yard near a running lawnmower on a hot summer day. His body temperature is 106°F, blood pressure is normal, and heart rate is 160 beats/min. Which of the following sets of changes is most likely to be present in this man?

	Sweating	Hyperventilation	Vasodilation of Skin
(A)	No	No	No
(B)	No	Yes	Yes
(C)	Yes	No	No
(D)	Yes	Yes	No
(E)	Yes	No	Yes
(F)	Yes	Yes	Yes

37. Erythrocytes are constantly dying and being replaced. Heme from the hemoglobin is converted to which of the following substances before being eliminated from the body?
    (A) Bilirubin
    (B) Cholesterol
    (C) Cholic acid
    (D) Globin
    (E) Verdigarbin

38. The ammonia released during deamination of amino acids is removed from the blood almost entirely by conversion into which of the following substances?
    (A) Ammonium
    (B) Carbon dioxide
    (C) Ornithine
    (D) Urea
    (E) Water

39. During strenuous exercise that lasts for more than 5 to 10 seconds but less than 1 to 2 minutes, most of the energy for the exercising skeletal muscles comes from which of the following sources?
    (A) Adenosine triphosphate (ATP) already present in the cells
    (B) Anaerobic energy from glycolysis
    (C) Oxidation of carbohydrates
    (D) Oxidation of lactic acid into glucose
    (E) Conversion of lactic acid into pyruvic acid, which is degraded and oxidized in the citric acid cycle

40. Which of the following accounts for the largest component of daily energy expenditure in a sedentary individual?
    (A) Nonexercise activity such as maintaining body posture and fidgeting
    (B) The thermogenic effect of eating meals
    (C) Basal metabolic rate (energy for the body to simply to exist)
    (D) Nonshivering thermogenesis necessary to maintain body temperature

Answers

1. (D) Triglycerides are hydrolyzed to glycerol and fatty acids. The fatty acids and glycerol are transported in the blood to the tissues, where they will be oxidized to provide energy. Almost all cells, with the exception of some brain tissue, can use fatty acids almost interchangeably with glucose for energy.
   TMP11 840

2. (E) Shortly after a meal, almost all the food metabolized is carbohydrate. When carbohydrates are metabolized, an average of 100 CO_2 molecules are formed for each 100 O_2 molecules consumed; therefore, the respiratory exchange ratio averages about 1.0.
   TMP11 867

3. (E) About 60 per cent of the body heat is lost by radiation. Loss of heat by radiation means loss in the form of infrared heat waves, which is a type of electromagnetic wave. All objects radiate heat waves; thus, heat waves are radiated from the walls of rooms and other objects toward the body, and the body radiates heat waves to all surrounding objects. If the temperature of the body is greater than the temperature of surrounding objects, more heat radiates from the body than is radiated to the body.
   TMP11 981

4. (C) Cholecystokinin is released mainly in response to fat entering the duodenum and has a direct effect on the feeding centers to reduce subsequent eating. Ghrelin is released by the stomach during fasting and stimulates appetite. Increased release of neuropeptide Y by neurons of the hypothalamus also stimulates appetite. Decreased levels of leptin and peptide YY would also stimulate appetite.
   TMP11 868-870

5. (E) When liver parenchymal cells are destroyed, they are replaced with fibrous tissue that eventually contracts around the blood vessels, thereby greatly impeding the flow of portal blood through the liver. This increase in vascular resistance leads to an increase in portal vein pressure, which in turn raises the capillary pressure of the splanchnic organs, causing excess amounts of fluid transudate to enter the abdomen.
   TMP11 860

6. (A) When the amount of adipose tissue increases (signaling excess energy storage), the adipocytes produce increased amounts of leptin, which is released into the blood. Leptin crosses the blood-brain barrier and acts on the hypothalamus to initiate multiple actions that decrease fat storage, including reducing appetite and increasing energy expenditure. None of the other substances are released by adipocytes in response to increased adiposity.
   TMP11 871

7. (B) Continual release of energy from glucose when energy is not needed by the cells would be an extremely wasteful process. Both ATP and adenosine diphosphate (ADP) are important in controlling the rate of chemical reactions in the energy metabolism sequence. When ATP is abundant within the cell, it helps control energy metabolism by inhibiting the conversion of fructose-6-phosphate to fructose-1,6-diphosphate. It does so by inhibiting the enzyme phosphofructokinase.
   TMP11 836

8. (B) Both ADP and AMP increase the activity of the enzyme phosphofructokinase and increase the conversion of fructose-6-phosphate to fructose-1,6-diphosphate.
   TMP11 836

9. (C) About 95 per cent of bile salts is reabsorbed from the small intestine; about half of this occurs by diffusion through the mucosa in the early portions of the small intestine, and the remainder by an active transport process through the intestinal mucosa in the distal ileum. The bile salts then enter the portal blood and pass back to the liver. This recirculation of bile salts is called the enterohepatic circulation.
   TMP11 850, 851

10. (A) The fatty acid molecule is degraded in the mitochondria by the progressive release of two-carbon segments in the form of acetyl coenzyme A. This process is called the beta-oxidation process for degradation of fatty acids.
    TMP11 861

11. (A) Damage to hepatic cells in cirrhosis of the liver leads to the development of obstructive jaundice. The rate of bilirubin formation is normal, but the bilirubin cannot pass from the blood into the intestines. Usually, the free bilirubin still enters the liver cells and becomes conjugated in the normal way. This conjugated bilirubin is then returned to the blood, probably by rupture of the congested bile canaliculi and direct emptying of the bile into the lymph leaving the liver.
    TMP11 864

12. (B) A leptin gene mutation that reduces the secretion of leptin by adipocytes would cause early-onset morbid obesity, because leptin has a powerful role in suppressing appetite. All the other changes indicated would reduce appetite and would not cause obesity.
    TMP11 873

13. (B) The ventromedial nuclei of the hypothalamus serve as a satiety center. Electrical stimulation of this region causes almost complete satiety, and destruction of the center causes voracious appetite and extreme obesity. The lateral nuclei of the hypothalamus serve as the feeding center; destruction of this region would cause decreased appetite and weight loss. The supraoptic nuclei of the hypothalamus function as osmoreceptors, regulating the release of antidiuretic hormone from the posterior pituitary.
    TMP11 867, 868

14. (E) Essentially all the albumin in the plasma is formed in the liver. One of the complications of

cirrhosis is the failure of liver parenchymal cells to produce adequate amounts of albumin, thus leading to decreased plasma colloid osmotic pressure and generalized edema. Under normal conditions, about 75 per cent of the plasma colloid osmotic pressure can be attributed to albumin produced in the liver.
TMP11 855

15. (B) Cachexia is a metabolic disorder of increased energy expenditure that leads to rapid weight loss that cannot be explained by reduced food intake alone. This often occurs in patients with AIDS and is believed to be caused by the increased formation of inflammatory cytokines, which increase energy expenditure and decrease appetite. Decreased action of the melanocortin system, increased ghrelin, and increased endorphins in the hypothalamus would tend to increase rather than reduce energy intake and body weight.
TMP11 874

16. (A) Hemolytic disease is the premature destruction of erythrocytes. Excessive amounts of hemoglobin released from the red blood cells leads to overproduction of bilirubin by phagocytes. This increase in bilirubin production can lead to the development of pigment stones in the gallbladder that are composed primarily of bilirubin.
TMP11 864

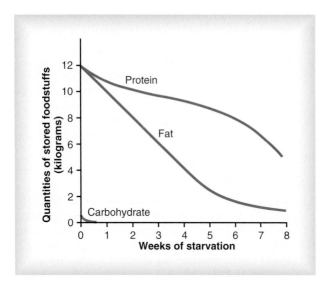

17. (A) The quantity of carbohydrate stored in the entire body is only a few hundred grams, which can supply the energy required for normal body functions for about a day. During starvation, carbohydrate stores are almost completely depleted after a day. Fat depletion begins to occur, but after 1 week, less than 10 per cent of the fat stores would be depleted. The amount of protein depletion during the first few days of starvation is very small, usually less than 10 per cent of the total protein stores. Thereafter, protein depletion occurs very slowly and only after most of the fat has been depleted.
TMP11 874-875

18. (A) The transport of glucose through the membranes of most cells is different from that which occurs through the gastrointestinal membrane or through the epithelium of the renal tubules. In both these latter cases, the glucose is transported by the mechanism of secondary active co-transport, in which active transport of sodium provides energy for absorbing glucose against a concentration difference. This sodium co-transport mechanism functions only in certain special epithelial cells that are specifically adapted for active absorption of glucose. At all other cell membranes, glucose is transported only from higher concentrations toward lower concentrations by facilitated diffusion made possible by the special binding properties of membrane glucose carrier protein.
TMP11 831

19. (B) None of the mechanisms of heat loss are effective when a person is placed in water that has a temperature greater than body temperature. Instead, the body will continue to gain heat until the body temperature becomes equal to the water temperature.
TMP11 891, 892

20. (D) The liver has a high blood flow, low vascular resistance, and low blood pressure. During resting conditions, about 27 per cent of the cardiac output flows through the liver, yet the pressure in the portal vein leading into the liver averages only 9 mm Hg. This high flow and low pressure indicate that the resistance to blood flow through the hepatic sinusoids is normally very low.
TMP11 860

21. (D) Under abnormal conditions, the cholesterol present in bile may precipitate, resulting in the formation of cholesterol gallstones. These account for about 80 per cent of all gallstones. Some of the risk factors for cholesterol gallstones include obesity, excess estrogen from pregnancy or hormone replacement, and gender. Women between 20 and 60 years of age are twice as likely to develop gallstones as men are.
TMP11 No discussion

22. (B) The degradation of amino acids occurs almost entirely in the liver, and it begins with deamination, which occurs mainly by the following transamination schema: The amino group from the amino acid is transferred to α-ketoglutaric acid, which then becomes glutamic acid. The glutamic acid then transfers the amino group to still other substances or releases it in the form of ammonia. In the process of losing the amino group, the glutamic acid once again becomes α-ketoglutaric acid, so that the cycle can repeat again and again.
TMP11 856

23. (C) This man is an alcoholic with cirrhosis of the liver. In this condition, the rate of bilirubin production is normal, and the free bilirubin still enters the liver cells and becomes conjugated in the usual way. The conjugated bilirubin is mostly returned to the

blood, probably by rupture of congested bile canaliculi, so that only small amounts enter the bile. The result is elevated levels of conjugated bilirubin in the plasma, with normal or near-normal levels of unconjugated bilirubin.
TMP11 863, 864

24. (C) Evaporation is the only mechanism of heat loss when the air temperature is greater than the body temperature. Each gram of water that evaporates from the surface of the body causes 0.58 kilocalorie of heat to be lost from the body. Even when a person is not sweating, water still evaporates *insensibly* from the skin and lungs at a rate of 450 to 600 ml/day, which amounts to about 12 to 16 kilocalories of heat loss per hour.
TMP11 892

25. (E) The skin temperature can alter slightly the set-point level for core temperature control by altering the set-point of the hypothalamic temperature control center. Pyrogens can increase the hypothalamic set-point temperature. Pyrogens can be proteins, breakdown products of proteins, and especially lipopolysaccharides released from bacterial cell membranes. Drugs such as aspirin that reduce the level of fever are called antipyretics.
TMP11 894, 895

26. (C) Some of the most important effects of ascorbic acid (vitamin C) deficiency include failure of wounds to heal and fragile blood vessels, which lead to small petechial hemorrhages throughout the body.
TMP11 877-878

27. (E) One of the basic functions of vitamin A is its use in the formation of retinal pigments of the eye, and deficiency of vitamin A can lead to night blindness.
TMP11 875

28. (E) When the hypothalamic set-point temperature is greater than the body temperature, the person feels cold, and the normal responses that cause elevation of body temperature occur. These include shivering and vasoconstriction as well as piloerection and epinephrine secretion. Shivering increases heat production. The increase in epinephrine secretion causes an immediate increase in the rate of cellular metabolism, which is an effect called *chemical thermogenesis*. Vasoconstriction of the skin blood vessels decreases heat loss through the skin.
TMP11 899

29. (B) When the hypothalamic set-point temperature is lower than the body temperature, the person feels hot, and the normal responses that cause the body temperature to decrease occur, including sweating and vasodilation. Sweating increases heat loss from the body by evaporation. Vasodilation of skin blood vessels facilitates heat loss from the body by increasing the skin blood flow.
TMP11 899

30. (A) When the hypothalamic set-point temperature is equal to the body temperature, the body exhibits neither heat loss nor heat conservation mechanisms, even when the body temperature is far above normal. Therefore, the person does not feel hot even when the body temperature is 104°F, as shown in the diagram.
TMP11 899

31. (B) Thiamine is needed for the final metabolism of carbohydrates and amino acids. Decreased utilization of these nutrients secondary to thiamine deficiency is responsible for many of the characteristics of beriberi, including peripheral vasodilation and edema, lesions of the central and peripheral nervous system, and gastrointestinal tract disturbances.
TMP11 875, 876

32. (E) Almost 90 per cent of the total adenosine triphosphate (ATP) produced by glucose metabolism is formed during oxidation of the hydrogen atoms released during the early stages of glucose degradation. This process is called oxidative phosphorylation. Only two ATP molecules are formed by glycolysis, and another two are formed in the citric acid cycle. ATP is not formed by glycogenesis or glycogenolysis.
TMP11 835

33. (C) Niacin, also called nicotinic acid, functions as a coenzyme and combines with hydrogen atoms as they remove food substrates by various types of dehydrogenases. When a deficiency of niacin exists, the normal rate of dehydrogenation is reduced, and oxidative and delivery of energy from foodstuffs cannot occur at a normal rate. This causes dermatitis, inflammation of the mucous membranes, and psychic disturbances, as well as other disorders of the clinical entity called pellagra.
TMP11 876

34. (B) The two end products of glycolysis—pyruvic acid and hydrogen atoms—combine with NAD^+ to form NADH and H^+. The buildup of either or both of these products would stop the glycolytic process and prevent the formation of ATP. Under anaerobic conditions, the majority of pyruvic acid is converted to lactic acid. Therefore, lactic acid represents a type of sinkhole into which the glycolytic end products can disappear.
TMP11 837

35. (B) Phosphocreatine contains high-energy phosphate bonds and is three to eight times as abundant as ATP or ADP in a cell. Creatine does not contain high-energy phosphate bonds.
TMP11 882

36. (B) This patient is suffering from heatstroke. Patients with heatstroke commonly exhibit tachypnea and hyperventilation caused by direct central nervous system stimulation, acidosis, or hypoxia. The blood vessels in the skin are vasodilated, and the skin is warm. Sweating ceases in patients with

true heatstroke, most likely because the high temperature itself causes damage to the anterior hypothalamic-preoptic area. The nerve impulses from this area are transmitted in the autonomic pathways to the spinal cord and then through sympathetic outflow to the skin to cause sweating.
   TMP11 899, 900

37. (A) Hemoglobin is metabolized by tissue macrophages (also called the reticuloendothelial system). The hemoglobin is first split into globin and heme, and the heme ring is opened to produce free iron and a straight chain of four pyrrole nuclei, from which bilirubin will eventually be formed. The free bilirubin is taken up by hepatic cells, and most of it is conjugated with glucuronic acid; the conjugated bilirubin passes into the bile canaliculi and then into the intestines.
   TMP11 863

38. (D) Two molecules of ammonia and one molecule of carbon dioxide combine to form one molecule of urea and one molecule of water. Essentially all urea formed in the human body is synthesized in the liver. In the absence of the liver or in serious liver disease, ammonia accumulates in the blood. The ammonia is toxic to the brain, often leading to a state called hepatic coma.
   TMP11 856

39. (B) Most of the extra energy required for strenuous activity that lasts for more than 5 to 10 seconds but less than 1 to 2 minutes is derived from anaerobic glycolysis. Release of energy by glycolysis occurs much more rapidly than oxidative release of energy, which is much too slow to supply the needs of the muscle in the first few minutes of exercise. ATP and phosphocreatine already present in the cells are rapidly depleted in less than 5 to 10 seconds. After the muscle contraction is over, oxidative metabolism is used to reconvert much of the accumulated lactic acid into glucose; the remainder becomes pyruvic acid, which is degraded and oxidized in the citric acid cycle.
   TMP11 883

40. (C) Basal metabolic rate counts for about 50 to 70 per cent of the daily energy expenditure in most sedentary individuals. Nonexercise activity, such as fidgeting or maintaining posture, accounts for approximately 7 per cent of the daily energy expenditure, and the thermic effect of food accounts for about 8 per cent. Nonshivering thermogenesis can occur in response to cold stress, but the maximal response in adults is less than 15 per cent of the total metabolic rate.
   TMP11 886-888

Endocrinology and Reproduction

1. What is the cause of involution of the corpus luteum?
   (A) Low levels of luteinizing hormone and follicle-stimulating hormone (FSH) in the blood
   (B) High levels of human chorionic gonadotropin in the blood
   (C) High levels of FSH secreted from the anterior pituitary gland
   (D) Onset of menstruation

2. Which of the following is inconsistent with the diagnosis of Graves' disease?
   (A) Increased heart rate
   (B) Exophthalmos
   (C) Increased plasma levels of triiodothyronine (T$_3$)
   (D) Increased plasma levels of thyroxine (T$_4$)
   (E) Increased plasma levels of thyroid-stimulating hormone

3. Which of the following statements about antidiuretic hormone is true?
   (A) It is synthesized in the posterior pituitary gland
   (B) It increases salt and water reabsorption in the collecting tubules and ducts
   (C) It stimulates thirst
   (D) It has opposite effects on urine and plasma osmolality

4. After menopause, hormone replacement therapy with estrogen-like compounds is effective in preventing the progression of osteoporosis. What is the mechanism of their protective effect?
   (A) They stimulate the activity of osteoblasts
   (B) They increase absorption of calcium from the gastrointestinal tract
   (C) They stimulate calcium reabsorption by the renal tubules
   (D) They stimulate parathyroid hormone secretion by the parathyroid gland

5. After birth, what causes closure of the foramen ovale?
   (A) Arterial P$_{O_2}$ increases
   (B) Plasma prostaglandin E$_2$ levels increase
   (C) Left atrial pressure becomes higher than right atrial pressure
   (D) Increased strength of contraction of the myocardium

Questions 6-8

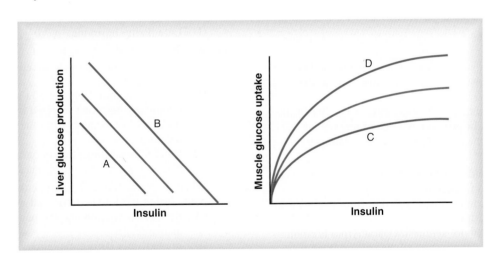

The red lines in the graphs above illustrate the normal relationships between plasma insulin concentration and glucose production in the liver and between plasma insulin concentration and glucose uptake in muscle.

6. In the above graphs, which lines most likely illustrate these relationships in a patient with type 2 diabetes?
   (A) A and C
   (B) A and D
   (C) B and C
   (D) B and D

7. In the above graphs, which lines most likely illustrate these relationships in a patient with acromegaly?
   (A) A and C
   (B) A and D
   (C) B and C
   (D) B and D

8. In the above graph on the right, line D most likely illustrates the influence of which of the following?
   (A) Exercise
   (B) Obesity
   (C) Growth hormone
   (D) Cortisol
   (E) Glucagon

9. One treatment for erectile dysfunction requires the injection of a substance into the corpora cavernosa of the penis. The injection of which of the following causes an erection?
   (A) Norepinephrine
   (B) A substance that releases nitric oxide
   (C) Thromboxane A$_2$, which is a vasoconstrictor prostaglandin
   (D) Angiotensin II

10. Which of the following statements concerning milk production by the breast is true?
    (A) It is stimulated by prolactin
    (B) It takes place in myoepithelial cells
    (C) It begins during the last month of pregnancy
    (D) It is not responsive to changes in demand for milk from the breast

11. If an antibody to human chorionic gonadotropin (HCG) is given during the first month of pregnancy, the pregnancy will be aborted. What is the explanation for this observation?
    (A) HCG stimulates the function of the corpus luteum
    (B) HCG stimulates the secretion of luteinizing hormone from the pituitary
    (C) HCG binds to progesterone receptors in the uterus
    (D) The excitability of the uterine smooth muscle is inhibited by HCG

12. Which of the following could be effective in initiating labor?
    (A) Administering progesterone to the mother
    (B) Administering luteinizing hormone to the mother
    (C) Administering an antagonist or blocker of the effects of prostaglandin E$_2$ to the mother
    (D) Mechanically dilating and stimulating the cervix

13. Why do children who are not exposed to ultraviolet light develop rickets?
    (A) They cannot absorb calcium from the gastrointestinal tract
    (B) They cannot synthesize parathyroid hormone
    (C) The metabolism of all the cells in bone is suppressed
    (D) They can form adequate amounts of 25-hydroxycholecalciferol but are unable to convert it to the active form, 1,25-dihydroxycholecalciferol

14. After birth, the pressure in the pulmonary artery decreases greatly. What is the cause of this?
    (A) Systemic arterial pressure increases
    (B) Ductus arteriosus closes
    (C) Left ventricular pressure increases
    (D) Pulmonary vascular resistance decreases

15. A 20-year-old woman reports to the clinic for a routine 6-month prenatal examination. She is feeling more tired than normal. Physical examination indicates that she does not have a goiter, and the remainder of the examination suggests that her thyroid status is normal. She has increased plasma levels of thyroxine-binding globulin, which is a normal finding during pregnancy. However, the physician suspects that the patient is euthyroid (neither hyper- nor hypothyroid) and orders blood studies. If this patient is euthyroid, which of the following laboratory findings would be expected?
    (A) Normal total (protein-bound plus free) thyroxine (T$_4$), normal thyroid-stimulating hormone (TSH)
    (B) Normal total T$_4$, high TSH
    (C) High total T$_4$, normal TSH
    (D) High total T$_4$, high TSH
    (E) High total T$_4$, low TSH

16. Spermatogenesis is regulated by a negative feedback control system in which follicle-stimulating hormone (FSH) stimulates the steps in sperm cell formation. What is the negative feedback signal associated with sperm cell production that inhibits pituitary formation of FSH?
    (A) Testosterone
    (B) Inhibin
    (C) Estrogen
    (D) Luteinizing hormone

17. Which of the following is true of ovulation?
    (A) It occurs when estrogen secretion from the follicle is rising
    (B) It occurs within 24 hours of a surge of luteinizing hormone secreted from the pituitary
    (C) It occurs immediately after the formation of the corpus luteum
    (D) It is followed immediately by a fall in the plasma concentration of progesterone

18. When do progesterone levels rise to their highest point during the female hormonal cycle?
    (A) Between ovulation and the beginning of menstruation
    (B) Immediately before ovulation
    (C) When the blood concentration of luteinizing hormone is at its highest point
    (D) When 12 primary follicles are developing to the antral stage

19. Some cells secrete chemicals into the extracellular fluid that act on cells in the same tissue. Which of the following refers to this type of regulation?
    (A) Neural
    (B) Endocrine
    (C) Neuroendocrine
    (D) Paracrine
    (E) Autocrine

20. Which of the following pairs is an example of the type of regulation referred to in question 19?
    (A) Somatostatin—growth hormone secretion
    (B) Somatostatin—insulin secretion
    (C) Dopamine—prolactin secretion
    (D) Norepinephrine—corticotropin-releasing hormone secretion
    (E) Corticotropin-releasing hormone—adrenocorticotropic hormone secretion

21. Estrogen is required for normal reproductive function in the male. Where is the principal site of estrogen synthesis in the male?
    (A) Leydig cells
    (B) Osteoblasts
    (C) Liver cells
    (D) Prostate cells

22. A professional athlete in her mid-20s suffers a spontaneous fracture of the tibia during a 400-meter race. Radiographs show signs of extensive demineralization of many bones in her skeleton. Which of the following facts elicited during the taking of her medical history may explain these observations?
    (A) She consumes a high-carbohydrate diet
    (B) Her grandmother suffered a hip fracture at age 79
    (C) Her blood pressure is greater than normal
    (D) She has not had a normal menstrual cycle for 4 years

23. In the circulatory system of a fetus, which of the following is greater before birth than after birth?
    (A) Arterial P_{O_2}
    (B) Right atrial pressure
    (C) Aortic pressure
    (D) Left ventricular pressure

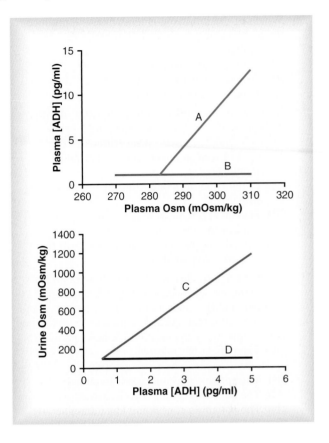

Questions 24–26

Match each of the patients described in questions 24 to 26 with the correct set of plasma values listed in the table below. Normal values are as follows: plasma aldosterone concentration, 10 ng/dl; plasma cortisol concentration, 10 μg/dl; plasma potassium concentration, 4.5 mEq/L.

	Aldosterone Concentration	Cortisol Concentration	Potassium Concentration
(A)	10.0	2.0	4.5
(B)	2.0	2.0	6.0
(C)	40.0	30.0	2.0
(D)	40.0	10.0	4.5
(E)	40.0	10.0	2.0

24. A patient with Addison's disease ( )

25. A patient with Conn's syndrome ( )

26. A patient on a low-sodium diet ( )

27. In the figures above, which lines most likely reflect the responses in a patient with nephrogenic diabetes insipidus?
    (A) A and C
    (B) A and D
    (C) B and C
    (D) B and D

28. Which of the following is greater after birth than before birth?
    (A) Flow through the foramen ovale
    (B) Pressure in the right atrium
    (C) Flow through the ductus arteriosus
    (D) Aortic pressure

29. What factor controls the rate of formation of 1,25-dihydroxycholecalciferol?
    (A) Amount of calcium in the diet
    (B) Concentration of parathyroid hormone in the plasma
    (C) Concentration of 25-hydroxycholecalciferol in the plasma
    (D) Rate of formation of vitamin D_3 in the skin
    (E) All of the above

30. Which of the following is most likely to produce the greatest increase in insulin secretion?
    (A) Amino acids
    (B) Amino acids and glucose
    (C) Amino acids and somatostatin
    (D) Glucose and somatostatin

31. In order for male differentiation to occur during embryonic development, testosterone must be secreted from the testes. What stimulates the secretion of testosterone during embryonic development?
    (A) Luteinizing hormone from the maternal pituitary gland
    (B) Human chorionic gonadotropin
    (C) Inhibin from the corpus luteum
    (D) Gonadotropin-releasing hormone from the embryo's hypothalamus

32. A patient has an elevated plasma thyroxine (T_4) concentration, a low plasma thyroid-stimulating hormone (TSH) concentration, and a thyroid gland that is smaller than normal. Which of the following is the most likely explanation for these findings?
    (A) The patient has a lesion in the anterior pituitary that prevents TSH secretion
    (B) The patient is taking propylthiouracil
    (C) The patient is taking thyroid extract
    (D) The patient is consuming large amounts of iodine
    (E) The patient has Graves' disease

33. Free ion activity of calcium in the extracellular fluid will be increased within 1 minute by which of the following?
    (A) Reduction in extracellular phosphate ion activity
    (B) Reduction in extracellular pH
    (C) Increase in extracellular P_{CO_2}
    (D) All of the above

34. Menstruation ends when the endometrium and epithelium begin to regrow and reline the surface of the uterus. What stimulates the regrowth of the cells of the epithelium?
    (A) Estrogen
    (B) Progesterone
    (C) Luteinizing hormone
    (D) Follicle-stimulating hormone

35. Which of the following anterior pituitary hormones plays a major role in the regulation of a nonendocrine target gland?
    (A) Adrenocorticotropic hormone
    (B) Thyroid-stimulating hormone
    (C) Prolactin
    (D) Follicle-stimulating hormone
    (E) Luteinizing hormone

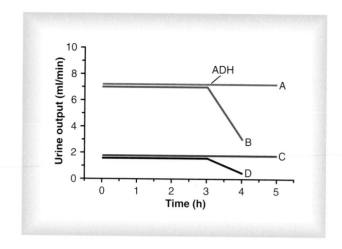

36. An experiment is conducted in which antidiuretic hormone (ADH) is administered at hour 3 to four subjects (A to D). In the figure above, which lines most likely reflect the response to ADH administration in a normal patient and in a patient with central diabetes insipidus?

	Normal	Central Diabetes Insipidus
(A)	B	A
(B)	B	D
(C)	D	A
(D)	D	B

37. A female athlete who took testosterone-like steroids for several months stopped having normal menstrual cycles. What is the best explanation for this observation?
    (A) Testosterone stimulates inhibin production from the corpus luteum
    (B) Testosterone binds to receptors in the endometrium, resulting in the endometrium's failure to develop during the normal cycle
    (C) Testosterone binds to receptors in the anterior pituitary that stimulate the secretion of follicle-stimulating hormone (FSH) and luteinizing hormone (LH)
    (D) Testosterone inhibits the hypothalamic secretion of gonadotropin-releasing hormone and the pituitary secretion of LH and FSH

38. In humans, which of the following are the major circulating adrenal steroids that produce the three main types of adrenal steroid actions?

	Glucocorticoid	Mineralocorticoid	Adrenal Androgen
(A)	Cortisol	Aldosterone	Testosterone
(B)	Cortisol	Aldosterone	Dehydroepiandrosterone
(C)	Cortisol	Deoxycorticosterone	Dehydroepiandrosterone
(D)	Corticosterone	Aldosterone	Dehydroepiandrosterone
(E)	Corticosterone	Deoxycorticosterone	Testosterone

39. Which of the following decreases the resistance in the arteries leading to the sinuses of the penis?
    (A) Stimulation of the sympathetic nerves innervating the arteries
    (B) Nitric oxide
    (C) Inhibition of activity of the parasympathetic nerves leading to the arteries
    (D) All of the above

40. A patient has a goiter associated with high plasma levels of both thyrotropin-releasing hormone (TRH) and thyroid-stimulating hormone (TSH). Her heart rate is elevated. This patient most likely has which of the following?
    (A) Endemic goiter
    (B) Hypothalamic tumor secreting large amounts of TRH
    (C) Pituitary tumor secreting large amounts of TSH
    (D) Graves' disease

41. A 40-year-old woman comes to the emergency room with a fracture in the neck of the femur. Radiographs reveal generalized demineralization of the bone in the area. Her plasma calcium ion concentration is significantly greater than normal: 12.2 mg/dl. Which of the following conditions is consistent with this presentation?
    (A) Osteoporosis
    (B) Rickets
    (C) Hyperparathyroidism
    (D) Renal failure

42. Which of the following is most likely to produce the greatest increase in glucagon secretion?
    (A) Amino acids
    (B) Amino acids and glucose
    (C) Amino acids and somatostatin
    (D) Glucose and somatostatin

43. A 46-year-old man has "puffy" skin and is lethargic. His plasma thyroid-stimulating hormone concentration is low and increases markedly when he is given thyrotropin-releasing hormone. Which of the following is the most likely diagnosis?
    (A) Hyperthyroidism due to a thyroid tumor
    (B) Hyperthyroidism due to an abnormality in the hypothalamus
    (C) Hypothyroidism due to an abnormality in the thyroid
    (D) Hypothyroidism due to an abnormality in the hypothalamus
    (E) Hypothyroidism due to an abnormality in the pituitary

44. Small stores of which of the following hormones are most likely to be found in the hormone's endocrine-producing gland?
    (A) Cortisol
    (B) Thyroxine (T_4)
    (C) Corticotropin-releasing hormone
    (D) Adrenocorticotropic hormone
    (E) Insulin

45. A man is taking a number of medications, one of which appears to be interfering with the emission phase of the sexual act. Which of the following medications could cause this problem?
    (A) A sympathetic nervous system transmitter blocker
    (B) Viagra, which prolongs the duration of action of nitric oxide
    (C) A drug that increases the release of nitric oxide
    (D) A testosterone-like androgen compound

46. In controlling aldosterone secretion, angiotensin II acts on which of the following structures?
    (A) Zona glomerulosa
    (B) Zona fasciculata
    (C) Zona reticularis
    (D) Adrenal medulla

47. Giving prostaglandin E_2 (PGE_2) to a pregnant woman may result in an abortion. What is the best explanation for this finding?
    (A) PGE_2 strongly stimulates uterine contraction
    (B) PGE_2 causes constriction of the arteries leading to the placenta
    (C) PGE_2 stimulates the release of oxytocin from the posterior pituitary
    (D) PGE_2 increases the secretion of progesterone from the corpus luteum

48. During the first few years after menopause, follicle-stimulating hormone (FSH) levels are normally extremely high. A 56-year-old woman completed menopause 3 years ago. However, she is found to have low levels of FSH in her blood. Which of the following is the best explanation for this finding?
    (A) She has been receiving hormone replacement therapy with estrogen and progesterone since she completed menopause
    (B) Her adrenal glands continue to produce estrogen
    (C) Her ovaries continue to secrete estrogen
    (D) She took birth control pills for 20 years before menopause

49. Which of the following pairs of hormones and the corresponding action is incorrect?
    (A) Glucagon—increased glycogenolysis in liver
    (B) Glucagon—increased glycogenolysis in skeletal muscle
    (C) Glucagon—increased gluconeogenesis
    (D) Cortisol—increased gluconeogenesis
    (E) Cortisol—decreased glucose uptake in muscle

50. A large dose of insulin is administered intravenously to a patient. Which of the following sets of hormonal changes is most likely to occur in the plasma in response to the insulin injection?

	Growth Hormone	Glucagon	Epinephrine
(A)	↑	↓	↔
(B)	↔	↑	↑
(C)	↑	↑	↑
(D)	↓	↑	↑
(E)	↓	↓	↔

51. Delayed breathing at birth is a common danger faced by newborn infants. What is a frequent cause of delayed breathing?
    (A) Fetal hypoxia during the birth process
    (B) Maternal hypoxia during the birth process
    (C) Fetal hypercapnia
    (D) Maternal hypercapnia

52. Which of the following hormones is largely unbound to plasma proteins?
    (A) Cortisol
    (B) Thyroxine (T_4)
    (C) Antidiuretic hormone
    (D) Estradiol
    (E) Progesterone

53. A 3-week-old infant is brought to the emergency room in a comatose condition. The history reveals that her parents have been feeding her concentrated, undiluted formula for 5 days. (Infant formula preparations are often sold in concentrated forms that must be properly diluted with water before feeding.) The infant's plasma osmolality is 352 mOsm/L (normal is 280 to 300 mOsm/L), and the osmolality of the urine is 497 mOsm/L. What is the explanation for the hyperosmotic condition of the plasma?
    (A) The infant has inappropriate antidiuretic hormone regulation
    (B) The infant has excessive secretion of aldosterone
    (C) The infant is unable to form a urine sufficiently concentrated to excrete the solute load from the formula without losing more water than required to maintain normal plasma osmolality
    (D) The infant has a renal collecting duct abnormality that prevents it from forming a concentrated urine

54. Why is milk produced only after delivery, not before?
    (A) Levels of luteinizing hormone and follicle-stimulating hormone are too low during pregnancy to support milk production
    (B) High levels of progesterone and estrogen during pregnancy suppress milk production
    (C) The alveolar cells of the breast do not reach maturity until after delivery
    (D) High levels of oxytocin are required for milk production to begin, and oxytocin is not secreted until the baby stimulates the nipple

55. In an experiment, patients in group 1 are given compound X, and patients in group 2 are given compound Y. After 1 week, group 1 patients have a lower metabolic rate and a larger thyroid gland than group 2 patients do. Identify compounds X and Y. (T_4, thyroxine; TRH, thyrotropin-releasing hormone; TSH, thyroid-stimulating hormone.)

	Compound X	Compound Y
(A)	TSH	Placebo
(B)	T_4	Placebo
(C)	Placebo	TSH
(D)	Placebo	T_4
(E)	Placebo	TRH

56. Which of the following increases the rate of excretion of calcium ions by the kidney?
    (A) Decrease in calcitonin concentration in the plasma
    (B) Increase in phosphate ion concentration in the plasma
    (C) Decrease in the plasma level of parathyroid hormone
    (D) Metabolic alkalosis

57. Over a period of several months, a 39-year-old woman has developed hyperpigmentation in association with an increase in blood pressure. Additionally, her blood glucose concentration has increased slightly. Which of the following is the most likely diagnosis?
    (A) Addison's disease
    (B) Conn's syndrome
    (C) Pituitary tumor secreting large amounts of adrenocorticotropic hormone
    (D) Adrenal tumor secreting large amounts of cortisol
    (E) Panhypopituitarism

58. A 25-year-old man is severely injured when hit by a speeding vehicle and loses 20 per cent of his blood volume. Which of the following sets of physiological changes would be expected to occur in response to the hemorrhage? (ADH, antidiuretic hormone)

	Atrial Stretch Receptor Activity	Arterial Baroreceptor Activity	ADH Secretion
(A)	↓	↓	↑
(B)	↓	↓	↓
(C)	↔	↑	↑
(D)	↑	↑	↑
(E)	↑	↑	↓

59. A patient with normal thyroid function has been given the wrong medication. Which of the following sets of changes would most likely be reported if this patient took propylthiouracil for several weeks? (T_4, thyroxine; TSH, thyroid-stimulating hormone)

	Thyroid Size	Plasma T_4 Concentration	Plasma TSH Concentration
(A)	↓	↓	↓
(B)	↓	↓	↑
(C)	↑	↓	↓
(D)	↑	↓	↑
(E)	↑	↑	↑

60. If a woman has a tumor secreting large amounts of estrogen from the adrenal gland, which of the following will occur?
    (A) Progesterone levels in the blood will be very low
    (B) She will secrete normal amounts of luteinizing hormone
    (C) She will have normal timing of ovulations
    (D) Her bones will begin to develop signs of osteoporosis early in life
    (E) None of the above

61. In a normal young man, what is the maximum pressure that can be achieved within the corpora cavernosa during a sexual experience?
    (A) 20 to 40 mm Hg
    (B) 60 to 80 mm Hg
    (C) 150 to 250 mm Hg
    (D) 400 to 600 mm Hg

Questions 62 and 63

	Hepatic Glucose Uptake	Muscle Glucose Uptake	Hormone-Sensitive Lipase Activity
(A)	↑	↑	↑
(B)	↑	↓	↑
(C)	↓	↑	↓
(D)	↑	↑	↓
(E)	↓	↑	↑

62. When compared with the postabsorptive state, which of the above sets of metabolic changes would most likely occur during the postprandial state? ( )

63. When compared with resting conditions, which of the above sets of metabolic changes would most likely occur during exercise? ( )

64. Very early in embryonic development, testosterone is formed within the male embryo. What is the function of this hormone at this stage of development?
    (A) Stimulation of bone growth
    (B) Stimulation of development of male sex organs
    (C) Stimulation of development of skeletal muscle
    (D) Inhibition of luteinizing hormone secretion

65. Which of the following changes would be expected to occur with increased binding of a hormone to plasma proteins?
    (A) Increase in plasma clearance of the hormone
    (B) Decrease in half-life of the hormone
    (C) Increase in hormone activity
    (D) Increase in degree of negative feedback exerted by the hormone
    (E) Increase in plasma reservoir for rapid replenishment of free hormone

66. A patient arrives in the emergency room apparently in cardiogenic shock due to a massive heart attack. His initial arterial blood sample reveals the following concentrations of ions:

Sodium	137 mmol/L
Bicarbonate	14 mmol/L
Free calcium	2.8 mmol/L
Potassium	4.8 mmol/L
pH	7.16

To correct the acidosis, the attending physician begins an infusion of sodium bicarbonate and after 1 hour takes another blood sample, which reveals the following values:

Sodium	138 mmol/L
Bicarbonate	22 mmol/L
Free calcium	2.3 mmol/L
Potassium	4.5 mmol/L
pH	7.34

What is the cause of the decrease in calcium ion concentration?
    (A) The increase in arterial pH resulting from the sodium bicarbonate infusion inhibited parathyroid hormone secretion
    (B) The increase in pH resulted in the stimulation of osteoblasts, which removed calcium from the circulation
    (C) The increase in pH resulted in an elevation in the concentration of HPO_4^-, which shifted the equilibrium between HPO_4^- and Ca^{++} toward $CaHPO_4$
    (D) The increase in arterial pH stimulated the formation of 1,25-dihydroxycholecalciferol, which resulted in an increased rate of absorption of calcium from the gastrointestinal tract

67. A 30-year-old woman is breast-feeding her infant. During suckling, which of the following hormonal responses is expected?
    (A) Increased secretion of antidiuretic hormone (ADH) from the supraoptic nuclei
    (B) Increased secretion of ADH from the paraventricular nuclei
    (C) Increased secretion of oxytocin from the paraventricular nuclei
    (D) Decreased secretion of neurophysin
    (E) Increased plasma levels of both oxytocin and ADH

68. A 30-year-old man has Conn's syndrome. Which of the following sets of physiological changes is most likely to occur in this patient compared with a healthy person?

	Arterial Pressure	Extracellular Fluid Volume	Sodium Excretion
(A)	↔	↔	↔
(B)	↑	↔	↔
(C)	↑	↑	↔
(D)	↔	↑	↓
(E)	↑	↑	↓

69. Why is it important to feed newborn infants every few hours?
    (A) The hepatic capacity to store and synthesize glycogen and glucose is not adequate to maintain the plasma glucose concentration in a normal range for more than a few hours after feeding
    (B) If adequate fluid is not ingested frequently, the plasma protein concentration will rise to greater than normal levels within a few hours
    (C) The function of the gastrointestinal system is poorly developed and can be improved by keeping food in the stomach at all times
    (D) The hepatic capacity to form plasma proteins is minimal and requires the constant availability of amino acids from food to avoid hypoproteinemic edema

70. A patient has a pituitary tumor that secretes large amounts of thyroid-stimulating hormone. Which of the following findings would most likely be reported for this patient?
    (A) Normal plasma levels of thyroxine (T_4)
    (B) Normal plasma levels of triiodothyronine (T_3)
    (C) Exophthalmos
    (D) Decreased respiratory rate
    (E) Goiter

71. RU486 causes abortion if it is administered before or soon after implantation. What is the specific effect of RU486?
    (A) It binds to luteinizing hormone receptors, stimulating the secretion of progesterone from the corpus luteum
    (B) It blocks progesterone receptors so that progesterone has no effect within the body
    (C) It blocks the secretion of follicle-stimulating hormone by the pituitary
    (D) It blocks the effects of oxytocin receptors in the uterine muscle

72. During the early phase of erection, arterial blood flow into the corpora cavernosa increases as much as 60-fold over that in the flaccid state. What is the best explanation for this increase in blood flow?
    (A) Arterial pressure increases due to sexual stimulation
    (B) The level of sympathetic stimulation to the arterioles supplying the corpora cavernosa increases
    (C) Resistance in the arterioles supplying the corpora cavernosa decreases
    (D) Formation of nitric oxide in the endothelial cells of the arterioles supplying the corpora cavernosa is inhibited by the increase in parasympathetic nervous system activity

73. If parathyroid hormone is infused intravenously into an animal, which of the following will be true 2 hours later?
    (A) Plasma phosphate ion concentrations will be elevated
    (B) Plasma calcium ion concentrations will be decreased
    (C) The rate of calcium excretion will be elevated
    (D) The rate of phosphate excretion in the urine will be increased

74. A 55-year-old man has developed the syndrome of inappropriate antidiuretic hormone secretion due to carcinoma of the lung. Which of the following physiological responses would be expected?
    (A) Increased plasma osmolality
    (B) Inappropriately low urine osmolality (relative to plasma osmolality)
    (C) Increased thirst
    (D) Decreased secretion of antidiuretic hormone from the pituitary gland

75. During pregnancy, the uterine smooth muscle is quiescent. As a result, forceful uterine contractions do not occur until the ninth month of gestation. Which of the following best explains this quiescence of the uterine smooth muscle?
    (A) Prostaglandin synthesis is inhibited by a factor from the placenta
    (B) Oxytocin levels are greater than normal
    (C) The very high levels of progesterone present during pregnancy suppress the activity of the uterine smooth muscle
    (D) Human chorionic gonadotropin exerts an inhibitory effect on the uterine smooth muscle

76. A 40-year-old man who is sodium-depleted is administered an angiotensin-converting enzyme (ACE) inhibitor for 2 weeks. Which of the following sets of physiological changes would most likely occur in this patient after taking the ACE inhibitor for 2 weeks?

	Plasma Aldosterone Concentration	Plasma Cortisol Concentration	Sodium Excretion
(A)	↔	↔	↔
(B)	↔	↓	↔
(C)	↓	↔	↑
(D)	↓	↓	↑
(E)	↓	↔	↔

77. A young woman is amenorrheic. Where in her body is progesterone being formed?
    (A) Corpus luteum
    (B) Pituitary gland
    (C) Endometrium
    (D) Primary follicles
    (E) None of the above

78. Before the preovulatory surge in luteinizing hormone, granulosa cells of the follicle secrete which of the following?
    (A) Testosterone
    (B) Progesterone
    (C) Estrogen
    (D) Inhibin

Questions 79 and 80

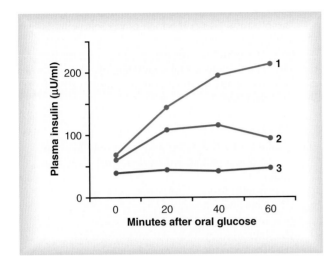

79. Based on the figure above, which set of curves most likely reflects the responses in a healthy individual and in patients with type 1 and type 2 diabetes mellitus (DM)?

	Healthy	Type 1 DM	Type 2 DM
(A)	3	2	1
(B)	1	2	3
(C)	1	3	2
(D)	2	1	3
(E)	2	3	1

80. Based on the figure above, which set of curves most likely reflects the responses in a healthy individual and in a patient in the early stages of Cushing's syndrome?

	Healthy	Cushing's Syndrome
(A)	3	2
(B)	1	2
(C)	1	3
(D)	2	1
(E)	2	3

81. Neonates that are kept in 100 per cent oxygen incubators for several days become blind when they are removed from the incubator, a condition referred to as retrolental fibroplasia. What is the explanation for the loss of sight?
   (A) The high concentration of oxygen stimulates the growth of fibrous tissue into the retina
   (B) The high concentration of oxygen causes rupture of blood vessels in the retina, resulting in fibrous infiltration of the vitreous humor
   (C) The high concentration of oxygen retards the growth of blood vessels in the retina, but when the oxygen therapy is stopped, the fall in oxygen concentration stimulates an overgrowth of blood vessels in the retina and vitreous humor, which later become densely fibrous and block the light from the pupil
   (D) The high concentration of oxygen destroys the retinal neurons

82. Which of the following peptide—second messenger pairs is incorrect?
   (A) Glucagon—cAMP
   (B) Insulin—cAMP
   (C) Thyroid-stimulating hormone—cAMP
   (D) Adrenocorticotropic hormone—cAMP
   (E) Antidiuretic hormone (V_2 receptor)—cAMP

83. Which of the following is produced by the trophoblast cells during the first 3 weeks of pregnancy?
   (A) Estrogen
   (B) Luteinizing hormone
   (C) Oxytocin
   (D) Human chorionic gonadotropin
   (E) None of the above

84. Which of the following findings is most likely in a patient who has myxedema?
   (A) Somnolence
   (B) Palpitations
   (C) Increased respiratory rate
   (D) Increased cardiac output
   (E) Weight loss

85. At birth, a large, well-nourished baby is found to have a plasma glucose concentration of 17 mg/dl (normal is 80 to 100 mg/dl) and a plasma insulin concentration twice the normal value. What is the explanation for these findings?
   (A) The neonate suffered from in utero malnutrition
   (B) The mother was malnourished during pregnancy
   (C) The mother is diabetic, with poorly controlled hyperglycemia
   (D) The mother is obese

86. Which of the following stimulates the secretion of parathyroid hormone (PTH)?
   (A) Decrease in extracellular calcium ion activity below the normal value
   (B) Calcitonin
   (C) Respiratory acidosis
   (D) PTH-releasing hormone from the hypothalamus

87. A 40-year-old woman is placed on a high-potassium diet for several weeks. Which of the following hormonal changes is most likely to occur?
   (A) Increased secretion of dehydroepiandrosterone
   (B) Increased secretion of cortisol
   (C) Increased secretion of aldosterone
   (D) Increased secretion of adrenocorticotropic hormone
   (E) Decreased secretion of corticotropin-releasing hormone

88. Which of the following sets of physiological changes is most likely to occur in a patient in the early stages of acromegaly?

	Somatomedin C Production	Somatostatin Secretion	Insulin Secretion
(A)	↑	↓	↔
(B)	↑	↑	↓
(C)	↑	↑	↑
(D)	↓	↓	↔
(E)	↓	↑	↑

89. If a woman hears her baby cry, she may experience milk ejection from the nipples even before the baby is placed to the breast. What is the explanation for this?
    (A) The sound of the hungry baby's cry elicits secretion of oxytocin from the posterior pituitary, which reaches the breast and causes contraction of the myoepithelial cells
    (B) The sound of the hungry baby's cry causes a reflex relaxation of the myoepithelial cells, allowing the milk to flow
    (C) The sound of the hungry baby's cry elicits a surge of prolactin from the anterior pituitary, which promptly stimulates milk production from the breast
    (D) The sound of the hungry baby's cry elicits sympathetic nervous system discharge that causes contraction of the myoepithelial cells

90. Which of the following hormones or physiological conditions would most likely increase growth hormone secretion?
    (A) Growth hormone
    (B) Somatostatin
    (C) Somatomedin C
    (D) Aging
    (E) Hypoglycemia

91. A young woman comes to the emergency room with a fracture in the neck of the femur. Physical examination and history reveal that she is 25 years old, 5 feet 7 inches tall, 93 pounds, heart rate 52, and blood pressure 145/78; she is apparently in excellent general health and physical condition. The fracture occurred while she was doing her daily 8-mile training run in preparation for a marathon event. Her diet is vegetarian. She does not smoke or drink alcohol, and she has been amenorrheic for the last 5 years. Radiographs of the fracture site reveal demineralization of all bones in the area. These findings are consistent with which of the following diagnoses?
    (A) Rickets due to malnutrition
    (B) Osteoporosis secondary to absence of estrogen due to amenorrhea
    (C) Metabolic acidosis with demineralization of the bone
    (D) Primary hypoparathyroidism

92. A neonate develops a jaundice condition with a bilirubin concentration of 10 mg/dl on day 2 (normal is 3 mg/dl at 2 days old). The neonatologist can be confident that the condition is not erythroblastosis fetalis if which of the following is true?
    (A) The bilirubin concentration rises no further
    (B) The hematocrit falls only slightly
    (C) The mother, father, and neonate are all Rh negative
    (D) The mother has no history of hepatic dysfunction

93. Which of the following findings would likely be reported in a patient with a deficiency in iodine intake?
    (A) Weight loss
    (B) Nervousness
    (C) Increased sweating
    (D) Increased synthesis of thyroglobulin
    (E) Tachycardia

94. Before intercourse, a woman irrigates her vagina with a solution that lowers the pH of the vaginal fluid to 4.5. What will be the effect on sperm cells in the vagina?
    (A) Their metabolic rate will increase
    (B) Their rate of movement will decrease
    (C) Their formation of prostaglandin E_2 will increase
    (D) Their rate of oxygen consumption will increase

95. Which of the following hormones has anabolic effects in muscle at physiological concentrations but is catabolic at very high levels?
    (A) Insulin
    (B) Growth hormone
    (C) Testosterone
    (D) Estrogen
    (E) Thyroxine (T_4)

96. Men who take large doses of testosterone-like androgenic steroids for long periods are sterile in the reproductive sense of the word. What is the explanation for this finding?
    (A) High levels of androgens bind to testosterone receptors in the Sertoli cells, resulting in overstimulation of inhibin formation
    (B) Overstimulation of sperm cell production results in the formation of defective sperm cells
    (C) High levels of androgen compounds inhibit the secretion of gonadotropin-releasing hormone by the hypothalamus, resulting in the inhibition of luteinizing hormone and follicle-stimulating hormone release by the anterior pituitary
    (D) High levels of androgen compounds produce hypertrophic dysfunction of the prostate gland

97. A 30-year-old woman is administered cortisone for the treatment of an autoimmune disease. Which of the following is most likely to occur?
    (A) Increased adrenocorticotropic hormone secretion
    (B) Increased cortisol secretion
    (C) Increased insulin secretion
    (D) Increased muscle mass
    (E) Hypoglycemia between meals

98. The function of which of the following is increased by an elevated parathyroid hormone concentration?
    (A) Osteoclasts
    (B) Hepatic formation of 25-hydroxycholecalciferol
    (C) Phosphate reabsorptive pathways in the renal tubules
    (D) All of the above

99. Which of the following statements about peptide or protein hormones is usually true?
    (A) They have longer half-lives than steroid hormones
    (B) They have receptors on the cell membrane
    (C) They have a slower onset of action than both steroid and thyroid hormones
    (D) They are not stored in endocrine-producing glands

100. Which of the following sets of physiological changes would be most likely to occur in a patient with acromegaly?

	Pituitary Mass	Kidney Mass	Femur Length
(A)	↓	↓	↑
(B)	↓	↑	↑
(C)	↑	↔	↔
(D)	↑	↑	↔
(E)	↑	↑	↑

101. Cortisol and growth hormone are most dissimilar in their metabolic effects on which of the following?
    (A) Protein synthesis in muscle
    (B) Glucose uptake in peripheral tissues
    (C) Plasma glucose concentration
    (D) Mobilization of triglycerides

102. Infants of mothers who had adequate nutrition during pregnancy do not require iron supplements or a diet rich in iron until about 3 months of age. Why is this?
    (A) Growth of the infant does not require iron until after the third month
    (B) The fetal liver stores enough iron to meet the infant's needs until the third month
    (C) Synthesis of new red blood cells begins after 3 months
    (D) Muscle cells that develop before the third month do not contain myoglobin

103. A college wrestler wishes to lose weight to compete in a lower weight class. He takes thyroxine (T_4) for several weeks and loses 20 pounds. Which of the following would be expected to occur as long as he continues the same dose of T_4?
    (A) Goiter
    (B) Exophthalmos
    (C) Myxedema
    (D) Tachycardia
    (E) Lethargy

104. Where does fertilization normally take place?
    (A) Uterus
    (B) Cervix
    (C) Ovary
    (D) Ampulla of the fallopian tubes

105. A patient comes to the emergency room and is found to have a slightly below-normal concentration of calcium in the blood (calcium ion activity = 0.9 mmol/L), a phosphate concentration approximately 50 per cent below normal ($HPO_4^- = 0.5$ mmol/L), and undetectable amounts of calcium ion in the urine. Which of the following would one expect to find in this patient?
    (A) Above-normal calcitonin concentration in the blood
    (B) Greater than normal parathyroid hormone concentration in the blood
    (C) Suppressed osteoclastic activity in the bone
    (D) Below-normal blood pH

106. Which of the following findings is most likely to occur in a patient who has uncontrolled type 1 diabetes mellitus?
    (A) Decreased plasma osmolality
    (B) Increased plasma volume
    (C) Increased plasma pH
    (D) Increased release of glucose from the liver
    (E) Decreased rate of lipolysis

107. Which of the following sets of physiological changes would be expected to occur in a patient with a mutation in the growth hormone receptor resulting in dwarfism?

	Femur Length	Growth Hormone Secretion	Somatomedin C Production
(A)	↓	↓	↓
(B)	↔	↓	↓
(C)	↓	↑	↑
(D)	↔	↑	↔
(E)	↓	↑	↓

108. Two days before the onset of menstruation, secretions of follicle-stimulating hormone (FSH) and luteinizing hormone (LH) reach their lowest levels. What is the cause of this low level of secretion?
    (A) The anterior pituitary gland becomes unresponsive to the stimulatory effect of gonadotropin-releasing hormone (GnRH)
    (B) Estrogen from the developing follicles exerts a feedback inhibition on the hypothalamus
    (C) The rise in body temperature inhibits hypothalamic release of GnRH
    (D) Secretion of estrogen, progesterone, and inhibin by the corpus luteum suppresses hypothalamic secretion of GnRH and pituitary secretion of FSH

109. In a radioimmunoassay, the displacement of a high percentage of radioactivity from the antibody by a plasma sample indicates which of the following?
    (A) Low levels of the measured hormone in the sample
    (B) High levels of the measured hormone in the sample
    (C) Excess levels of radioactivity in the assay system
    (D) Nonspecificity of the antibody for the hormone

110. A baby is born with a penis, a scrotum with no testes, no vagina, and XX chromosomes. This condition is referred to as hermaphroditism. Which of the following could cause this abnormality?
    (A) Abnormally high levels of human chorionic gonadotropin production by the trophoblast cells
    (B) Abnormally low rates of estrogen production by the placenta
    (C) Abnormally high levels of luteinizing hormone in the maternal blood
    (D) Abnormally high levels of testosterone in the maternal blood

111. Which of the following contributes to "sodium escape" in Conn's syndrome?
    (A) Decreased plasma levels of atrial natriuretic peptide
    (B) Increased plasma levels of angiotensin II
    (C) Decreased sodium reabsorption in the collecting tubules
    (D) Increased arterial pressure

112. A scientist studying developmental physiology performs an experiment in which a substance is given to pregnant rats who give birth to pups that have XY chromosomes but female genital organs. What was the substance given to the rats?
    (A) An antibody that blocked the effect of human chorionic gonadotropin in the embryo and fetus
    (B) A large quantity of estrogen-like compounds
    (C) Follicle-stimulating hormone
    (D) Testosterone

113. An experiment is conducted in which patients in group 1 are given compound X, and patients in group 2 are given compound Y. After 3 weeks, studies show that patients in group 1 have a higher rate of adrenocorticotropic hormone (ACTH) secretion and a lower blood glucose concentration than those in group 2. Identify compounds X and Y.

	Compound X	Compound Y
(A)	Cortisone	Placebo
(B)	Cortisol	Placebo
(C)	Placebo	Cortisol
(D)	ACTH	Placebo
(E)	Placebo	ACTH

114. In the early stages of type 2 diabetes mellitus, which of the following findings is most likely?
    (A) Abnormally high postprandial blood levels of insulin
    (B) Abnormally low postprandial blood levels of glucose
    (C) Decreased body mass
    (D) Increased insulin sensitivity
    (E) Ketoacidosis

115. Which of the following metabolic substrates is preferentially metabolized by growth hormone?
    (A) Fats
    (B) Proteins
    (C) Glycogen
    (D) Glucose

116. A man suffers from a disease that destroyed only the motor neurons of the spinal cord below the thoracic region. Which aspect of sexual function would not be possible?
    (A) Arousal
    (B) Erection
    (C) Lubrication
    (D) Ejaculation

117. A sustained program of lifting heavy weights will increase bone mass. What is the mechanism of this effect of weightlifting?
    (A) Elevated metabolic activity stimulates parathyroid hormone secretion
    (B) Mechanical stress on the bones increases the activity of osteoblasts
    (C) Elevated metabolic activity results in an increase in dietary calcium intake
    (D) Elevated metabolic activity results in stimulation of calcitonin secretion

118. Levels of transcortin are elevated in a pregnant woman. Which of the following laboratory findings would be expected in this patient?
    (A) Increased total (protein-bound plus free) plasma cortisol concentration
    (B) Increased free (non-protein-bound) plasma cortisol concentration
    (C) Decreased total plasma cortisol concentration
    (D) Decreased free plasma cortisol concentration
    (E) Little or no change in total plasma cortisol concentration

119. Birth control pills containing combinations of synthetic estrogen and progesterone compounds given for the first 21 days of the menstrual cycle are effective in preventing pregnancy. What is the explanation for their efficacy?
    (A) They prevent the preovulatory surge of luteinizing hormone secretion from the pituitary gland
    (B) They prevent development of the ovarian follicles
    (C) They suppress the function of the corpus luteum soon after it forms
    (D) They prevent normal development of the endometrium

120. Which of the following physiological responses is greater for triiodothyronine (T_3) than for thyroxine (T_4)?
    (A) Secretion rate from the thyroid
    (B) Plasma concentration
    (C) Plasma half-life
    (D) Affinity for nuclear receptors in target tissues
    (E) Latent period for onset of action in target tissues

121. A "birth control" compound for men has been sought for several decades. Which of the following would provide effective sterility?
    (A) A substance that mimics the actions of luteinizing hormone
    (B) A substance that blocks the actions of inhibin
    (C) A substance that blocks the actions of follicle-stimulating hormone
    (D) A substance that mimics the actions of gonadotropin-releasing hormone

122. In order for milk to flow from the nipple of the mother into the mouth of the nursing infant, which of the following must occur?
    (A) Myoepithelial cells must relax
    (B) Prolactin levels must fall
    (C) Oxytocin secretion from the posterior pituitary must take place
    (D) The baby's mouth must develop a strong negative pressure over the nipple
    (E) All of the above

123. Failure of the ductus arteriosus to close is a common developmental defect. Which of the following would likely be present in a 12-month-old infant with patent ductus arteriosus?
    (A) Below-normal arterial Po_2
    (B) Below-normal arterial Pco_2
    (C) Greater than normal arterial blood pressure
    (D) Lower than normal pulmonary arterial pressure

124. Which of the following statements about antidiuretic hormone and thyrotropin is accurate?
    (A) Both are synthesized in the hypothalamus
    (B) Both are stored in the pituitary gland
    (C) Both are secreted into the median eminence
    (D) Both are highly bound to plasma proteins

125. The placenta does which of the following?
    (A) Develops from the granulosa cells
    (B) Secretes luteinizing hormone
    (C) Secretes estrogen
    (D) Allows direct mixing of maternal and fetal blood
    (E) None of the above

126. Why is osteoporosis much more common in elderly women than in elderly men?
    (A) Men continue to produce testosterone throughout their lifetime, whereas women cease estrogen production after menopause
    (B) Women consume less dietary calcium than men
    (C) Gastrointestinal absorption of calcium is more effective in men than in women
    (D) The bones of women contain less calcium than those of men even before menopause

127. When compared with the late-evening values typically observed in normal subjects, plasma levels of both adrenocorticotropic hormone and cortisol would be expected to be higher in which of the following individuals?
    (A) Normal subjects after waking in the morning
    (B) Normal subjects administered dexamethasone
    (C) Patients with Cushing's syndrome (adrenal adenoma)
    (D) Patients with Addison's disease
    (E) Patients with Conn's syndrome

128. Which of the following would produce opposite directional changes in insulin and glucagon secretion?
    (A) Amino acids
    (B) Somatostatin
    (C) Early-stage type 2 diabetes mellitus
    (D) Increased sympathetic activity

129. Which blood vessel in the fetus has the highest Po_2?
    (A) Ductus arteriosus
    (B) Ductus venosus
    (C) Ascending aorta
    (D) Left atrium

130. A 59-year-old woman has osteoporosis, hypertension, hirsutism, and hyperpigmentation. Magnetic resonance imaging indicates that the pituitary gland is not enlarged. Which of the following conditions is most consistent with these findings?
    (A) Pituitary adrenocorticotropic hormone (ACTH)–secreting tumor
    (B) Ectopic ACTH-secreting tumor
    (C) Inappropriately high secretion rate of corticotropin-releasing hormone
    (D) Adrenal adenoma
    (E) Addison's disease

131. Which of the following is an inappropriate hypophysial hormone response to the hypothalamic hormone listed? (ACTH, adrenocorticotropic hormone; CRH, corticotropin-releasing hormone; GH, growth hormone; GnRH, gonadotropin-releasing hormone; LH, luteinizing hormone; TRH, thyrotropin-releasing hormone; TSH, thyroid-stimulating hormone)

	Hypothalamic Hormone	Hypophysial Hormone Secretion
(A)	Somatostatin	↓ GH
(B)	Dopamine	↑ Prolactin
(C)	GnRH	↑ LH
(D)	TRH	↑ TSH
(E)	CRH	↑ ACTH

132. Extracellular calcium concentration remains only slightly below normal for many months even when dietary calcium intake is minimal. What accounts for this ability to maintain calcium concentration in the extracellular fluid?
    (A) Only a slight reduction in plasma calcium concentration stimulates large, sustained increases in parathyroid hormone secretion
    (B) Osteoclasts stimulated by high levels of parathyroid hormone remove calcium from the large quantity stored in the bone, thereby maintaining the near-normal extracellular calcium level
    (C) Renal excretion of calcium is greatly reduced under the influence of high concentrations of parathyroid hormone
    (D) All of the above

133. A patient is administered sufficient thyroxine (T_4) to increase plasma levels of the hormone several-fold. Which of the following sets of changes is most likely in this patient after several weeks of T_4 administration?

	Respiratory Rate	Heart Rate	Plasma Cholesterol Concentration
(A)	↑	↑	↑
(B)	↑	↑	↓
(C)	↑	↓	↑
(D)	↓	↓	↑
(E)	↓	↑	↓

134. During the latter stages of pregnancy, many women experience an increase in body hair growth in a masculine pattern. What is the explanation for this?
    (A) The ovaries secrete some testosterone along with the large amounts of estrogen produced late in pregnancy
    (B) The fetal ovaries and testes secrete androgenic steroids
    (C) The maternal and fetal adrenal glands secrete large amounts of androgenic steroids that are used by the placenta to form estrogen
    (D) The placenta secretes large amounts of estrogen, some of which is metabolized to testosterone

135. What is the cause of menopause?
    (A) Reduced levels of gonadotropic hormones secreted from the anterior pituitary gland
    (B) Reduced responsiveness of the follicles to the stimulatory effects of gonadotropic hormones
    (C) Reduced rate of secretion of progesterone from the corpus luteum
    (D) Reduced numbers of follicles available in the ovary for stimulation by gonadotropic hormones

136. Release of which of the following hormones is an example of neuroendocrine secretion?
    (A) Growth hormone
    (B) Cortisol
    (C) Oxytocin
    (D) Prolactin
    (E) Adrenocorticotropic hormone

137. During the week following ovulation, the endometrium increases in thickness to 5 to 6 millimeters. What stimulates this increase in thickness?
    (A) Luteinizing hormone
    (B) Estrogen from the corpus luteum
    (C) Progesterone from the corpus luteum
    (D) Follicle-stimulating hormone

138. Which of the following sets of metabolic changes would most likely occur in response to cortisol?

	Plasma Glucose Concentration	Lipolysis	Nitrogen Balance
(A)	↓	↑	−
(B)	↓	↑	+
(C)	↑	↓	+
(D)	↑	↑	−
(E)	↑	↓	+

139. Inhibition of the iodide pump would be expected to cause which of the following changes?
    (A) Increased synthesis of thyroxine (T_4)
    (B) Increased synthesis of thyroglobulin
    (C) Increased metabolic rate
    (D) Decreased thyroid-stimulating hormone secretion
    (E) Extreme nervousness

140. Before implantation, the blastocyst obtains its nutrition from the uterine endometrial secretions. How does the blastocyst obtain nutrition during the first week after implantation?
    (A) It continues to derive nutrition from endometrial secretions
    (B) The cells of the blastocyst contain stored nutrients that are metabolized for nutritional support
    (C) The placenta provides nutrition derived from maternal blood
    (D) The trophoblast cells digest the nutrient-rich endometrial cells and then absorb their contents for use by the blastocyst

141. Which of the following increases the rate of deposition and decreases the rate of absorption of bone?
    (A) Elevation of parathyroid hormone concentration
    (B) Elevation of estrogen concentration
    (C) Elevation of extracellular hydrogen ion concentration
    (D) Reduction in mechanical stress on the bone

142. Which of the following pituitary hormones has a chemical structure most similar to that of antidiuretic hormone?
    (A) Oxytocin
    (B) Adrenocorticotropic hormone
    (C) Thyroid-stimulating hormone
    (D) Follicle-stimulating hormone
    (E) Prolactin

143. What is the most common cause of respiratory distress syndrome in neonates born at 7 months' gestation?
    (A) Pulmonary edema due to pulmonary arterial hypertension
    (B) Formation of a hyaline membrane over the alveolar surface
    (C) Failure of the alveolar lining to form adequate amounts of surfactant
    (D) Excessive permeability of the alveolar membrane to water

144. Which of the following steroid hormones cannot be synthesized to any appreciable degree in the zona fasciculata?
    (A) Aldosterone
    (B) Cortisol
    (C) Corticosterone
    (D) Dehydroepiandrosterone
    (E) Deoxycorticosterone

145. A 45-year-old woman has a mass in the sella turcica that compresses the portal vessels, disrupting pituitary access to hypothalamic secretions. The secretion rate of which of the following hormones would most likely increase in this patient?
    (A) Adrenocorticotropic hormone
    (B) Growth hormone
    (C) Prolactin
    (D) Luteinizing hormone
    (E) Thyroid-stimulating hormone

146. A man who has been exposed to high levels of gamma radiation is sterile due to destruction of the germinal epithelium of the seminiferous tubules, although he has normal levels of testosterone. Which of the following would be found in this patient?
    (A) Normal secretory pattern of gonadotropin-releasing hormone
    (B) Normal levels of inhibin
    (C) Suppressed levels of follicle-stimulating hormone
    (D) Absence of Leydig cells

147. A patient has hypothyroidism due to a primary abnormality in the thyroid gland. Increased plasma levels of which of the following would most likely be reported?
    (A) Cholesterol
    (B) Thyroxine-binding globulin
    (C) Reverse triiodothyronine (RT_3)
    (D) Diiodotyrosine
    (E) Iodide

Questions 148 and 149

An experiment was conducted in which rats were injected with one of two hormones or saline (control) for 2 weeks. Autopsies were then performed, and organ weights were measured (in milligrams).

	Control	Hormone 1	Hormone 2
Pituitary	12.9	8.0	14.5
Thyroid	250	500	245
Adrenal glands	40	37	85
Body weight	300	152	175

148. Hormone 1 is which of the following?
    (A) Thyroid-releasing hormone
    (B) Thyroid-stimulating hormone (TSH)
    (C) Thyroxine (T_4)
    (D) Adrenocorticotropic hormone (ACTH)
    (E) Cortisol

149. Hormone 2 is which of the following?
    (A) TSH
    (B) T_4
    (C) Corticotropin-releasing hormone
    (D) ACTH
    (E) Cortisol

Answers

1. (A) The development and continued function of the corpus luteum is dependent on stimulation by luteinizing hormone and follicle-stimulating hormone. When the gonadotropic hormones in the blood fall to low levels, the corpus involutes and menstruation begins.
    TMP11 1115

2. (E) In Graves' disease, thyroid-stimulating immunoglobulins bind to cell membrane receptors, causing the thyroid to produce excessive amounts of thyroid hormones (T_3 and T_4). As a result of negative feedback, increased plasma levels of T_3 and T_4 suppress the secretion of thyroid-stimulating hormone. In addition, increased plasma levels of immunoglobulins often cause exophthalmos, and an increased heart rate is a common response to high circulating levels of thyroid hormones.
    TMP11 940

3. (D) Antidiuretic hormone (ADH) increases the permeability of the collecting tubules and ducts to water, but not to sodium, which in turn increases water reabsorption and decreases water excretion.

As a result, urine concentration increases, and the retained water dilutes the plasma. ADH is synthesized in the supraoptic and paraventricular nuclei of the hypothalamus and has no direct effect on the thirst center.
TMP11 349-351, 359, 927, 928

4. (A) Estrogen compounds are believed to have an osteoblast-stimulating effect. When the amount of estrogen in the blood falls to very low levels after menopause, the balance between the bone-building activity of the osteoblasts and the bone-degrading activity of the osteoclasts is tipped toward bone degradation. When estrogen compounds are added as part of hormone replacement therapy, the bone-building activity of the osteoblasts is increased to balance the osteoclastic activity.
TMP11 927, 1017

5. (A) After birth, the pressure in the right atrium falls due to a reduction in pulmonary vascular resistance, and the left atrial pressure increases due to an increase in systolic arterial resistance and pressure. Consequently, the small valve that lies over the foramen ovale on the left side of the atrial septum closes over the opening.
TMP11 1046

6. (C) Type 2 diabetes mellitus is characterized by diminished sensitivity of target tissues to the metabolic effects of insulin; that is, there is insulin resistance. As a result, hepatic uptake of glucose is impaired, and glucose release is enhanced. In muscle, the uptake of glucose is impaired.
TMP11 963, 964, 974

7. (C) In acromegaly, high plasma levels of growth hormone cause insulin resistance. Consequently, there is increased glucose production by the liver and impaired glucose uptake by peripheral tissues.
TMP11 974

8. (A) During exercise, glucose utilization by muscle is increased, which is largely independent of insulin.
TMP11 963

9. (B) The arteries leading to the sinuses of the corpora cavernosa are normally constricted. For erection to take place, the arteries must dilate. Normally, the release of nitric oxide causes vasodilatation in these arteries. Thus, a substance that stimulates the release of nitric oxide in sufficient quantities will lead to erection.
TMP11 1002

10. (A) Prolactin promotes milk production by the alveolar cells of the breast. This hormone is secreted by the mother's anterior pituitary gland, and its concentration in the blood rises steadily from the fifth week of pregnancy until the birth of the baby, at which time it is 10 to 20 times the normal nonpregnant level.
TMP11 1039

11. (A) HCG is secreted from the trophoblast cells. It binds to luteinizing hormone receptors on the cells of the corpus luteum, thereby stimulating estrogen and progesterone secretion during the first weeks of pregnancy. Without HCG, involution of the corpus luteum would occur, followed by menstruation and abortion of the pregnancy.
TMP11 1032

12. (D) Obstetricians frequently induce labor by rupturing the membranes so that the baby's head stretches the cervix more forcefully than usual, or they irritate it in other ways.
TMP11 1036, 1037

13. (A) Exposure of the skin to ultraviolet light results in conversion of 7-dehydrocholesterol to vitamin D_3, which is subsequently converted to 1,25-dihydroxycholecalciferol, the active form of vitamin D_3 required to stimulate the absorption of calcium from the gastrointestinal tract. Without exposure to ultraviolet light, no 1,25-dihydroxycholecalciferol can be formed, and calcium reabsorption from the gut will be severely impaired, resulting in rickets.
TMP11 983, 991

14. (D) The pulmonary vascular resistance greatly decreases as a result of expansion of the lungs. In the unexpanded fetal lungs, the blood vessels are compressed because of the small volume of the lungs. Immediately on expansion, these vessels are no longer compressed, and the resistance to blood flow decreases severalfold.
TMP11 1046

15. (C) T_4 is highly bound to plasma proteins, especially to thyroxine-binding globulin, which increases during pregnancy. An increase in thyroxine-binding globulin tends to decrease free T_4, which leads to an increase in TSH secretion, causing the thyroid to increase thyroid hormone secretion. Increased secretion of thyroid hormones continues until free T_4 returns to normal levels. At this time, plasma levels of TSH are normal, because there is no further stimulus for TSH secretion. However, total T_4 (bound plus free) is elevated. Because free T_4 (and not bound T_4) enters cells and produces biological effects, and because the concentration of T_4 is normal, the patient would be euthyroid.
TMP11 934, 938, 939

16. (B) The Sertoli cells of the seminiferous tubules secrete inhibin at a rate proportional to the rate of production of sperm cells. Inhibin has a direct inhibitory effect on anterior pituitary secretion of FSH. FSH binds to specific receptors on the Sertoli cells, causing the cells to grow and secrete substances that stimulate sperm cell production. The secretion of inhibin thereby provides the negative feedback control signal from the seminiferous tubules to the pituitary gland.
TMP11 1007

17. (B) The rate of secretion of luteinizing hormone (LH) from the anterior pituitary increases markedly, rising 6- to 10-fold and peaking about 12 hours before ovulation. In response to the increase in LH concentration, the follicle undergoes changes that lead to ovulation. If the surge in LH secretion does not occur, ovulation will not take place.
TMP11 1014, 1015, 1021

18. (A) The corpus luteum is the only source of progesterone production, except for minute quantities secreted from the follicle before ovulation. The corpus luteum is functional between ovulation and the beginning of menstruation, during which time the concentration of luteinizing hormone (LH) is suppressed below the level achieved during the pre-ovulatory LH surge.
TMP11 1019

19. (D) Paracrine communication refers to cell secretions that diffuse into the extracellular fluid to affect neighboring cells.
TMP11 905

20. (B) The delta cells of the pancreas secrete somatostatin, which inhibits the secretion of insulin and glucagon from the pancreatic beta and alpha cells, respectively. Choice D is an example of neural communication, and the remaining choices are examples of neuroendocrine communication.
TMP11 905, 971

21. (C) Large amounts of estrogen are formed from testosterone and androstanediol in the liver, accounting for as much as 80 per cent of the total male estrogen production.
TMP11 1004

22. (D) The spontaneous fracture of the tibia and the findings of extensive demineralization of the bones suggest that the young woman has osteoporosis. This disease usually begins in women after menopause, and it is believed to be due to low levels of estrogen. This woman's lack of menstrual cycles for 4 years indicates that she may have had very low levels of estrogen during that time, leading to osteoporosis.
TMP11 1017

23. (B) Right atrial pressure falls dramatically after the onset of breathing due to a reduction in pulmonary vascular resistance, pulmonary arterial pressure, and right ventricular pressure.
TMP11 1046, 1047

24. (B) Secretion of adrenal cortical hormones is deficient in patients with Addison's disease. Consequently, low plasma levels of both aldosterone and cortisol would be reported. As a result of the low plasma levels of aldosterone, plasma potassium concentration would be increased.
TMP11 957

25. (E) Patients with Conn's syndrome have tumors of the zona glomerulosa that secrete large amounts of aldosterone. Consequently, plasma levels of aldosterone are elevated, causing hypokalemia. The secretion of cortisol from the zona fasciculata is normal.
TMP11 959

26. (D) Aldosterone secretion is elevated when dietary sodium intake is low, but cortisol secretion is normal. Although aldosterone increases the rate of potassium secretion by the principal cells of the collecting tubules, this effect is offset by a low distal tubular flow rate. Consequently, there is little change in either potassium excretion or plasma potassium concentration.
TMP11 368-371, 950, 951

27. (B) In patients with nephrogenic diabetes insipidus, the kidneys do not respond appropriately to antidiuretic hormone (ADH), and the ability to form concentrated urine is impaired. In contrast, there is a normal ADH secretory response to changes in plasma osmolality.
TMP11 357-359, 928

28. (D) Owing to the loss of blood flow through the placenta, systemic vascular resistance doubles at birth. This increases the aortic pressure as well as the pressure in the left ventricle and left atrium.
TMP11 1046, 1047

29. (B) The rate of the reaction in the cortex of the kidney that results in the formation of 1,25-dihydroxycholecalciferol is very tightly controlled by the concentration of parathyroid hormone.
TMP11 984

30. (B) Both amino acids and glucose stimulate insulin secretion. Further, amino acids strongly potentiate the glucose stimulus for insulin secretion. Somatostatin inhibits insulin secretion.
TMP11 968, 969, 971

31. (B) Human chorionic gonadotropin also binds to luteinizing hormone receptors on the interstitial cells of the testes of the male fetus, resulting in the production of testosterone in male fetuses up to the time of birth. This small secretion of testosterone is what causes the fetus to develop male sex organs instead of female sex organs.
TMP11 1032

32. (C) If a subject were taking sufficient amounts of exogenous thyroid extract to increase plasma levels of T_4 above normal, feedback would cause TSH secretion to decrease. Low plasma levels of TSH would result in atrophy of the thyroid gland. In Graves' disease, the same changes in plasma levels of T_4 and TSH would be present, but the thyroid gland would not be atrophied. In fact, goiter is often present in patients with Graves' disease. A lesion in the anterior pituitary that prevents TSH secretion or the taking of propylthiouracil or large amounts of iodine would be associated with low plasma levels of T_4.
TMP11 938, 939

33. (B) If extracellular pH is reduced, the additional hydrogen ion in solution will bind with negatively charged phosphate ions and negatively charged portions of protein molecules, thereby reducing the number of potential ionic partners for positively charged calcium ions. As a result, the free calcium ion activity in the solution will increase.
TMP11 979

34. (A) After menstruation, only a thin layer of epithelium remains, and the only epithelial cells left are those in the deeper portions of the glands in crypts of the endometrium. Under the influence of estrogen, which is secreted in increasing quantities by the follicles during the first part of the monthly cycle, epithelial cells and endometrial cells proliferate rapidly.
TMP11 1018, 1019

35. (C) The major target tissue for prolactin is the breast, where it stimulates the secretion of milk. The other anterior pituitary hormones (adrenocorticotropic hormone, thyroid-stimulating hormone, follicle-stimulating hormone, and luteinizing hormone) stimulate hormones from endocrine glands.
TMP11 907

36. (D) In patients with central diabetes insipidus, there is an inappropriately low secretion rate of ADH in response to changes in plasma osmolality, but there is no impairment in the renal response to ADH. Because plasma levels of ADH are depressed, there is an impaired ability to concentrate urine, and a large volume of dilute urine is excreted. Loss of water tends to increase plasma osmolality, which stimulates the thirst center. This leads to a very high rate of water turnover.
TMP11 357-359, 928

37. (D) The cells of the anterior pituitary that secrete LH and FSH, and the cells of the hypothalamus that secrete gonadotropin-releasing hormone, are inhibited by both estrogen and testosterone. The steroids taken by the woman caused sufficient inhibition to result in cessation of the monthly menstrual cycle.
TMP11 1007, 1020

38. (B) Aldosterone and cortisol account for more than 90 to 95 per cent of all mineralocorticoid and glucocorticoid activity, respectively. Most adrenal androgenic activity is due to the secretion of dehydroepiandrosterone.
TMP11 944, 945

39. (B) Nitric oxide is the vasodilator that is normally released, causing vasodilatation in these arteries.
TMP11 1002

40. (B) A hypothalamic tumor secreting large amounts of TRH would stimulate the pituitary gland to secrete increased amounts of TSH. As a result, the secretion of thyroid hormones would increase, and this would result in an elevated heart rate. In comparison, a patient with either a pituitary tumor secreting large amounts of TSH or Graves' disease would have low plasma levels of TRH because of feedback. Both TRH and TSH levels would be elevated in endemic goiter, but the heart rate would be depressed because of the low rate of T_4 secretion.
TMP11 937-942

41. (C) Demineralization of the bone could be caused by any of the choices, but only an elevated parathyroid hormone concentration would result in both demineralization and elevated plasma calcium concentration. The elevated parathyroid hormone concentration results in overstimulation of the osteoclasts, loss of calcium from bone, stimulation of calcium absorption from the renal tubular fluid and inhibition of calcium excretion, and stimulation of the formation of 1,25-dihydroxycholecalciferol, which increases the rate of calcium absorption from the gastrointestinal tract.
TMP11 990

42. (A) Amino acids stimulate glucagon as well as insulin secretion. Glucose and somatostatin inhibit glucagon secretion.
TMP11 971

43. (D) Lethargy and myxedema are signs of hypothyroidism. Low plasma levels of thyroid-stimulating hormone indicate that the abnormality is in either the hypothalamus or the pituitary gland. Because the pituitary was responsive to the administration of thyrotropin-releasing hormone (TRH), this suggests that pituitary function is normal and that the hypothalamus is producing insufficient amounts of TRH.
TMP11 938, 939, 941, 942

44. (A) Steroid hormones are not stored to any appreciable extent in their endocrine-producing glands. This is true for cortisol, which is produced in the adrenal cortex. In contrast, there are appreciable stores of thyroid and peptide hormones in their endocrine-producing glands.
TMP11 908

45. (A) Emission is stimulated by sympathetic nervous system impulses that leave the cord at T-12 to L-2 and pass to the genital organs through the hypogastric and pelvic sympathetic nervous plexus.
TMP11 1002

46. (A) The cells of the zona glomerulosa secrete most of the aldosterone. These cells have receptors for angiotensin II, which is a major controller of aldosterone secretion.
TMP11 950

47. (A) The fetal portion of the placenta releases prostaglandins in high concentrations at the time of labor. This release is associated with deterioration of the placenta. Prostaglandins, especially PGE_2, strongly stimulate uterine smooth muscle.
TMP11 1036

48. (A) After menopause, the absence of feedback inhibition by estrogen and progesterone results in extremely high rates of FSH secretion. Women taking estrogen as part of hormone replacement therapy for symptoms associated with post-menopausal conditions have suppressed levels of FSH owing to the inhibitory effect of estrogen.
TMP11 1022

49. (B) Glucagon stimulates glycogenolysis in the liver, but it has no physiological effects in muscle. Both glucagon and cortisol increase gluconeogenesis, and cortisol impairs glucose uptake by muscle.
TMP11 951, 970

50. (C) Injection of insulin leads to a decrease in blood glucose concentration. Hypoglycemia stimulates the secretion of growth hormone, glucagon, and epinephrine, all of which have counter regulatory effects to increase glucose levels in the blood.
TMP11 924, 971, 972

51. (A) Prolonged fetal hypoxia during delivery can cause serious depression of the respiratory center. Hypoxia may occur during delivery because of compression of the umbilical cord, premature separation of the placenta, excessive contraction of the uterus, or excessive anesthesia of the mother.
TMP11 1044

52. (C) In general, peptide hormones are water soluble and are not highly bound by plasma proteins. Antidiuretic hormone, a neurohypophysial peptide hormone, is virtually unbound by plasma proteins. In contrast, steroid and thyroid hormones are highly bound to plasma proteins.
TMP11 909, 910

53. (C) Functional development of the kidneys is not complete until about the end of the first month of life. The kidneys of a neonate can concentrate urine to only about 1.5 times the osmolality of plasma (in contrast to 3 to 4 times plasma osmolality in an adult). If the undiluted formula had a very high osmotic concentration, the neonate would be unable to excrete the solute in a sufficiently concentrated urine to prevent the development of hyperosmolality of the plasma.
TMP11 1043

54. (B) Although estrogen and progesterone are essential for the physical development of the breast during pregnancy, a specific effect of both these hormones is to inhibit the actual secretion of milk. Even though prolactin levels are increased 10- to 20-fold at the end of pregnancy, the suppressive effects of estrogen and progesterone prevent milk production until after the baby is born. Immediately after birth, the sudden loss of both estrogen and progesterone secretion from the placenta allows the lactogenic effect of prolactin to promote milk production.
TMP11 1039

55. (D) Administration of T_4 in amounts that increase plasma levels of the hormone above normal would be expected to increase the metabolic rate and decrease TSH secretion. Decreased plasma levels of TSH lead to atrophy of the thyroid gland. Thus, patients in group 1 would have a lower metabolic rate and a larger thyroid than patients in group 2, who were administered T_4.
TMP11 935, 938, 939

56. (C) The concentration of parathyroid hormone strongly regulates the absorption of calcium ion from the renal tubular fluid. A reduction in hormone concentration reduces calcium reabsorption and increases the rate of calcium excretion in the urine. The other choices have little effect on or decrease calcium excretion.
TMP11 987

57. (C) Because adrenocorticotropic hormone (ACTH) or fragments of its prohormone stimulate the formation of melanin by melanocytes in the skin, hyperpigmentation is commonly observed in patients with pituitary tumors secreting large amounts of ACTH. Increased plasma levels of ACTH also stimulate the adrenal glands to secrete increased amounts of cortisol, which tends to increase the blood glucose concentration. The blood glucose concentration would also tend to be elevated if an adrenal tumor were secreting large amounts of cortisol, but because of feedback, plasma ACTH levels would be suppressed, and hyperpigmentation would not be observed.
TMP11 956, 958

58. (A) Hemorrhage decreases the activation of stretch receptors in the atria and arterial baroreceptors. Decreased activation of these receptors increases ADH secretion.
TMP11 360, 929

59. (D) Propylthiouracil blocks several of the early steps in the synthesis of thyroid hormones but does not prevent the formation of thyroglobulin in follicular cells. Therefore, if propylthiouracil were administered to a normal patient, plasma levels of T_4 would fall, and decreased feedback inhibition would lead to an increase in TSH secretion. High plasma levels of TSH would cause hypertrophy of the thyroid gland, even though the production of thyroid hormones is depressed.
TMP11 939

60. (A) The high concentration of estrogen resulting from the adrenal tumor suppresses the surge of luteinizing hormone secretion from the anterior pituitary, and as a result, ovulation does not occur. If ovulation does not occur, progesterone production does not take place.
TMP11 1020

61. (C) Arterial resistance leading into the corpora cavernosa is greatly reduced during erection, while venous resistance leading from the sinuses is

extremely high due to compression of the veins against the fibrous tissue surrounding the sinuses. Therefore, pressure in the sinuses during erection is at least equal to systolic arterial pressure. However, contraction of the skeletal muscles in the floor of the perineum that overlies portions of the corpora cavernosa can compress the sinuses, increasing the pressure to levels that are substantially higher than systolic pressure.
TMP11 1002

62. (D) After eating a meal, insulin secretion is increased. As a result, there is an increased rate of glucose uptake by both the liver and muscle. Insulin also inhibits hormone-sensitive lipase, which decreases hydrolysis of triglycerides in fat cells.
TMP11 936-965, 969

63. (E) During exercise, glucose uptake by muscle is enhanced, which tends to decrease the blood glucose concentration. Insulin secretion is depressed during exercise, whereas the secretion of glucagon and epinephrine is elevated. Therefore, hepatic glucose uptake is impaired, and the activity of hormone-sensitive lipase is increased.
TMP11 963-965, 970

64. (B) The primary function of testosterone in the embryonic development of males is to stimulate formation of the male sex organs.
TMP11 1004

65. (E) Protein-bound hormones are biologically inactive and cannot be metabolized. Thus, an increase in protein binding would tend to decrease hormone activity and plasma clearance and increase the half-life of the hormone. Free hormone is also responsible for negative feedback inhibition of hormone secretion. Therefore, a sudden increase in hormone binding to plasma proteins would decrease negative feedback. Protein binding of hormones does, however, provide a reservoir for the rapid replacement of free hormone.
TMP11 909-910

66. (C) The reduction in hydrogen ion indicated by the elevation in pH increases the concentration of negatively charged phosphate ion species available for ionic combination with calcium ions. Consequently, free calcium ion concentration is reduced.
TMP11 989

67. (C) During suckling, stimulation of receptors on the nipples increases neural input to both the supraoptic and paraventricular nuclei. Activation of these nuclei leads to the release of oxytocin and neurophysin from secretion granules in the posterior pituitary gland. Suckling does not stimulate the secretion of appreciable amounts of ADH.
TMP11 928

68. (C) In Conn's syndrome, large amounts of aldosterone are secreted. Because aldosterone causes

sodium retention, hypertension is a common finding in patients with this condition. However, the degree of sodium retention is modest, as is the resultant increase in extracellular fluid volume. This occurs because the rise in arterial pressure offsets the sodium-retaining effects of aldosterone, limiting sodium retention and permitting daily sodium balance to be achieved.
TMP11 947, 948, 959

69. (A) Because the liver functions imperfectly during the first weeks of life, the glucose concentration in the blood is unstable and falls to very low levels within a few hours after feeding.
TMP11 1047

70. (E) A pituitary tumor secreting large amounts of thyroid-stimulating hormone would be expected to stimulate the thyroid gland, leading to goiter and a high secretion rate of thyroid hormones. High plasma levels of thyroid hormones would increase the respiratory rate but would not cause exophthalmos. Immunoglobulins cause exophthalmos.
TMP11 936-940

71. (B) Progesterone is required to maintain the decidual cells of the endometrium. If progesterone levels fall, as they do during the last days of a nonpregnant menstrual cycle, menstruation will follow within a few days, with loss of pregnancy. Administration of a compound that blocks the progesterone receptor during the first few days after conception will terminate the pregnancy.
TMP11 1033

72. (C) During the early phase of erection, the resistance of the arterioles supplying the corpora cavernosa decreases to very low levels due to the vasodilatation induced by nitric oxide.
TMP11 1002

73. (D) Administration of parathyroid hormone causes rapid loss of phosphates in the urine, owing to the hormone's ability to diminish proximal tubular reabsorption of phosphate ions.
TMP11 986

74. (D) An inappropriately high rate of antidiuretic hormone (ADH) secretion from the lung promotes excess water reabsorption, which tends to produce a concentrated urine and a decrease in plasma osmolality. Low plasma osmolality suppresses both thirst and ADH secretion from the pituitary gland.
TMP11 379, 928

75. (C) A specific effect of progesterone is to decrease the contractility of the pregnant uterus, thus preventing uterine contractions, which would cause spontaneous abortion.
TMP11 1033

76. (E) During sodium depletion, the renin-angiotensin system is activated, and the high levels of circulating angiotensin II stimulate the adrenal glands to

secrete increased amounts of aldosterone. In contrast, angiotensin II has no effect on cortisol secretion, and sodium depletion is associated with normal plasma levels of cortisol. Consequently, reducing plasma levels of angiotensin II by administering an ACE inhibitor would decrease plasma aldosterone to normal levels but would have no effect on plasma cortisol concentration. Because high plasma levels of aldosterone promote sodium retention, reducing aldosterone levels by administering an ACE inhibitor would tend to produce a natriuresis and a decrease in arterial pressure. In time, the opposing effects of reduced arterial pressure and aldosterone secretion on sodium excretion would offset each other, and sodium balance would eventually be achieved at a lower arterial pressure.
TMP11 948, 950, 951

77. (E) Progesterone is formed mainly in the corpus luteum. If the woman is not having menstrual cycles, she is not ovulating, and corpus luteum formation will not take place.
TMP11 1015

78. (C) Follicle-stimulating hormone stimulates the granulosa cells of the follicle to secrete estrogen.
TMP11 1013

79. (E) In response to increased blood levels of glucose, plasma insulin concentration normally increases during the 60-minute period following oral intake of glucose. In type 1 diabetes mellitus, insulin secretion is depressed. In contrast, in type 2 diabetes mellitus, insulin resistance is a common finding and, at least in the early stages of the disease, there is an abnormally high rate of insulin secretion.
TMP11 975

80. (D) In Cushing's syndrome, high plasma levels of cortisol impair glucose uptake in peripheral tissues, which tends to increase plasma levels of glucose. As a result, the insulin response to oral intake of glucose is enhanced.
TMP11 974, 975

81. (C) Too much oxygen in the incubator stops the growth of new blood vessels in the retina. Then when oxygen therapy is stopped, an overgrowth of blood vessels occurs, with a great mass of vessels growing all through the vitreous humor. Later the vessels are replaced by a mass of fibrous tissue, causing permanent blindness.
TMP11 1051

82. (B) Peptide hormones generally produce biological effects by binding to receptors on the cell membrane. In turn, the cytoplasmic generation of "second messengers" mediates the hormonal response. Many hormones use the adenylyl cyclase–cAMP and the phospholipase C second messenger systems to produce alterations in target tissue activity. Although insulin binds to surface receptors in the production of biological effects, it does not work through either of these two second messenger systems.
TMP11 913, 962, 963

83. (D) Human chorionic gonadotropin is secreted from the trophoblast cells beginning shortly after the blastocyst implants in the endometrium.
TMP11 1032

84. (A) Somnolence is a common feature of hypothyroidism. Palpitations, increased respiratory rate, increased cardiac output, and weight loss are all associated with hyperthyroidism.
TMP11

85. (C) An infant born of an untreated diabetic mother will have considerable hypertrophy and hyperfunction of the islets of Langerhans in the pancreas. As a consequence, the infant's blood glucose concentration may fall to lower than 20 mg/dl shortly after birth.
TMP11 1050

86.(A) Secretion of parathyroid hormone is regulated by changes in extracellular calcium concentration. Increases in the secretion rate are stimulated by decreases in extracellular calcium ion concentration.
TMP11 988

87. (C) Potassium is a potent stimulus for aldosterone secretion, as is angiotensin II. Therefore, a patient consuming a high-potassium diet would exhibit high circulating levels of aldosterone.
TMP11 950

88. (C) The adult form of excess growth hormone secretion is called acromegaly and is usually associated with a pituitary tumor. Increased plasma levels of growth hormone stimulate the liver and other tissues to produce somatomedin C. As a result of feedback, increased plasma levels of somatomedin C cause the hypothalamus to increase the secretion of growth hormone–inhibiting hormone, somatostatin. Elevated plasma levels of growth hormone also tend to increase plasma glucose concentration, which favors an increase in insulin secretion.
TMP11 923-926

89. (A) Neural projections from higher centers of the brain to the hypothalamus can elicit the secretion of oxytocin into the blood from the posterior pituitary gland. Upon reaching the breast, oxytocin stimulates contraction of the myoepithelial cells, forcing milk from the alveoli and ducts to the nipple.
TMP11 1040

90. (E) Acute hypoglycemia is a potent stimulus for growth hormone secretion. The other four choices would be expected to decrease growth hormone secretion.
TMP11 924, 925

91. (B) Estrogen causes increased osteoblastic activity in the bones. In young women, normal levels of

estrogen maintain the metabolic activity of the bone, allowing continued skeletal strength. When estrogen levels fall to very low levels, as occurs after menopause, osteoclastic activity exceeds the bone-building effects of the osteoblasts, increasing the risk of osteoporosis. This young woman is not having normal menstrual cycles and therefore is not producing estrogen. As a result, she has developed osteoporosis and skeletal weakness, resulting in the fracture.
TMP11 1017

92. (C) In order for erythroblastosis fetalis to occur, the baby must inherit Rh-positive red blood cells from the father. If the mother is Rh negative, she then becomes immunized against the Rh-positive antigen in the red blood cells of the fetus, and her antibodies destroy fetal red blood cells, releasing large quantities of bilirubin into the fetus's plasma.
TMP11 1048

93. (D) Because iodine is needed to synthesize thyroid hormones, the production of thyroid hormones is impaired if iodine is deficient. As a result of feedback, plasma levels of thyroid-stimulating hormone increase and stimulate the follicular cells to increase the synthesis of thyroglobulin. This results in a goiter. Increased metabolic rate, sweating, nervousness, and tachycardia are all common features of hyperthyroidism, not hypothyroidism due to iodine deficiency.
TMP11 941, 942

94. (B) Sperm cell motility decreases as pH is reduced below 6.8. At a pH of 4.5, sperm cell motility is significantly reduced. However, the buffering effect of sodium bicarbonate in the prostatic fluid raises the pH somewhat, allowing the sperm cells to regain some mobility.
TMP11 999

95. (E) Thyroid hormones are essential for normal growth, but inappropriately high plasma levels of the hormones cause excessive protein catabolism and muscle weakness.
TMP11 937

96. (C) Testosterone secreted by the testes in response to luteinizing hormone (LH) inhibits hypothalamic secretion of gonadotropin-releasing hormone (GnRH), thereby inhibiting anterior pituitary secretion of LH and follicle-stimulating hormone. Taking large doses of testosterone-like steroids also suppresses the secretion of GnRH and the pituitary gonadotropic hormones, resulting in sterility.
TMP11 1007

97. (C) Steroids with potent glucocorticoid activity tend to increase plasma glucose concentration. As a result, insulin secretion is stimulated. Increased glucocorticoid activity also diminishes muscle protein. Because of feedback, cortisone administration leads to a decrease in adrenocorticotropic hormone

secretion and, therefore, a decrease in plasma cortisol concentration.
TMP11 951, 952, 955

98. (A) An increase in the concentration of parathyroid hormone results in the stimulation of existing osteoclasts and, over longer periods, increases the number of osteoclasts present in the bone.
TMP11 987

99. (B) In general, peptide hormones produce biological effects by binding to receptors on the cell membrane. Peptide hormones are stored in secretion granules in their endocrine-producing cells and have relatively short half-lives because they are not highly bound to plasma proteins. Protein hormones often have a rapid onset of action because, unlike steroid and thyroid hormones, protein synthesis is usually not a prerequisite to produce biological effects.
TMP11 906, 909, 910, 912-915

100. (D) A pituitary tumor secreting growth hormone is likely to present as an increase in pituitary gland size. The anabolic effects of excess growth hormone secretion lead to enlargement of the internal organs, including the kidneys. Because acromegaly is the state of excess growth hormone secretion after epiphyseal closure, increased femur length does not occur.
TMP11 927

101. (A) Growth hormone and cortisol have opposite effects on protein synthesis in muscle. Growth hormone is anabolic and promotes protein synthesis in most cells of the body, whereas cortisol decreases protein synthesis in extrahepatic cells, including muscle. Both hormones impair glucose uptake in peripheral tissues and, therefore, tend to increase plasma glucose concentration. Both hormones also mobilize triglycerides from fat stores.
TMP11 922, 923, 951, 952

102. (B) If the mother has had adequate amounts of iron in her diet, the infant's liver usually has enough stored iron to form blood cells for 4 to 6 months after birth. However, if the mother has had insufficient iron, the infant may develop severe anemia after about 3 months of life.
TMP11 1044, 1049

103. (D) Elevated plasma levels of thyroid hormone increase the metabolic rate and tend to decrease body weight. Excess thyroid hormone also increases heart rate. Goiter and exophthalmos are often associated with hyperthyroidism, but they are not caused by increased plasma levels of thyroid hormone. Myxedema and lethargy are symptoms of hypothyroidism.
TMP11 936-937, 940

104. (D) Fertilization of the ovum normally takes place in the ampulla of one of the fallopian tubes.
TMP11 1027

105. (B) The below-normal plasma calcium concentration in this patient would be expected to strongly stimulate the secretion of parathyroid hormone, which in turn would be expected to increase the rate of excretion of phosphate ions by the kidney and reduce the rate of calcium ion excretion into the urine. Therefore, all the findings can be attributed to a greater than normal parathyroid hormone concentration.
TMP11 989

106. (D) Because insulin secretion is deficient in type 1 diabetes mellitus, there is increased (not decreased) release of glucose from the liver. Low plasma levels of insulin also lead to a high rate of lipolysis; increased plasma osmolality, hypovolemia, and acidosis are all symptoms of uncontrolled type 1 diabetes mellitus.
TMP11 972-974

107. (E) In contrast to most forms of dwarfism in which there is a deficiency in growth hormone secretion, in dwarfism associated with a mutation in the growth hormone receptor the rate of growth hormone secretion is elevated. These patients are unable to form somatomedin C. Consequently, linear growth is impaired.
TMP11 926

108. (D) Estrogen and, to a lesser extent, progesterone secreted by the corpus luteum during the luteal phase have strong feedback effects on the anterior pituitary gland to maintain low secretory rates of both FSH and LH. In addition, the corpus luteum secretes inhibin, which inhibits the secretion of FSH.
TMP11 1015

109. (B) In a radioimmunoassay, there is too little antibody to completely bind the radioactively tagged hormone and the hormone in the fluid to be assayed. Thus, there is competition between the labeled and endogenous hormone for binding sites on the antibody. Increased amounts of endogenous hormone in a plasma sample would displace radioactively labeled hormone from the antibody.
TMP11 915, 916

110. (D) If a pregnant woman bearing a female child has high blood levels of androgenic hormones early in pregnancy, the child will be born with male genitalia, resulting in a type of hermaphroditism.
TMP11 1049

111. (D) Under chronic conditions, the effects of high plasma levels of aldosterone to promote sodium reabsorption in the collecting tubules are sustained. However, persistent sodium retention does not occur, because of concomitant changes that promote sodium excretion. These include increased arterial pressure and increased plasma levels of atrial natriuretic peptide and decreased plasma angiotensin II concentration.
TMP11 948, 949

112. (A) In order for a male embryo to develop male genitalia, testosterone must be present in the embryo. Normally, human chorionic gonadotropin (HCG) secreted by the trophoblast cells stimulates testosterone secretion from the testes. Giving an antibody that blocks HCG would prevent testosterone secretion, resulting in the development of female genitalia in a male fetus.
TMP11 1004

113. (C) Increased plasma levels of cortisol tend to increase plasma glucose concentration and inhibit adrenocorticotropic hormone (ACTH) secretion. Therefore, if cortisol were administered to patients in group 2, the patients in group 1 would have lower plasma glucose concentrations and higher plasma levels of ACTH.
TMP11 951, 955, 956

114. (A) Obesity and insulin resistance are common features of type 2 diabetes mellitus. Because the blood glucose concentration tends to be elevated, especially after a meal, postprandial blood levels of insulin are also elevated. Ketoacidosis is usually not present in the early stages of type 2 diabetes mellitus.
TMP11 974, 975

115. (A) Fats are readily oxidized by growth hormone. In contrast, growth hormone decreases carbohydrate utilization and promotes the incorporation of amino acids into proteins.
TMP11 922, 923

116. (D) The motor neurons of the spinal cord of the thoracic and lumbar regions are the sources of innervation for the skeletal muscles of the perineum involved in ejaculation.
TMP11 1002

117. (B) Bone is deposited in proportion to the compressional load that the bone must carry. Continual mechanical stress stimulates osteoblastic deposition and calcification of bone.
TMP11 981

118. (A) Cortisol is highly bound to plasma proteins, particularly transcortin. Increased plasma levels of transcortin, such as occur during pregnancy, tend to decrease free cortisol concentration, but feedback results in increased adrenocorticotropic hormone secretion, which stimulates cortisol secretion until free plasma levels of the steroid return to normal levels. Thus, in a steady state, total plasma cortisol concentration (bound plus free) is elevated, but free cortisol concentration is normal.
TMP11 947, 955, 956

119. (A) Administration of either estrogen or progesterone in appropriate quantities during the first half of the menstrual cycle can inhibit ovulation by preventing the preovulatory surge of luteinizing hormone secretion by the anterior pituitary gland, which is essential for ovulation.
TMP11 1021, 1024

120.(D) In target tissues, nuclear receptors for thyroid hormones have a greater affinity for T_3 than for T_4. The secretion rate, plasma concentration, half-life, and onset of action are all greater for T_4 than for T_3.
TMP11 933, 934

121. (C) Blocking the action of follicle-stimulating hormone on the Sertoli cells of the seminiferous tubules interrupts the production of sperm. Choice C is the only option that is certain to provide sterility.
TMP11 1007

122. (C) Oxytocin is secreted from the posterior pituitary gland and carried in the blood to the breast, where it causes the cells that surround the outer walls of the alveoli and ductile system to contract. Contraction of these cells raises the hydrostatic pressure of the milk in the ducts to 10 to 20 mm Hg. Consequently, milk flows from the nipple into the baby's mouth.
TMP11 1040

123. (A) If the ductus arteriosus remains patent, poorly oxygenated blood from the pulmonary artery flows into the aorta, giving the arterial blood an oxygen level that is below normal.
TMP11 1046, 1047

124. (B) Antidiuretic hormone (ADH) and thyroid-stimulating hormone (TSH) are stored in the posterior and anterior lobes of the pituitary gland, respectively. Although TSH is also synthesized in the anterior pituitary gland, this is not the case for ADH, which is synthesized in the hypothalamus. Both hormones are peptides, and neither is bound to any appreciable degree by plasma proteins.
TMP11 919, 920, 927, 928, 938

125. (C) The placenta secretes both estrogen and progesterone from the trophoblast cells.
TMP11 1029, 1030

126. (A) Testosterone stimulates the cellular functions of bone that lead to bone formation. Testosterone secretion from the interstitial cells declines with age, but it continues at sufficient levels to stimulate bone formation throughout a man's lifetime. Conversely, estrogen production in women falls to zero after menopause, leaving the bones without the stimulatory effect of estrogen. As a result, osteoporosis is common in women after menopause.
TMP11 991, 992

127. (A) In healthy patients, the secretory rates of adrenocorticotropic hormone (ACTH) and cortisol are low in the late evening but high in the early morning. In patients with Cushing's syndrome (adrenal adenoma) or in patients administered dexamethasone, plasma levels of ACTH are very low and are certainly not higher than normal early-morning values. In patients with Addison's disease, plasma levels of ACTH are elevated as a result of deficient adrenal secretion of cortisol. The secretion of ACTH and cortisol would be expected to be normal in Conn's syndrome.
TMP11 956-959

128. (D) Activation of the sympathetic nervous system has reciprocal effects on insulin and glucagon secretion. Sympathetic activation decreases insulin secretion and increases glucagon secretion. Amino acids stimulate the secretion of both hormones, and in type 2 diabetes mellitus, the plasma levels of both insulin and glucagon are elevated.
TMP11 968-971, 974, 975

129. (B) Blood returning from the placenta through the umbilical vein passes through the ductus venosus. The blood coming from the placenta has the highest concentration of oxygen found in the fetus.
TMP11 1046

130. (B) Osteoporosis, hypertension, hirsutism, and hyperpigmentation are all symptoms of Cushing's syndrome associated with high plasma levels of ACTH. If the high plasma ACTH levels were the result of either a pituitary adenoma or an abnormally high rate of corticotropin-releasing hormone secretion from the hypothalamus, the patient would likely have an enlarged pituitary gland. In contrast, the pituitary gland would not be enlarged if an ectopic tumor were secreting high levels of ACTH.
TMP11 958, 959

131. (B) Prolactin secretion is inhibited, not stimulated, by the hypothalamic release of dopamine into the median eminence. Growth hormone is inhibited by the hypothalamic inhibiting hormone somatostatin. The secretion of luteinizing hormone, thyroid-stimulating hormone, and adrenocorticotropic hormone are all under the control of the releasing hormones indicated.
TMP11 921

132. (D) During prolonged calcium deficiency, the plasma calcium concentration begins to fall. However, as it falls, parathyroid hormone secretion increases sharply, thereby stimulating osteoclastic degradation of bone and liberating calcium to the extracellular fluid. At the same time, the elevated parathyroid hormone concentration strongly stimulates calcium reabsorption from the tubular fluid of the kidneys and reduces calcium excretion to very low levels.
TMP11 1089

133. (B) Increased heart rate, increased respiratory rate, and decreased cholesterol concentration are all responses to excess thyroid hormone.
TMP11 936, 937

134. (C) Estrogen secreted by the placenta is not synthesized from basic substrates in the placenta. Instead, it is formed almost entirely from androgenic steroid compounds that are formed in both the mother's and the fetus's adrenal glands. These

androgenic compounds are transported by the blood to the placenta and converted by the trophoblast cells to estrogen compounds. Their concentration in the maternal blood may also stimulate hair growth on the body.
TMP11 1033

135. (D) By age 45 years, only a few primordial follicles remain in the ovaries to be stimulated by gonadotropic hormones, and the production of estrogen decreases as the number of follicles approaches zero. When estrogen production falls below a critical value, it can no longer inhibit the production of gonadotropic hormones from the anterior pituitary. Follicle-stimulating hormone and luteinizing hormone are produced in large quantities, but as the remaining follicles become atretic, production by the ovaries falls to zero.
TMP11 1022

136. (C) The secretion of chemical messengers (neurohormones) from neurons into the blood is referred to as neuroendocrine secretion. Thus, in contrast to the local actions of neurotransmitters at nerve endings, neurohormones circulate in the blood before producing biological effects at target tissues. Oxytocin is synthesized from magnocellular neurons whose cell bodies are located in the paraventricular and supraoptic nuclei and whose nerve terminals terminate in the posterior pituitary gland. Target tissues for circulating oxytocin are the breast and uterus, where the hormone plays a role in lactation and parturition, respectively.
TMP11 905, 927, 928

137. (C) Progesterone secreted in large quantities from the corpus luteum causes marked swelling and secretory development of the endometrium.
TMP11 1018, 1019

138. (D) Cortisol tends to increase plasma glucose concentration and promotes lipolysis. Additionally, in most tissues, cortisol diminishes the tissue stores of proteins, resulting in a negative nitrogen balance.
TMP11 951, 952

139. (B) Inhibition of the iodide pump decreases the synthesis of thyroid hormones but does not impair the production of thyroglobulin by follicular cells. Decreased plasma levels of thyroid hormones result in a low metabolic rate and lead to an increase in thyroid-stimulating hormone (TSH) secretion. Increased plasma levels of TSH stimulate the follicular cells to synthesize more thyroglobulin. Nervousness is a symptom of hyperthyroidism and is not caused by thyroid hormone deficiency.
TMP11 932-935

140. (D) As the blastocyst implants, the trophoblast cells invade the decidua, digesting and imbibing it. The stored nutrients in the decidual cells are used by the embryo for growth and development. During the first week after implantation, this is the only means by which the embryo can obtain nutrients.

The embryo continues to obtain at least some of its nutrition in this way for up to 8 weeks, although the placenta begins to provide nutrition after about the 16th day beyond fertilization (a little more than 1 week after implantation).
TMP11 1029

141. (B) Elevation of estrogen concentration stimulates osteoblastic activity and reduces the rate of degradation of bone by osteoclasts.
TMP11 982, 1017

142. (A) Both antidiuretic hormone and oxytocin are peptides containing nine amino acids. Their chemical structures differ in only two amino acids.
TMP11 928

143. (C) One of the most characteristic findings in respiratory distress syndrome is failure of the respiratory epithelium to secrete adequate quantities of surfactant into the alveoli. Surfactant decreases the surface tension of the alveolar fluid, allowing the alveoli to open easily during inspiration. Without sufficient surfactant, the alveoli tend to collapse, and there is a tendency to develop pulmonary edema.
TMP11 1045

144. (A) The enzyme aldosterone synthase is not present in the zona fasciculata. Consequently, aldosterone is not synthesized in these cells of the adrenal cortex.
TMP11 944, 945

145. (C) The primary controllers of adrenocorticotropic hormone (ACTH), growth hormone, luteinizing hormone (LH), and thyroid-stimulating hormone (TSH) secretion from the pituitary gland are hypothalamic releasing hormones. They are secreted into the median eminence and subsequently flow into the hypothalamic-hypophysial portal vessels before bathing the cells of the anterior pituitary gland. Conversely, prolactin secretion from the pituitary gland is influenced primarily by the hypothalamic inhibiting hormone dopamine. Consequently, obstruction of blood flow through the portal vessels would lead to reduced secretion of ACTH, growth hormone, LH, and TSH but increased secretion of prolactin.
TMP11 921

146. (A) Gamma radiation destroys the cells undergoing the most rapid rates of mitosis and meiosis, the germinal epithelium of the testes. The man described is said to have normal testosterone levels, suggesting that the secretory patterns of gonadotropin-releasing hormone and luteinizing hormone are normal and that his interstitial cells are functional. Because he is not producing sperm, the levels of inhibin secreted by the Sertoli cells would be maximally suppressed, and his levels of follicle-stimulating hormone would be strongly elevated.
TMP11 1007

147. (A) Increased plasma cholesterol concentration is commonly observed in hypothyroidism.
TMP11 936

148. (B) In this experiment, the size of the thyroid gland increased because thyroid-stimulating hormone (TSH) causes hypertrophy and hyperplasia of its target gland and increased secretion of thyroid hormones. Increased plasma levels of thyroid hormones inhibit the secretion of thyrotropin-releasing hormone, which decreases stimulation of the pituitary thyrotropes, resulting in a decrease in the size of the pituitary gland. Higher plasma levels of thyroid hormones also increase metabolic rate and decrease body weight.
TMP11 936-939, 951, 952, 955, 956

149. (C) In this experiment, the size of the pituitary and adrenal glands increased because corticotropin-releasing hormone stimulates the pituitary corticotropes to secrete adrenocorticotropic hormone, which in turn stimulates the adrenals to secrete corticosterone and cortisol. Higher plasma levels of cortisol increase protein degredation and lipolysis and, therefore, decrease body weight.
TMP11 936-939, 951, 952, 955, 956

Sports Physiology

1. Which of the following causes excess muscle mass in the average male compared with the average female?
   (A) Increased testosterone secreted in the male
   (B) Increased estrogen secreted in the female
   (C) Higher exercise levels in the male
   (D) Greater glycogen deposition by the male

2. What is the definition of the power of a muscle?
   (A) Maximum weight it can lift
   (B) Force required to stretch it after it has contracted
   (C) Work the muscle can perform per unit of time
   (D) Length of time a muscle can lift a given amount of weight

3. If a person runs a 10-kilometer race, what is the source of most of the adenosine triphosphate (ATP) produced?
   (A) Stored ATP
   (B) Phosphagen system
   (C) Glycogen–lactic acid system
   (D) Phosphocreatine system
   (E) Metabolism of glucose, fat, and amino acids

4. Which of the following athletes is able to exercise the longest before exhaustion occurs?
   (A) One on a high-fat diet
   (B) One on a high-carbohydrate diet
   (C) One on a mixed carbohydrate-fat diet
   (D) One on a high-protein diet
   (E) One on a mixed protein-fat diet

5. If muscle strength is increased with resistive training, which of the following conditions is most likely to occur?
   (A) Decrease in the number of myofibrils
   (B) Increase in mitochondrial enzymes
   (C) Decrease in the components of the phosphagen energy system
   (D) Decrease in stored triglycerides

6. Which of the following statements comparing slow-twitch and fast-twitch muscle fibers is most accurate?
   (A) Fast-twitch fibers are less dependent on the phosphagen and glycogen–lactic acid systems
   (B) Slow-twitch fibers are surrounded by more mitochondria
   (C) Slow-twitch fibers have less myoglobin
   (D) Slow-twitch fibers are surrounded by fewer capillaries
   (E) Fast-twitch fibers are smaller in diameter

7. Which of the following statements about respiration in exercise is most accurate?
   (A) Maximum oxygen consumption of a male marathoner is less than that of an untrained average male
   (B) Maximum oxygen consumption can be increased about 100 per cent by training
   (C) Maximum oxygen diffusing capacity of a male marathoner is much greater than that of an untrained average male
   (D) Blood levels of oxygen and carbon dioxide are abnormal during exercise

8. Tobacco smoking causes which of the following effects on the pulmonary system?
   (A) Dilatation of terminal bronchioles
   (B) Decreased air flow resistance
   (C) Decreased fluid secretion in the bronchial tree
   (D) Paralyzed cilia on the respiratory epithelial cells

9. Which of the following statements about athletes who run marathons compared with nonathletes is most accurate?
   (A) Stroke volume in the marathoner is about 50 per cent greater at rest
   (B) Percentage increase in heart rate during maximum exercise is much less in the marathon runner
   (C) Maximum cardiac output is only 3 to 4 per cent greater in the marathon runner
   (D) Resting heart rate in the marathon runner is significantly higher

10. Which of the following is most likely to occur in athletes who use androgens to increase performance?
    (A) Decreased high-density blood lipoproteins
    (B) Decreased low-density blood lipoproteins
    (C) Increased testicular function
    (D) Decreased incidence of hypertension

Answers

1. (A) The increased muscle mass in males is caused by testosterone, which is secreted by the male testes. This produces a powerful anabolic effect, causing greatly increased deposition of protein everywhere in the body, but especially in the muscles. In females, estrogen causes a greater deposition of fat, not protein.
   TMP11 1055

2. (C) The power of a muscle is the work the muscle can perform in a unit of time. This is determined not only by the strength of the muscle contraction but also by the distance of contraction and the number of times it contracts each minute. The power is generally measured in kilogram-meters per minute. This is equivalent to a muscle lifting 1 kilogram of weight to a height of 1 meter in 1 minute.
   TMP11 1056

3. (E) When a person runs a long-distance race, such as 10 kilometers, the phosphagen system can supply energy for only 8 to 10 seconds. The phosphagen system is ATP and the phosphocreatine system combined. The glycogen–lactic acid system supplies energy for only 1.3 to 1.6 minutes. Therefore, the aerobic system, which consists of the metabolism of glucose, fats, and amino acids, supplies most of the energy in long-term exercise.
   TMP11 1056

4. (B) An athlete on a high-carbohydrate diet stores nearly twice as much glycogen in the muscles compared with an athlete on a mixed carbohydrate-fat diet. This glycogen is converted to lactic acid and supplies four adenosine triphosphate (ATP)

molecules for each molecule of glucose. It also forms ATP 2.5 times as rapidly as oxidative metabolism in the mitochondria. This extra energy from glycogen significantly increases the amount of time an athlete can exercise.
TMP11 1057, 1058

5. (B) During resistive training, muscles that are contracted with at least a 50 per cent maximum force at least three times weekly experience an optimal increase in muscle strength. This causes muscle hypertrophy, and several changes occur. There is an increase in the number of myofibrils and up to a 120 per cent increase in mitochondrial enzymes. The components of the phosphagen energy system can increase as much as 60 to 80 per cent, and stored glycogen can increase up to 50 per cent. Also, a 75 to 100 per cent increase in stored triglycerides can occur.
TMP11 1060

6. (B) The basic differences between fast-twitch and slow-twitch fibers are the following: Fast-twitch fibers are more dependent on anaerobic metabolism, and slow-twitch fibers are more dependent on aerobic metabolism. Fast-twitch fibers are more dependent on the phosphagen and glycogen–lactic acid systems than slow-twitch fibers are. Slow-twitch fibers are organized for endurance and depend on aerobic metabolism; therefore, they have many more mitochondria and more myoglobin, which combines with oxygen in the muscle fiber. The number of capillaries that supply the oxygen is much greater in the vicinity of slow-twitch fibers than fast-twitch fibers.
TMP11 1060, 1061

7. (C) During exercise, the maximum oxygen consumption of a male marathoner is much greater than that of an untrained average male. However, athletic training increases maximum oxygen consumption by only about 10 per cent. Therefore, the maximum oxygen consumption in marathoners is probably

partly genetically determined. These runners also have a large increase in maximum oxygen diffusing capacity, and their blood levels of oxygen and carbon dioxide remain relatively normal during exercise.
TMP11 1061, 1062

8. (D) Tobacco smoking decreases an athlete's pulmonary ventilatory ability for several reasons. First, nicotine constricts the terminal bronchioles of the lungs, which increases the resistance to air flow in and out of the lungs. Second, the smoke has an irritating effect in the bronchiolar trees, which increases fluid secretion. Third, nicotine paralyzes the cilia on the surfaces of the respiratory epithelial cells, which normally beat continually to remove excess fluid and foreign particles.
TMP11 1062

9. (A) When comparing a marathoner and a nonathlete, there are several differences in the responses of the heart. In a marathoner, stroke volume is much higher at rest, and the heart rate is much lower. The heart rate can increase approximately 270 per cent in a marathoner during maximum exercise, which is a much greater percentage than occurs in a nonathlete. In addition, the maximum increase in cardiac output is approximately 30 per cent greater in a marathoner.
TMP11 1062-1064

10. (A) Use of male sex hormones (androgens) or other anabolic steroids to increase muscle strength can enhance athletic performance under some conditions, but it can have adverse effects on the body. Anabolic steroids increase the risk of cardiovascular damage because they increase the incidence of hypertension, decrease high-density blood lipoproteins, and increase low-density blood lipoproteins. These factors all promote heart attacks and strokes. These androgenic substances also decrease testicular function, which decreases the formation of sperm and the body's production of natural testosterone.
TMP11 1066